Surgery of the Autonomic Nervous System

Surgery of the Autonomic Nervous System

Edited by

Jonathan A. Hyam
Victor Horsley Department of Neurosurgery,
National Hospital for Neurology and Neurosurgery,
Queen Square, University College London Hospitals, UK

Erlick A. C. Pereira
Department of Neurosurgery,
Oxford University Hospitals NHS Trust, UK

Alexander L. Green
Nuffield Department of Surgical Sciences,
University of Oxford, UK

OXFORD
UNIVERSITY PRESS

OXFORD
UNIVERSITY PRESS

Great Clarendon Street, Oxford, OX2 6DP,
United Kingdom

Oxford University Press is a department of the University of Oxford.
It furthers the University's objective of excellence in research, scholarship,
and education by publishing worldwide. Oxford is a registered trade mark of
Oxford University Press in the UK and in certain other countries

First Edition published in 2016

Impression: 1

Published in the United States of America by Oxford University Press
198 Madison Avenue, New York, NY 10016, United States of America

British Library Cataloguing in Publication Data
Data available

Library of Congress Control Number: 2015951913

ISBN 978–0–19–968640–7

Printed and bound by
CPI Group (UK) Ltd, Croydon, CR0 4YY

Foreword

Over a decade ago I spotted blood pressure changes in an awake patient during an operation electrically stimulating the brainstem to relieve chronic pain. I encouraged my then registrar, Alex Green, to study the phenomenon, which had up until that point been just a footnote in an obscure neurosurgical textbook. He went on to build a career researching the effects of deep-brain stimulation upon autonomic function and in turn supervised both Jonathan Hyam elucidating its interactions with breathing and Erlick Pereira investigating its cardiovascular and analgesic mechanisms. The paediatrician and renowned educationalist, Maria Montessori, once commented that 'the greatest sign of success for a teacher . . . is to be able to say, "The children are now working as if I did not exist."' It is, therefore, with immense pride that I foreword a book co-edited independently of me by three of the most prolific academic surgeons I have mentored. All commenced research under my wing in their spare time as junior registrars and each emerged half a decade later a mature and talented neurosurgeon with doctorates, national and international prizes, and nearly two-hundred scientific papers between them. *Surgery of the Autonomic Nervous System* encapsulates their efforts to consolidate expert opinion from a nexus of overlapping specialties (neurological, vascular, cardiac, thoracic, anaesthetic, surgical, and medical) and sciences (neural, physiological, biochemical, engineering, and computational) into an emerging discipline characterized by exciting new therapies. It is a testament to their visionary perspective that the book transcends not just so many subjects, but so many disorders of autonomic function carefully crystallized into a veritable almanac for the autonomic surgeon-scientist. Of course, the specialist 'autonomic surgeon' does not as yet exist, let alone the autonomic surgeon-scientist! I sincerely hope that this volume and its eclectic, well-referenced, and generously illustrated chapters may one day soon inspire its creation. It is worth debating, finally, whether overwhelming pride, dogged intransigence, sheer phlegmatism, or inspired genius have motivated my delegating this foreword to the book's most junior co-author. Perhaps I should become known as the Montessorian Professor . . .

Professor Tipu Aziz
Professor of Neurosurgery
The Nuffield Department of Clinical Neurosciences, Oxford, UK

Contents

About the Editors

Jonathan Hyam is a Consultant Brain & Spine Neurosurgeon at The National Hospital for Neurology & Neurosurgery, Queen Square, and an Honorary Senior Lecturer in Neurosurgery at the Institute of Neurology, University College London. His specialist expertise is Deep Brain Stimulation for Parkinson's disease, tremor, and dystonia, as well as surgical and minimal-access treatments for headache and spinal pain.

In 2011 he received America's Congress of Neurological Surgeons' Resident Prize for Stereotactic & Functional Neurosurgery in Washington, DC. He was awarded a PhD from Oxford University in Neurosurgery and Physiology, and a Diploma in Microscopic Neurosurgery from The Yasargil Neurosurgery Laboratory of the University of Zurich. He is an invited specialist advisor to NICE on behalf of the British Society for Stereotactic & Functional Neurosurgery.

Jonathan Hyam was awarded the prestigious Arris & Gale Lectureship from the Royal College of Surgeons of England in honour of his contribution to the understanding of how deep brain stimulation can influence the heart, lungs, and pain pathways, and how these can be benefited using neurosurgery.

Alexander Green is an Academic Neurosurgeon at the University of Oxford. His main academic interest is neuromodulation with a particular focus on control of the autonomic nervous system and the application of neuromodulation to control autonomic function. He has published over 140 peer-reviewed articles, authored 2 books (including this one), and numerous book chapters. At the time of writing, he is President of the British Society for Stereotactic and Functional Neurosurgery and an advisor to a number of bodies including the National Institute for Health and Care Excellence (NICE), NHS England and Industry.

Erlick Pereira is a Neurosurgeon in London and Honorary Clinician in Oxford. He studied medicine at Somerville College, Oxford University after natural sciences (experimental psychology) at Trinity College, Cambridge. He has published over 100 papers and 20 book chapters and won awards from both the American Association and Congress of Neurological Surgeons. He is an affiliated Professor at the University of Porto and Hunterian Professor of the Royal College of Surgeons of England. His doctoral thesis in deep brain surgery for pain and autonomic function was advised by Alexander Green. He is a Fellow of the Royal College of Surgeons of England and Senior Fellow of the Higher Education Academy. His clinical interests are functional neurosurgery including deep brain stimulation and complex spinal surgery. His academic interests include novel indications of deep brain stimulation such as chronic pain, stroke and spinal cord injury, and neuroimaging the spinal cord.

Contributors

Stana Bojanic
Consultant Neurosurgeon,
Department of Neurosurgery,
John Radcliffe Hospital,
Oxford, UK

Emma V. Carrington
Clinical Research Fellow,
National Centre for Bowel Research
and Surgical Innovation,
The Royal London Hospital,
London, UK

Kenneth F. Casey
Associate Professor,
Department of Neurosurgery,
Michigan State University,
East Lansing, USA;
Associate Professor,
Department of Physical Medicine
and Rehabilitation,
Wayne State University,
Detroit, USA

Roberto Cordella
Department of Neurosurgery,
Fondazione Istituto Neurologico
"Carlo Besta", Milan,
Italy

Mike J. L. DeJongste
Department of Cardiology,
Thoraxcenter,
University Medical Center Groningen,
University of Groningen,
The Netherlands

Murray Esler
Baker IDI Heart & Diabetes Institute,
Melbourne, Australia

Robert D. Foreman
George Lynn Cross Research
Professor of Physiology,
Adjunct Professor of Anesthesiology,
University of Oklahoma Health
Sciences Center
Oklahoma City, OK

Angelo Franzini
Department of Neurosurgery,
Fondazione Istituto Neurologico
"Carlo Besta", Milan, Italy

Samer Ghostine
Neurosurgery Department,
University of California in Irvine,
Orange, USA

Alexander L. Green
Nuffield Department of Surgical Sciences,
University of Oxford,
UK

Gerbrand J. Groen
Department of Anesthesiology,
Pain Center,
University Medical Center Groningen,
University of Groningen,
The Netherlands

Gert Holstege
Centre for Clinical Research,
The University of Queensland,
Australia

Emma H. Horrocks
Clinical Research Fellow,
National Centre for Bowel Research
and Surgical Innovation,
The Royal London Hospital,
London, UK

Jonathan A. Hyam
Victor Horsley Department of Neurosurgery,
National Hospital for Neurology and Neurosurgery,
Queen Square, University College London, UK

Peter J. Jannetta
Vice Chairman, Academic Affairs,
Department of Neurosurgery,
Allegheny Hospital, Pittsburgh, PA
Professor of Neurosurgery,
Drexel University School of Medicine,
Philadelphia, USA

J. Patrick Johnson
The Spine Center,
Cedars-Sinai Medical Center,
Los Angeles, USA

Philip E. V. Van Kerrebroeck
Department of Urology and Pelvic Care,
Maastricht University Medical Centre,
The Netherlands

Charles Knowles
Professor of Surgical Research,
National Centre for Bowel Research and Surgical Innovation,
The Royal London Hospital,
London, UK

Abraham A. Kroon
Department of Medicine,
Maastricht University Medical Center and Cardiovascular Research Institute Maastricht (CARIM), Maastricht,
The Netherlands

Michiel Kuijpers
Department of Cardiothoracic Surgery, Thoraxcenter,
University Medical Center Groningen,
University of Groningen,
The Netherlands

Peter W. de Leeuw
Department of Medicine,
Maastricht University Medical Center and Cardiovascular Research Institute Maastricht (CARIM), Maastricht,
The Netherlands

Massimo Leone
Department of Neurology,
Fondazione Istituto Neurologico "Carlo Besta", Milan,
Italy

Thelma Lovick
School of Physiology,
Pharmacology and Neuroscience
University of Bristol
UK

Joseph R. Madsen
Director, Epilepsy Surgery Program,
Department of Neurosurgery,
Boston Children's Hospital,
Harvard Medical School,
Boston, USA

Tom A. T. Marcelissen
Department of Urology,
Maastricht University Medical Centre,
The Netherlands

Manjit S. Matharu
Headache Group, Institute of Neurology and The National Hospital for Neurology and Neurosurgery, Queen Square,
London, UK

Tim McCormick
Consultant Anaesthetist,
Oxford Pain Management Centre,
Churchill Hospital, Oxford

Giuseppe Messina
Department of Neurosurgery,
Fondazione Istituto Neurologico "Carlo Besta", Milan,
Italy

Sarah Miller
Headache Group,
Institute of Neurology and
The National Hospital for
Neurology and Neurosurgery,
Queen Square,
London, UK

Erlick A. C. Pereira
Nuffield Department of Surgical Sciences,
University of Oxford,
UK

Brian Perri
The Spine Center,
Cedars-Sinai Medical Center,
Los Angeles, USA

Benjamin I. Rapoport
Department of Neurological Surgery,
Weill Cornell Medical College,
New York-Presbyterian Hospital,
New York, USA

Michele Rizzi
Department of Neurosurgery,
Fondazione Istituto Neurologico
"Carlo Besta", Milan,
Italy

Christian E. Sampson
Assistant Professor of Surgery,
Harvard Medical School,
Brigham & Women's Hospital,
Boston, USA

Srinath Samudrala
The Spine Center, Cedars-Sinai Medical
Center, Los Angeles,
USA

Markus Schlaich
Dobney Chair in Clinical Research,
School of Medicine and Pharmacology,
Royal Perth Hospital Unit,
Faculty of Medicine,
Dentistry & Health Sciences,
The University of Western Australia,
Perth, Australia; Neurovascular
Hypertension & Kidney Disease
Laboratory, Baker IDI Heart
& Diabetes Institute,
Melbourne, Australia

Khawar Siddique
The Spine Center,
Cedars-Sinai Medical Center,
Los Angeles, USA

Martijn A. C. Smits
Department of Urology and Pelvic Care,
Maastricht University Medical Centre,
The Netherlands

Edy E. Soffer
Department of Medicine,
University of Southern California
Los Angeles, USA

Noel N. Thin
Clinical Research Fellow,
National Centre for Bowel Research
and Surgical Innovation,
The Royal London Hospital,
London, UK

Shoshanna Vaynman
The Spine Center,
Cedars-Sinai Medical Center,
Los Angeles, USA

Laurence Watkins
Division of Neurosurgery,
Institute of Neurology and The National
Hospital for Neurology and Neurosurgery,
Queen Square, London, UK

Chapter 1

Neural control of the heart and cardiovascular system

Jonathan A. Hyam and Alexander L. Green

Key points

1. Sites from all levels of the brain and spinal cord are involved in the neural control of blood pressure.
2. Multiple feedback and feedforward mechanisms maintain beat-to-beat cardiovascular control.
3. Central command provides a feedforward, top-down control over cardiovascular performance in relation to anticipated requirements.
4. The periaqueductal grey is involved in the 'fight-or-flight' response and can produce rapid pressor or depressor changes in cardiovascular performance.
5. The rostroventrolateral medulla (RVLM) is the final outflow from the brain mediating sympathetic drive.

Introduction

The accurate matching of cardiovascular performance to the metabolic requirements of the body is crucial to sustain individual organ systems and, therefore, the entire body itself. Cardiovascular performance is mediated by changes in the heart and peripheral vessels in addition to circulating volume, the latter governed by the kidneys. All of these structures have a rich autonomic innervation. Arterial blood pressure is determined by the rate and contractility of the heart, the volume of venous return and end-diastolic filling of the heart, and the resistance produced by the diameter of vessels within the peripheral vascular tree (represented mathematically in Fig. 1.1). Although the heart has its own autorhythmicity and will beat regularly even if separated from the rest of the body, and will eject blood with a varying contractility according to each end-diastolic volume, cardiovascular performance is dependent on outside effectors to enable it to respond sufficiently to the body's varying requirements. Slow changes in cardiovascular performance

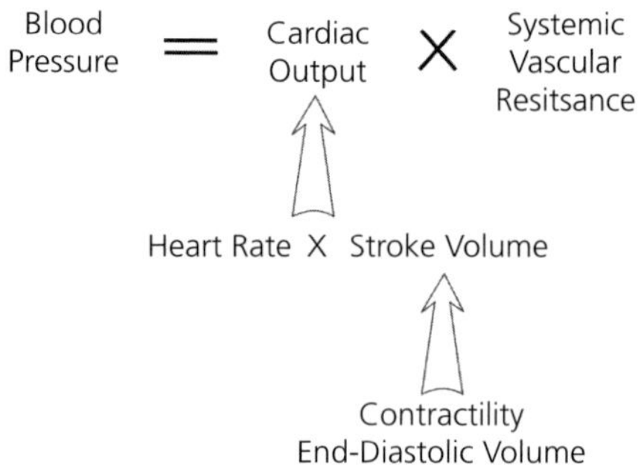

Fig. 1.1 Mathematical relationships linking cardiovascular parameters to blood pressure magnitude.

can be effected via alteration of circulating volume by renal volume control mechanisms/ the renin–angiotensin system and also by the effects of circulating catecholamines, such as adrenaline (epinephrine). Rapid adjustments in response to the external environment on a beat-to-beat basis, however, are neutrally mediated and can be sustained over long periods of time. This chapter describes the neural pathways and key reflexes via which cardiovascular performance is controlled.

Central and intra-thoracic cardiovascular autonomic architecture

The neural complex controlling cardiovascular performance comprises the central autonomic network (CAN), intra-thoracic extracardiac ganglia within the sympathetic chain, the intra-thoracic intrinsic cardiac ganglionated plexus at the heart, and the final effector neurones (see Fig. 1.2). Within these structures, beat-to-beat modulation of the cardiovascular system is achieved by integration of afferent information from cardiovascular afferents of the heart and various locations in the cardiovascular system, with non-cardiac afferent information from all over the body within the central nervous system and intra-thoracic peripheral ganglia. Subsequent processing within these structures is translated into the efferent output to modulate changes in heart, blood vessel, and adrenal medulla performance within seconds (1).

Central autonomic network

Multiple sites constitute the CAN, from the level of the spinal cord through to the cortex. It is reciprocally connected to numerous other systems, such as the pain and motor pathways in addition to reticular and forebrain monoamine and cholinergic attentional, motivational, emotional, and sleep–wake cycle pathways (2). The CAN is, therefore, not only affected by the activity of these pathways but can modulate them also. The CAN receives afferent input from all over the body, which it processes, and then, by virtue of its direct connections to descending sympathetic and parasympathetic motor pathways, produces an appropriate coordinated cardiovascular output. Brain areas at every level contribute to the CAN, such as the anterior cingulate gyrus of the cerebral cortex, the hypothalamus of

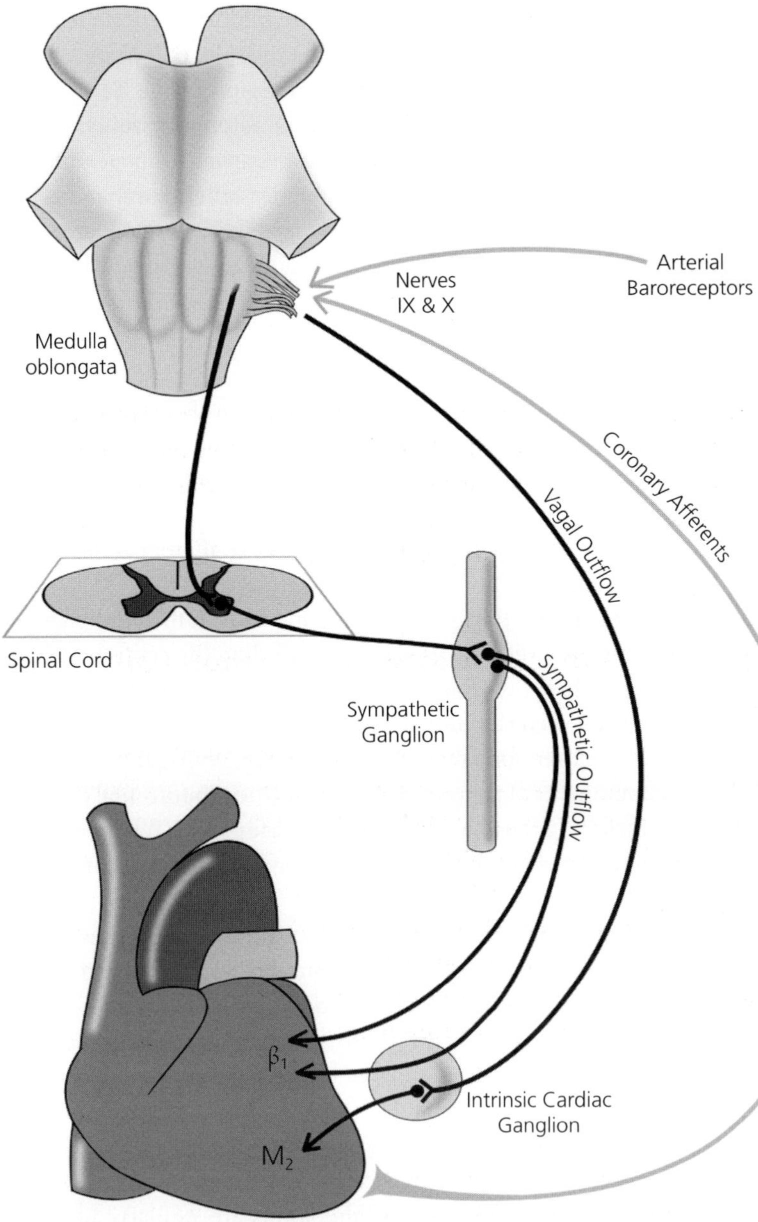

Fig. 1.2 Schematic demonstrating the sympathetic and parasympathetic (vagal) outflow to the heart. Post-ganglionic sympathetic fibres run directly to cardiac β_1-adrenergic receptors and also indirectly via intrinsic cardiac ganglia where they contribute to processing with parasympathetic and local circuit neurones. Vagal outflows synapse at the intrinsic cardiac ganglia before sending post-ganglionic efferents to muscurinic M_2 receptors.

the diencephalon, the periaqueductal grey (PAG) of the midbrain, parabrachial nucleus of the pons, the nucleus tractus solitarius (NTS) of the medulla oblongata, and, for cardiovascular sympathetic outflow, the intermediolateral region of the T1–5 spinal cord. Fig. 1.3 displays the areas involved in the modulation of autonomic function. Labelling studies in which pseudorabies virus was injected into the ventricular myocardium stained parasympathetic cardiac vagal motor neurones and higher order command cells within constituent areas of the CAN, such as the NTS, nucleus ambiguus (NA), area postrema, locus coeruleus, parabrachial nuclei (PBN), PAG, hypothalamus, amygdala, insula, and frontal cortices (3).

Cortical control of the cardiovascular system

Higher cortical areas play important roles in the reception of cardiovascular afferent information, integration and processing of information from multiple other neural pathways, and the modulation of cardiovascular function via direct and indirect pathways to autonomic motor circuits.

The insula is the primary viscerosensory cortex receiving afferent information from throughout the cardiovascular system. It receives projections from the NTS in addition to other sites within the CAN, such as the hypothalamus and PBN. It then provides descending projections to multiple sites within the network, including the central nucleus of the amygdala and, via the hypothalamus, the rostroventrolateral medulla (RVLM). Through these connections, the insula itself can initiate responses that can be translated into alterations of cardiovascular function (for a review see Benarroch 1997 (2)).

The amygdala and components of the prefrontal cortex (the orbitofrontal cortex and the medial frontal cortex, including the anterior cingulate cortex (ACC)) have also been implicated in the descending control of the cardiovascular system and their modulation has even caused asystole.

The ACC sits at the intersection of motor control, cognition, and arousal state. Paus describes it as having the potential to translate intentions into actions (5). Pyramidal neurones of the ACC project directly and indirectly to subcortical sites that confer autonomic control, such as the hypothalamus (5) and PAG (6), allowing it to influence autonomic outflow. Pool and Ransohoff electrically stimulated the ACC intra-operatively in humans undergoing surgery for psychiatric disease and elicited a variety of changes in systolic and diastolic blood pressure, respiratory rate, and heart rate (7). Gentil et al. also stimulated the ACC during limbic surgery and found consistent increase in skin conductance activity, an autonomic surrogate (8). Cardiovascular alterations are similarly seen in animal studies (9–12). Exercise and mental stressor tasks in which increased heart rate and arterial blood pressure were produced were associated with increased ACC regional cerebral blood flow (13), whilst fMRI studies have shown increased blood oxygen level dependent (BOLD) signal in the ACC during autonomic challenges, such as posture, respiratory, and isometric exercise, as well as cognitive tasks such as Stroop (14). Cingulate lesion studies in humans have demonstrated derangement of autonomic drive, particularly sympathetic. Patients with unilateral and bilateral cingulotomies had attenuated electrodermal activity during a reaction time task (15) and patients with ACC lesions after subtotal resection surgery for glioma were unable to generate a normal cardiovascular drive during cognitive effort with a reduction in sympathetic activity (14).

The amygdala plays a major role in the modulation of autonomic, cardiovascular, and endocrine responses (16). As a constituent of the limbic system, the amygdala is a site where emotional stimuli, such as anxiety and fear, can be integrated with autonomic responses to produce appropriate emotional behaviour (17–20). The central nucleus of the amygdala shares an important connection with the lateral area of the hypothalamus, whereby cardiovascular responses to conditioned stimuli are conferred. The amygdala also projects to other CAN sites, including the PBN, NTS, and dorsal motor nucleus of the vagus nerve (DMNX) (18). Afferents are received by the amygdala from various parts of the cardiovascular autonomic network, namely baroreceptors from the periphery (demonstrated in cats and suspected in humans), as well as the ACC and insula of the CAN (18, 21). Electrical stimulation of the amygdala causes changes in cardiovascular performance that are dependent on the conscious state of the animal. A pressor response occurs in awake animals, manifesting as increases in heart rate and blood pressure, compared to an opposite, depressor, response during sleep or anaesthesia (22–24).

Forebrain regions, especially the insula, appear to be lateralized in terms of cardiovascular control. Stimulation experiments in animals and humans have shown polar effects, depending on which hemisphere is targeted. Hilz et al. performed intracarotid amobarbital injection to reduce hemispheric activity. They found a decrease in blood pressure and the high frequency (purely parasympathetic) component of heart rate variability (HRV) with right-sided inactivation compared to an increase in blood pressure, heart rate, and the low frequency (sympathetic and probably also partly parasympathetic) component of HRV (25). Muscle sympathetic nerve activity recorded from peroneal nerves in humans also supports a right-sided lateralization of sympathetic outflow (26). In the rat, cells associated with baroreceptors were found clustered within the right posterior insula (27). Insular infarct in humans has been associated with cardiovascular derangement, such as hypertensive episodes, when occurring in the right hemisphere (28, 29), with pathological sympathetic activation most excessively seen after middle cerebral artery infarctions, which involve the right insula (30). Further, regulation of vagal activity is suggested to be driven by the left cerebral cortex (31). An inflexible model of lateralized cardiovascular control, however, has been downplayed as even simple tasks are associated with dynamic cortical activations with varied spatial and temporal distributions (32, 33). Thayer and Lane propose that a dynamic systems' framework exists, whereby the network is flexible and different components can be recruited according to particular challenges. The resulting 'emergent' functional networks are self-regulated, adaptable, and specific to an individual context (33, 34).

The cortex exerts a fine control over cardiovascular activity via multiple layers of tonic inhibition. In this way, sympathetic-mediated cardio-acceleratory, inotropic, and vasoconstrictive drive is held in check by higher neural centres. The prefrontal cortex provides an important tonic inhibition over the amygdala. This is mediated via GABAergic neurones. Discontinuation of amygdala inhibition leads to increased cardiovascular activity, such as heart rate, through multiple mechanisms, including inhibition of vagal outflow by NTS inhibition and activation of tonically active sympathoexcitatory RVLM neurones directly or indirectly, via relaxation of their inhibition (35, 33). The inhibitory influence exerted by the prefrontal cortex on the autonomic nervous system represents one of a host of systems in which it exerts regulatory control, such as executive and affective functions. These processes are associated with changes in heart rate and HRV (36), and the prefrontal cortex is likely to play an important role in Thayer and Lane's Neurovisceral Integration Model of physiological, cognitive, and affective processes related to each other to serve goal-directed behaviour (33).

Subcortical control of the cardiovascular system

Multiple areas within the diencephalon, midbrain, and pons are involved in the neurocircuitry of cardiovascular control. The hypothalamus and PAG are crucial components of the network, exerting potent influences on autonomic outflow.

The hypothalamus has been called the mediator of forebrain autonomic responses (18). It influences not only the neural circuitry to the heart and vascular tree, but also modulates circulating volume via the kidney. The lateral hypothalamic area (LHA) produces cardiovascular pressor or depressor effects, depending on which of its subdivisions is stimulated. Subdivisions of the LHA project directly and indirectly onto other sites within the CAN, such as the insula, with direct projections to the sympathetic intermediolateral regions of the spinal cord (37–39). The paraventricular nucleus of the hypothalamus (PVH) provides important modulation of sodium excretion, and therefore circulating volume, via renal sympathetic outflow. The autonomic neurones within the PVH show marked activation during water deprivation in rats (40). The PVH receives a representation of circulating body water and salt levels via afferents from plasma and intracranial sodium receptors and, via the NTS, hepatic osmoreceptors and plasma volume receptors. The PVH then activates the renal sympathetic system via a direct outflow to the RVLM and in this way contributes to the slower changes in cardiovascular dynamics (for a review see Guyenet 2006 (41)).

The PAG (and periventricular grey, which will be considered as the same structure) is engaged in a variety of processes, including vocalization (42, 43), opiate and non-opiate mediated analgesia (44), fear and anxiety (44, 45), and reproductive behaviour (46). Its importance in autonomic and cardiovascular control is well documented in animals and humans. In 1935, Kabat showed that PAG stimulation could alter blood pressure in the cat (47). The columns of the PAG are functionally distinct and opposite. Activation of the dorsomedial and dorsolateral columns evokes the 'fight or flight' response and activation of the lateral and ventrolateral columns produces passive coping responses, (48, 49). This was perhaps the first evidence that the role of the PAG in autonomic control is as a 'higher' centre to influence the cardiovascular system in times of environmental stress, such as during an attack or an emotional situation or pain.

PAG neurones project onto cardiac vagal preganglionic neurones in the NA, DMNX, and the NTS (50). The PAG also has reciprocal connections with a number of higher centres involved in cardiovascular regulation, particularly the hypothalamus. Many of the descending connections from the hypothalamus pass through and are influenced by PAG. For example, the hypotensive response elicited by lateral hypothalamus stimulation can be attenuated by lidocaine injection into the PAG (52). In addition, the PAG has direct reciprocal connections with the amygdala, prefrontal cortex, and insula (52, 53). As with PAG connections to lower centres, these 'higher' connections also exhibit specificity with particular columns of the PAG. Thus, the role of PAG in autonomic regulation is probably as an 'integrator' of emotional/higher influence on cardiovascular control, similar to its role in pain control.

Medullary control of the cardiovascular system

A number of key components of the cardiovascular neurocircuitry are contained within the medulla oblongata. Most important to the beat-to-beat control of cardiovascular function are the NTS, NA, DMNX, and RVLM.

The NTS is crucial to not only the receipt of autonomic and somatic afferents from the thoracolumbar (sympathetic) and craniosacral (parasympathetic) levels to the CAN, but also in the selection of sympathetic or parasympathetic efferent outflows. The NTS is the principle site of termination of cardiovascular afferents. The glossopharyngeal (IXth) and vagus (Xth) nerves deliver information from arterial baroreceptors from the aortic arch and carotid sinus, cardiac baroreceptors from the walls of the ventricles and atria, and arterial chemoreceptors from the aortic and carotid bodies (54) to the NTS, which it then relays rostrally to multiple other CAN sites. Visceral and somatic second-order neurones (54) with plasma electrolyte, humoral, and cerebrospinal fluid chemical information from the area postrema, in the floor of the fourth ventricle, also input to the NTS (56). In this way the NTS receives a moment-to-moment representation of the cardiovascular status of the body and its circulating constituents. Once this information is processed by the rest of the CAN and integrated with information from elsewhere in the brain, such as pain or threat, for example, the NTS is the gateway to either sympathetic or parasympathetic outflows. NTS output to the RVLM modulates sympathetic drive via the intermediolateral region of the spinal cord and onwards to the sympathetic trunk. Output to the NA or DMNX facilitates parasympathetic drive via the vagus nerve (1) (see Fig. 1.3).

The RVLM is recognized to be a key regulator of arterial blood pressure (56, 57) and a component of the cardiovascular sympathetic outflow. It contains the neurones responsible for the tonic excitation of preganglionic vasomotor efferents (2). Direct RVLM stimulation produces elevations in sympathetic nerve activity and cardiovascular parameters, namely heart rate, catecholamines levels, and blood pressure. Projections from the NTS, amygdala, hypothalamus, PAG, and dorsal horn of the spinal cord innervate the RVLM, which then provides a large projection to the sympathetic intermediolateral spinal cord region. It is pivotal to several circuits, including the defence reaction and the somatosympathetic and baroreceptor reflexes (2). The latter also relies on its GABAergic input from the caudal ventrolateral medulla (CVLM). The RVLM has a complex neurochemical composition and contains a group of adrenaline-synthesizing cells known as C1 cells, one of

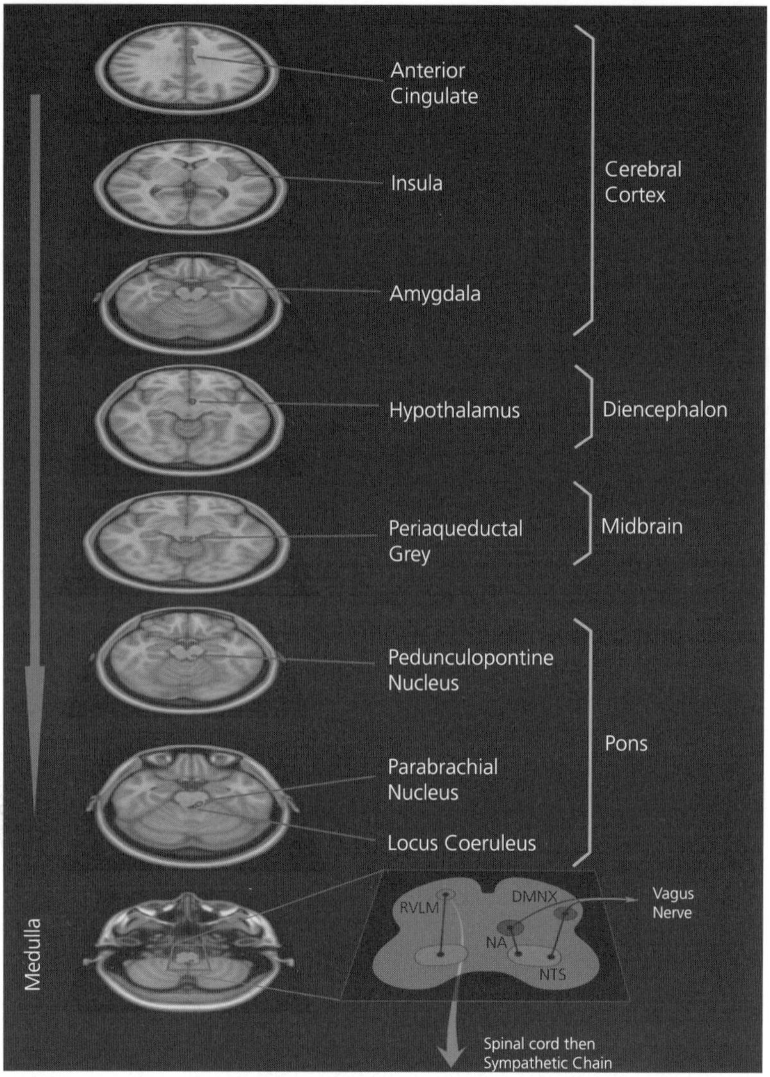

Fig. 1.3 The efferent outflow through the central autonomic network.

only three such cell groups in the central nervous system (58). A large proportion of C1 cells are baroreceptor-sensitive and are the main determinants of background sympathetic tone, but some also project onto the hypothalamic centres governing sodium and water balance (41). Other non-baroreceptor-sensitive C1 cells project onto chromaffin cells in the adrenal medulla, which secrete adrenaline, whilst others are involved in the activation of stress responses by the hypothalamic–pituitary axis (41, 59). The diverse output from the RVLM is suspected to be organized topographically, such that different populations of neurones control particular organs; for example, the heart, kidneys, or skeletal muscle arteries (41).

Sympathetic efferents

The final effectors of the cardiovascular sympathetic outflow are three classes of efferent neurones, named according to the stimulus to which they are sensitive (see Fig. 1.4). Glucosensitive efferents are activated by physical activity and hypoglycaemia to stimulate the adrenal medulla to secrete adrenaline (60). Thermosensitive efferents are activated by emotional stimuli, hypothermia, and hyperventilation to stimulate cutaneous vasoconstriction (61). The largest group, however, are the barosensitive cardiovascular efferents. The burst pattern of the barosensitive efferents is synchronized with respiration and pulse rate, and shows a continuous activity even during rest, conferring an ongoing 'sympathetic tone' on their target tissues (41). Barosensitive efferents innervate the heart, kidneys, adrenal medulla, and non-cutaneous arterioles. Whilst distension of carotid and aortic stretch receptors inhibit barosensitive efferent activity, their outflow is not influenced by the baroreceptor reflex arc alone. Distension of lung intraparenchymal stretch receptors also inhibit barosensitive efferent output, whereas their outflow is increased by stretch and metabolic receptors of exercising muscle (63), both peripheral and central chemoreceptors, and cutaneous nociceptors (61, 64). Importantly, their pattern of outflow to the kidneys is different under certain circumstances to their other targets. An increase in circulating volume with atrial stretch receptor distension causes a renal sympathetic efferent inhibition, which facilitates blood volume homeostasis (64, 65) (see Guyenet 2006 for a review (41)).

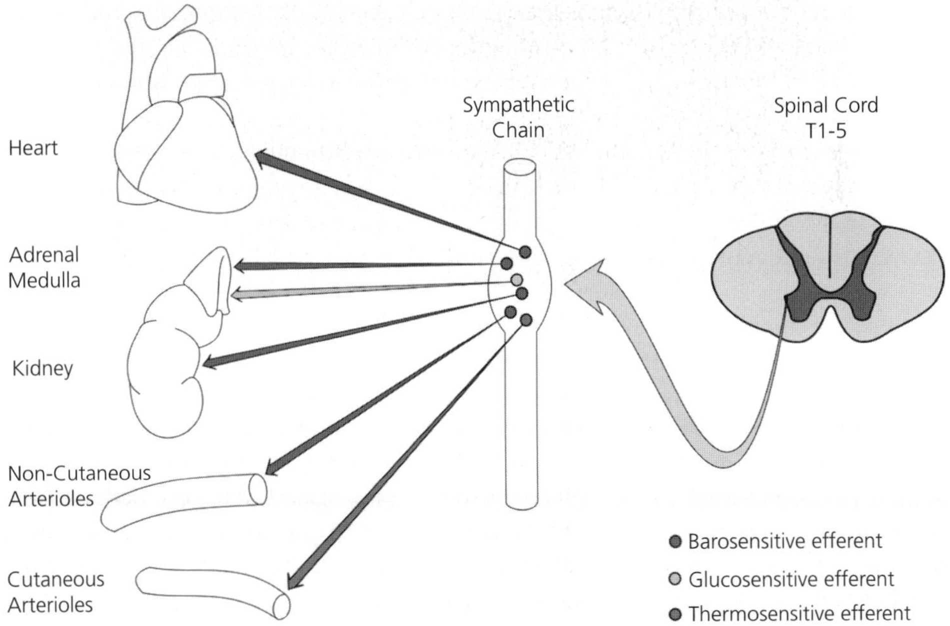

Fig. 1.4 Schematic to demonstrate the three classes of sympathetic efferents and their end-organ targets. (See Plate 1.)

Neural determinants of cardiovascular performance

The sympathetic efferents and their associated final effectors have an efferent role in control of cardiovascular performance, but how they orchestrate and fine-tune the end-organs' activity to produce the required local and systemic perfusion depends on a dynamic balance of multiple feedback and feedforward mechanisms, some simple reflexes, others much more complex processes. The response to external disturbances that may threaten circulatory homeostasis can occur rapidly from beat-to-beat via the neural circuitry and also more slowly over minutes-to-hours-to-days via neural and humoral processes. We shall discuss the neutrally mediated short- and long-term determinants of cardiovascular performance, as these processes provide opportunities for modulation by surgical techniques.

Baroreceptor reflex

The baroreceptor reflex is a short-term feedback loop and is the major compensatory mechanism to alterations in arterial blood pressure. Such stimuli include postural change and loss of circulating blood volume through haemorrhage. Arterial baroreceptors are located in the carotid sinus and aortic arch, and distension of the arterial walls stimulates these stretch receptors to fire. Changes in arterial blood pressure between 50 and 150 mmHg can de signalled (66). Afferent information is projected onto the NTS via the glossopharyngeal and vagus nerves (67). Thomas Willis, the seventeenth-century Oxford University anatomist, recognized the importance of the vagus nerve to cardiac activity and observed a 'great trembling' of the heart in the dog after transection of the vagus nerves. He recognized that the vagus nerves branched off to the aortic arch 'so that it may react to changes in the pulse' (68). Within the baroreceptor reflex circuit, the NTS projects to the RVLM indirectly via the CVLM. In response to baroreceptor stimulation, the NTS stimulates the CVLM to inhibit the RVLM's tonic sympathetic outflow. At the same time, the NTS excites the NA and DMNX, thus producing an increase in parasympathetic tone via vagal outflow, with a simultaneous reduction in sympathetic tone. Therefore, increases in blood pressure are counteracted by a shift in the autonomic balance towards parasympathetic activity, resulting in a reduction of heart rate via the sinoatrial node and negative inotropic and vasodilatory effects. Conversely, low arterial pressure and reduced baroreceptor stimulation results in the easing of sympathetic outflow via the RVLM and a reduction in vagal stimulation, with a resulting tendency towards tachycardia, increased cardiac contractility and vasoconstriction.

Baroreflex sensitivity can be modulated depending on the situation. Situations requiring different cardiovascular drives to satisfy metabolic demands can be catered for and the set-point of the feedback arc altered appropriately. In middle-aged and healthy young adults, the postural challenge of standing is associated with a decrease in baroreflex sensitivity (69, 70). The reflex is likely to be influenced by descending pathways from higher brain centres, such as the hypothalamus and forebrain areas (56).

The baroreceptor reflex plays a dominant role in the rapid prevention of wide fluctuations in arterial blood pressure. Baroreceptor denervation in dogs results in increased blood pressure variability without affecting the long-term absolute level. Cowley et al. therefore proposed that the baroreceptor reflex is not primarily responsible for setting the chronic level of systemic arterial pressure, but to minimize variation (71). It is the short-term variations in blood pressure that have been recently shown to be important in cardiovascular disease. Systolic blood pressure variability within the same medical clinic visit is a strong predictor of stroke, heart failure, and myocardial infarction (72). Impairment of baroreceptor mechanisms often accompanies cardiovascular diseases, such as hypertension, ischaemic heart disease, and heart failure (73). Therefore, there is a wealth of evidence that the integrity and sensitivity of this reflex is enormously important to circulatory homeostasis and end-organ preservation.

Chemoreceptor reflex

The chemoreceptor reflex is a second short-term feedback pathway that confers rapid cardiovascular adjustments. Chemoreceptors are located in the aortic and carotid bodies, and are sensitive primarily to arterial blood's oxygen partial pressure, rising in activity as it oxygen levels decrease. Similarly to the baroreceptor reflex, their afferents project onto the NTS via the glossopharyngeal and vagus nerves. Unlike the baroreceptor reflex, the NTS then projects directly (and indirectly via the Kölliker–Fuse nucleus) onto the RVLM (56). These inputs to the RVLM are excitatory, in contrast to the inhibitory input via the CVLM in the baroreceptor reflex. Therefore, sympathetic drive is increased by chemoreceptor stimulation causing vasoconstriction in vascular beds (excluding those in the heart and brain) and increased ventilation rate, therefore effecting a restriction of oxygen consumption in non-vital tissues and increased oxygen intake, respectively (56).

Feedback and feedforward pathways associated with exercise

The performance of skeletal exercise introduces an extra level of complexity to the regulation of cardiovascular function. Increased metabolic demands of exercising tissue elevate the requirements of the local and systemic circulation. Therefore, increases in heart rate, contractility, and peripheral resistances conferring elevations in arterial blood pressure are needed. Several mechanisms exist to match cardiovascular performance to tissue requirements.

Baroreceptor reflex

The baroreceptor reflex must alter its set-point to make allowances for the new desired elevated blood pressures (74), else as soon as a rise in arterial pressure is sensed, the RVLM and sympathetic outflow will be inhibited, frustrating efforts to increase tissue perfusion. The baroreceptors' aim of maintaining the blood pressure status quo must be tempered. Baroreflex sensitivity, therefore, decreases to facilitate the new cardiovascular targets.

Central command

The term central command was coined by Goodwin et al. in 1972 (75). It is a top-down feedforward mechanism by which higher brain areas modulate cardiorespiratory responses during exercise and was originally termed 'cortical irradiation' by Krogh and Lindhard in 1913 (76). It is classically defined as 'a feedforward mechanism involving parallel activation of motor and cardiovascular centres' (77). Central command provides a mechanism by which to plan and execute the necessary alteration in cardiorespiratory function to achieve sufficient local tissue perfusion, oxygen intake, and carbon dioxide venting in proportion to the task to be undertaken in order to create and maintain optimal conditions for exercise. The cardiovascular component of central command has been shown to be functionally independent of the motor tasks themselves. Thornton et al. and Williamson et al. demonstrated that hypnotized subjects who imagined performing exercises of different magnitudes exhibited changes in cardiovascular variables proportional to the imagined work, despite the absence of actual muscle activity. Changes in heart rate and blood pressure correlated to the degree of exercise imagined; for example, increasing whilst 'cycling' uphill and decreasing whilst 'cycling' downhill (78, 79). Therefore, the perception of the magnitude of physical effort required is sufficient alone to drive cardiorespiratory changes.

It is rational physiologically for cardiorespiratory performance to be driven in a similar top-down manner and by similar centres as those coordinating exercising motor performance. Until recently, interrogation of the neurocircuitry of central command in the human has been limited to non-invasive neuro-imaging studies, which reflect changes in metabolic or vascular activity. The insula, ACC, other medial prefrontal areas, and the thalamus have been implicated by functional magnetic resonance imaging (fMRI) and positron emission tomography studies (13, 78, 81). The first invasive neurophysiological evidence, in which neuronal activity was directly evaluated in humans, implicated two subcortical sites: the subthalamic nucleus (STN) of the diencephalon, a site with important associative, limbic, and motor connections (82–85), and the PAG. Recordings from deep-brain macroelectrodes within the STN and PAG demonstrated changes in local field potential power during the anticipation of exercise and during exercise performance itself, with a parallel increase in cardiorespiratory variables (86). Further, direct electrical stimulation of both sites in awake humans via deep-brain electrodes causes changes in heart rate, blood pressure, and heart rate variability (87–91). Therefore, a network extending from multiple cortical areas through the diencephalon and brainstem is proposed to initiate cardiovascular performance changes according to expected exercise demands, even before the exercise is commenced.

Exercise pressor reflex

The exercise pressor reflex is another feedback mechanism via which cardiovascular performance is regulated according to skeletal muscle metabolic requirements (92, 93). This reflex was first demonstrated in 1937 by Alum and Smirk when elevations in arterial blood pressure were maintained after exercise had ceased due to inflation of a tourniquet proximal to the exercising muscle, preventing escape of local muscle metabolites (94). Peripheral neural drive from exercising muscle is generated by mechanoreflex and metaboreflex receptors, which are mechanically (stretch and pressure) and chemically sensitive, respectively. The afferent limb of the reflex consists of Group III and Group IV primary afferent neurones, which transmit mechanical and chemical information, respectively (95–98). Chemical stimuli from muscle metabolism include lactic acid, prostaglandins, hydrogen ions, adenosine, and ATP analogues. The afferents project onto the dorsal horn of the spinal cord and ascend to the brainstem, with the NTS the most likely central integrating site of the reflex (99). Other sites implicated in the pathway are the RVLM, CVLM, NA, and the PAG (for a review see Smith et al. 2006 (93)). Stimulation of the afferent limb of the pathway results in an increase in sympathetic drive and an inhibition of parasympathetic outflow (96), thereby elevating cardiovascular parameters to meet the perfusion demands of the exercising tissue.

Mechanisms associated with behaviour

Behavioural factors, such as anxiety, sleep, and panic, confer a range of effects on cardiovascular performance. Various behaviours are associated with cardiovascular changes over the short term, whereas others may be effected on a long-term basis.

The 'defence' reaction was described in the rat in 1956 by Hunsperger (100). This is an integrated response that is associated with survival in the wild. There are two main phenotypic responses, depending on the evaluation of the external situation. If escape from danger is possible, the response involves a 'fight or flight' reaction that includes raised blood pressure and heart rate, non-opioid mediated analgesia, and emotional effects such as fear (101, 102) in association with other effects such as vocalization, pupillary changes, micturition, and changes in skeletal blood flow (103). Conversely, if escape is not possible and it is safer to remain undetected, the reaction consists of a depression of cardiovascular parameters, such as lowered blood pressure and heart rate, opioid-mediated analgesia, and a 'withdrawal reaction', as well as fear (104, 105). It was soon established that the PAG is an important area involved in the defence reaction. Stimulation of the dorsomedial and dorsolateral columns evokes the 'fight or flight' response, whereas activation of the lateral and ventrolateral columns produces the passive coping responses (49, 101).

Cardiovascular performance in response to a perceived threat incorporates a variety of components of the CAN and forebrain structures. Arnsten and Goldman-Rakic proposed that the prefrontal cortex, an important source of inhibition of multiple pathways, including of sympathetic tone, is taken 'offline' when threat exists in order to allow more habitual responses to regulate behaviour of survival value (106). Therefore, the amygdala and subcortical structures can rapidly execute non-volitional behaviours without conscious deliberative processes causing a delay in the response (16). Not all prefrontal areas are inhibited, however.

The ACC is recognized to be active in situations where the rapid activation of motor and cardiorespiratory systems is critical. An example of such a situation is 'circa strike', the reaction to an imminent threat. This ecologically important state results in behaviour that facilitates avoidance and escape with activation of critical midbrain regions, such as the dorsal PAG, with facilitation of the 'flight or fight' response, whilst forebrain circuits are simultaneously inhibited (107). During the performance of a maze task involving an artificial intelligence predator, Mobbs et al. demonstrated increased dorsal ACC and midbrain blood oxygen level-dependent signal on fMRI during circa strike threat in humans and also increased skin conductance level, a presumed autonomic sympathetic arousal state surrogate marker (108). There was also a simultaneous decrease in the ACC/midbrain coupling with other components of the CAN, namely the amygdala and hypothalamus. In contrast, when the threat was remote rather than imminent, the subgenual ACC, amygdala, and hypothalamus were active instead. As the ACC is recognized to reside at the intersection of the brain's cognitive, motor, and arousal pathways, it makes biological sense for it to be central to the orchestration of such survival responses for the purposes of gain or self-preservation.

Conclusions

The neural control of the heart and cardiovascular system is highly complex and dynamic. Structures from all levels of the brain and spinal cord are involved in the relay and processing of multimodal information from throughout the body and the modulation of appropriate cardiovascular performance. Multiple feedback and feedforward mechanisms exist to ensure cardiovascular responses are tailored according to the individual's requirements. Some operate rapidly on a beat-to-beat basis, whereas others are responsible for slower changes. Understanding of the anatomy and physiology of this system provides the opportunity for various components to be influenced by surgical modulation therapies.

References

1 **Schmidt RF, Thews G**. Human Physiology. Springer-Verlag, New York, 1983.

2 **Benarroch EE**. Central Autonomic Network: Functional Organization and Clinical Correlations. Futura: Armonk, New York, 1997.

3 **Ter Horst GJ, Postema F**. Forebrain parasympathetic control of heart activity: retrograde transneuronal viral labelling in rats. Am J Physiol 1997;**273**:2926–2930.

4 **Paus T**. Primate anterior cingulate cortex: where motor control, drive and cognition interface. Nat Rev Neurosci 2001;**2**:417–24.

5 **Ongur D, An X, Price JL**. Prefrontal cortical projections to the hypothalamus in macaque monkey. J Comp Neurol 1998;**401**:480–505.

6 **An X, Bandler R, Ongur D, Price JL**. Prefrontal cortical projections to longitudinal columns in the midbrain periaqueductal grey in macaque monkeys. J Comp Neurol 1998;**401**:455–79.

7 **Pool JL, Ransohoff J**. Autonomic effects on stimulating rostral portion of cingulate gyri in man. J Neurophysiol 1949;**12**:385–92.

8 **Gentil AF, Eskandar EN, Marci CD, Evans KC, Dougherty DD**. Physiological response to brain stimulation during limbic surgery: further evidence of anterior cingulate modulation of autonomic arousal. Biol Psychiatr 2009;**66**(7):695–701.

9 **Burns SM, Wyss JM**. The involvement of the anterior cingulate cortex in blood pressure control. Brain Res 1985;**340**:71–77.

10 **Chefer SI, Talan MI, Engel BT**. Central neural correlates of learned heart rate control during exercise: central command demystified. J Appl Physiol 1997;**83**:1448–53.

11 **Kaada BR**. Somato-motor, autonomic and electrocorticographic responses to electrical stimulation of rhinencephalic and other structures in primates, cat and dog. Acta Phsyiologica Scandinavica 1951;**24**(Suppl 83):1–285.

12 **Kaada BR, Pribram KH, Epstein JA**. Respiratory and vascular responses in monkeys from temporal pole, insula orbital surface and cingulate gyrus. J Neurophysiol 1949;**12**:347–56.

13 **Critchley HD, Corfield DR, Chandler P, Mathias CJ, Dolan RJ**. Cerebral correlates of autonomic cardiovascular arousal: a functional neuroimaging investigation in humans. J Physiol 2000;**523**(1):259–70.

14 **Critchley HD, Mathias CJ, Josephs O et al**. Human cingulate cortex and autonomic control: converging neuroimaging and clinical evidence. Brain 2003;**126**:2139–52.

15 **Zahn TP, Grafman J, Tranel D**. Frontal lesions and electrodermal activity: effects of significance, Neuropsychologica 1999;**37**:1227–41.

16 **Thayer JF, Lane RD**. Caude Bernard and the heart-brain connection: further elaboration of a model of neurovisceral integration. Neurosci Behav Rev 2009;**33**:81–88.

17 **Cechetto DF, Gelb AW**. The amygdala and cardiovascular control. J Neurosurg Anesthesiol 2001;**13**:329–32.

18 **Cechetto DF**. Forebrain control of healthy and diseased hearts. In: Armour JA, Ardell JL (eds) Basic and Clinical Neurocardiology. Oxford University Press: New York; 2004;220–51.

19 **Davis M**. The role of the amygdala in fear and anxiety. Annu Rev Neurosci 1992;**15**:353–75.

20 **Kaada BR**. Stimulation and regional ablation of the amygdaloid complex with reference to functional representations. In: Eleftheriou BE (ed.) The Neurobiology of the Amygdala. Plenum Press: New York; 1972;205–82.

21 **Cechetto DF, Calaresu FR**. Central pathways relaying cardiovascular afferent information to amygdala. Am J Physiol 1985;**248**:R38–R45.

22 **Frysinger RC, Marks JD, Trelease RB, Shechtman VL, Harper RM**. Sleep states attenuate the pressor response to cenytral amygdala stimulation. Exp Neurol 1984;**83**:604–17.

23 **Galeno TM, Brody MB**. Hemodynamic responses to Amygdaloid stimulation in spontaneously hypertensive rats. Am J Physiol 1983;**245**:R281–86.

24 **Gelsema AJ, McKitrick DJ, Calaresu FR**. Cardiovascular responses to chemical and electrical stimulation of amygdala in rats. Am J Physiol 1987;**253**:R712–18.

25 **Hilz MJ, Dutsch M, Perrine K, Nelson PK, Rauhut U, Devinsky O**. Hemispheric influence on autonomic and baroreflex sensitivity. Ann Neurol 2001;**49**(5):575–84.

26 **Diedrich A, Porta A, Barbic F et al**. Lateralization of expression of neural sympathetic activity to the vessels and effect of carotid baroreceptor stimulation. Am J Physiol Heart Circ Physiol 2009;**296**:1758–65.

27 **Zhang Z, Oppenheimer SM**. Characterization, distribution and lateralization of baroreceptor-related neurons in the rat insular cortex. Brain Res 1997;**760**:243–50.

28 **Cereda C, Ghika J, Maeder P, Bogousslavsky J**. Strokes restricted to the insular cortex. Neurology 2002;**59**(12):1950–55.

29 **Colivicchi F, Bassi A, Santini M, Caltagirone C**. Prognostic implications of right-sided insular damage, cardiac autonomic derangement, and arrhythmias after acute ischemic stroke. Stroke 2005;**36**(8):1710–15.

30 **Meyer S, Strittmatter M, Fisher C, Georg T, Schmitz B**. Lateralization in autonomic dysfunction in ischemic stroke involving the insular cortex. Neuroreport 2004;**15**(2):357–61.

31 **Craig AD**. Forebrain emotional asymmetry: a neuroanatomical basis? Trends Cognit Sci 2005;**19**:566–71.

32 **Gevins A, Smith ME, McEvoy LK, Leong H, Le J**. Electroencephalographic imaging of higher brain function. Philos Trans R Soc Lond B 1999;**354**:1125–34.

33 **Thayer JF, Lane RD**. Claude Bernard and the heart-brain connection: further elaboration of a model of neurovisceral integration. Neurosci Behav Rev 2009;**33**(2):81–88.

34 **Thayer JF, Lane RD**. A model of neurovisceral integration in emotion regulation and dysregulation. J Affect Disord 2000;**61**:201–16.

35 **Saha S**. Role of the central nucleus of the amygdala in the control of blood pressure: Descending pathways to medullary cardiovascular nuclei. Clin Exp Pharmacol Physiol 2005;**32**:450–56.

36 **Thayer JF, Brosschot JF**. Psychosomatics and psychopathology: looking up and down from the brain. Psychoneuroendocrinology 2005;**30**:1050–58.

37 **Allen GV, Cechetto DF**. Functional and anatomical organization of cardiovascular pressor and depressor sites in the lateral hypothalamic area: I. Descending projections. J Comp Neurol 1992;**315**:313–32.

38 **Allen GV, Cechetto DF**. Functional and anatomical organization of cardiovascular pressor and depressor sites in the lateral hypothalamic area: II. Ascending projections. J Comp Neurol 1992;**330**:421–38.

39 **Cechetto DF, Saper CB**. Neurochemical organization of the hypothalamic projections to the spinal cord in the rat. J Comp Neurol 1988;**272**:579–604.

40 **Stocker SD, Hunwick KJ, Toney GM**. Hypothalamic paraventricular nucleus differentially supports lumbar and renal sympathetic outflow in water-deprived rats. J Physiol 2005;**563**(Pt 1):249–63.

41 **Guyenet PG**. The sympathetic control of blood pressure. Nat Rev Neurosci 2006;**7**:335–46.

42 **Brown TG**. Note on physiology of basal ganglia and midbrain of anthropoid ape especially in reference to act of laughter. J Physiol 1915;**49**:195–207.

43 **Kyuhou S, Gemba H**. Two vocalization-related subregions in the midbrain periaqueductal gray of the guinea pig. Neuroreport 1998;**9**:1607–10.

44 **Bandler R, Carrive P**. Integrated defence reaction elicited by excitatory amino acid microinjection in the midbrain periaqueductal grey region of the unrestrained cat. Brain Res 1988;**439**:95–106.

45 **Nashold BS Jr, Wilson WP, Slaughter DG**. Sensations evoked by stimulation in the midbrain of man. J Neurosurg 1969;**30**:14–24.

46 **Van der Horst VG, Holstege G**. Sensory and motor components of reproductive behavior: pathways and plasticity. Behav Brain Res 1998;**92**:157–67.

47 **Kabat H, Magoun HW, Ranson SW**. Electrical stimulation of Points in the forebrain and midbrain. The resultant alteration in blood pressure. Arch Neurol Psychiatr 1935;**34**:931–55.

48 **Carrive P, Bandler R**. Viscerotopic organization of neurones subserving hypotensive reactions within the midbrain periaqueductal grey: a correlative functional and anatomical study. Brain Res 1991b;**541**:206–15.

49 **Bittencourt AS, Carobrez AP, Zamprogno LP, Tufik S, Schenberg LC**. Organization of single components of defensive behaviors within distinct columns of periaqueductal gray matter of the rat: role of N-methyl-D-aspartic acid glutamate receptors. Neuroscience 2001;**125**:71–89.

50 **Farkas E, Jansen AS, Loewy AD**. Periaqueductal gray matter projection to vagal preganglionic neurones and the nucleus tractus solitaries. Brain Res 1997;**764**:257–61.

51 **Pajolla GP, Tavares RF, Pelosi GG, Correa FM**. Involvement of the periaqueductal gray in the hypotensive response evoked by L-glutamate microinjection in the lateral hypothalamus of unanesthetized rats. Autonom Neurosci 2005;**22**:84–93.

52 **Rizvi TA, Ennis M, Behbehani MM, Shipley MT**. Connections between the central nucleus of the amygdala and the midbrain periaqueductal gray: topography and reciprocity. J Comp Neurol 1991;**303**:121–31.

53 **Bandler R, Keay KA, Floyd N, Price J**. Central circuits mediating patterned autonomic activity during active vs. passive emotional coping. Brain Res Bull 2000;**53**:95–104.

54 **Dampney RAL**. Functional organization of central pathways regulating the cardiovascular system. Physiol Rev 1994;**74**(2):323–64.

55 **Loewy AD, Spyer KM**. Central Regulation of Autonomic Functions. Oxford University Press: Oxford, UK; 1990.

56 **Dampney RAL, Coleman MJ, Fontes MAP et al.** Central mechanisms underlying short- and long-term regulation of the cardiovascular system. Clin Exp Pharmacol Physiol 2002;**29**:261–68.

57 **Ross CA, Ruggiero DA, Park DH, et al.** Tonic vasomotor control by the rostral ventrolateral medulla: effect of electrical or chemical stimulation of the area containing C1 adrenaline neurons on arterial pressure, heart rate, and plasma catecholamines and vasopressin. J Neurosci 1984;**4**:474–94.

58 **Hokfelt T, Fuxe K, Goldstein M, Johansson O.** Immunohistochemical evidence for the existence of adrenaline neurons in the rat brain. Brain Res 1974;**66**:235–51.

59 **Ritter S, Bugarith K, Dinh TT.** Immunotoxic destruction of distinct catecholamine subgroups produces selective impairment of glucoregulatory responses and neuronal activation. J Comp Neurol 2001;**432**:197–216.

60 **Cao WH, Morrison SF.** Differential chemoreceptor reflex responses of adrenal preganglionic neurons. American Journal Physiology: Regulatory, Intergr Comp Physiol 2001;**281**:R1825–32.

61 **Janig W, Habler JH.** Neurophysiological analysis of target-related sympathetic pathways—from animal to huma: similarities and differences. Acta Physiologica (London) 2000;**524**:279–92.

62 **Guo ZL, Lai H, Longhurst JC.** Medullary pathways involved in cardiac sympathoexcitatory reflexes in the cat. Brain Res 2002;**925**:55–6.

63 **Sinoway LI, Li J.** A perspective on the muscle reflex: implications for congestive cardiac failure. J Appl Physiol 2005;**99**:5–22.

64 **Coote JH.** A role of the paraventricular nucleus of the hypothalamus in the autonomic control of heart and kidney. Exp Physiol 2005;**90**:169–73.

65 **Ramchandra R, Barrett CJ, Guild SJ, Malpas SC.** Evidence of differential control of renal and lumbar sympathetic nerve activity in conscious rabbits. Am J Physiol 2006;**290**:R701–08.

66 **Kirchheim HR.** Systemic arterial baroreceptor reflexes. Physiol Rev 1976;**56**:100–76.

67 **Wieling W, Karemaker JM.** Measurement of heart rate and blood pressure to evaluate disturbances in neurocardiovascular control. In: Mathias C, Bannister R (eds) Autonomic Failure: A Textbook of Clinical Disorders of the Autonomic Nervous System, 4th edn; Oxford University Press: New York; 2001.

68 **Finger S.** Origins of Neuroscience. Oxford University Press: New York; 1994.

69 **Bahjaoui-Bouhaddi M, Henriet MT, Cappelle S, Dumoulin G, Regnard J.** Active standing and passive tilting similarly reduce the slope of spontaneous baroreflex in healthy subjects. Physiol Res 1998;**47**:227–35.

70 **Cooper VL, Hainsworth R.** Carotid baroreceptor reflexes in humans during orthostatic stress. Exp Physiol 2001;**86**:677–81.

71 **Cowley AW Jr, Liard JF, Guyton AC.** Role of baroreceptor reflex in daily control of arterial blood pressure and other variables in dogs. Circ Res 1973;**32**:564–76.

72 **Rothwell PM, Howard SC, Dolan E et al.** Prognistic significance of visit-to-visit variability, maximum systolic blood pressure, and episodic hypertension. Lancet 2010;**375**:895–905.

73 **Eckberg DL, Sleight P (eds) Human Baroreflexes in Health and Disease.** Clarendon Press: Oxford; 1992.

74 **Potts JT, Shi XR, Raven PB.** Carotid baroreflex responsiveness during dynamic exercise in humans. Am J Physiol 1993;**265**:H1928–38.

75 **Goodwin GM, McCloskey DI, Mitchell JH.** Cardiovascular and respiratory responses to changes in central command during isometric exercise at a constant muscle tension. J Physiol 1972;**226**:173–90.

76 **Krogh A, Lindhard J.** The regulation of respiration and circulation during the initial stages of muscular work. J Physiol 1913;**47**:112–36

77 **Williamson JW, Fadel PJ, Mitchell JH**. New insights into central cardiovascular control during exercise in humans: a central command update. Exp Physiol 2006;**91**(1):51–58.

78 **Thornton JM, Guz A, Murphy K et al.** Identification of higher brain centres that may encode the cardiorespiratory response to exercise in humans. J Physiol 2001;**533**(3):823–36.

79 **Williamson JW, McColl R, Mathews D, Mitchell JH, Raven PB, Morgan WP**. Hypnotic manipulation of effort sense during dynamic exercise: cardiovascular responses and brain activation. J Appl Physiol 2001;**90**:1392–99.

80 **Williamson JW, McColl R, Mathews D, Mitchell JH, Raven PB, Morgan WP**. Brain activation by central command during actual and imagined handgrip under hypnosis. J Appl Physiol 2002;**92**:1317–24.

81 **Williamson JW, McColl R, Mathews D**. Evidence for central command activation of the human insular cortex during exercise. J Appl Physiol 2003;**94**:1726–34.

82 **Hamani C, Saint-Cyr JA, Fraser J, Kaplitt M, Lozano AM**. The subthalamic nucleus in the context of movement disorders. Brain 2004;**127**:4–20.

83 **Joel D, Weiner I**. The connections of the primate subthalamic nucleus: indirect pathways and the open-interconnected scheme of basal gangliathalamocortical circuitry. Brain Res Rev 1997;**23**:62–78.

84 **Parent A, Hazrati LN**. Functional anatomy of the basal ganglia. II. The place of subthalamic nucleus and external pallidum in basal ganglia circuitry. Brain Res Brain Res Rev 1995;**20**:128–54.

85 **Shink E, Bevan MD, Bolam JP, Smith Y**. The subthalamic nucleus and the external pallidum: two tightly interconnected structures that control the output of the basal ganglia in the monkey. Neuroscience 1996;**73**:335–57.

86 **Green AL, Wang S, Purvis S et al.** Identifying cardiorespiratory neurocircuitry involved in central command during exercise in humans. J Physiol 2007;**578**(2):605–12.

87 **Green AL, Hyam JA, Williams C, Wang S, Shlugman D, Stein JF, Paterson DJ, Aziz TZ**. Intra-operative deep brain stimulation of the periaqueductal grey matter modulates blood pressure and heart rate variability in humans. Neuromodulation 2010;**13**:174–81

88 **Green AL, Wang S, Owen SLF et al.** Deep brain stimulation can regulate arterial blood pressure in awake humans. Neuroreport 2005;**16**(16):1741–45.

89 **Green AL, Wang S, Owen SLF, Paterson DJ, Stein JF, Aziz TZ**. Controlling the heart via the brain: a potential new therapy for orthostatic hypotension. Neurosurgery 2006;**58**:1176–83.

90 **Pereira EAC, Lu G, Wang S et al.** Ventral periaqueductal grey stimulation alters heart rate variability in humans with chronic pain. Exp Neurol 2010;**223**:574–81.

91 **Thornton JM, Aziz T, Schlugman D, Paterson DJ**. Electrical stimulation of the midbrain increases heart rate and arterial blood pressure in awake humans. J Physiol 2002;**539**(Pt 2):615–21.

92 **Green AL, Paterson DJ**. Identification of neurocircuitry controlling cardiovascular function in humans using functional neurosurgery: implications for exercise control. Exp Physiol 2008;**93**(9):1022–28.

93 **Smith SA, Mitchell JH, Garry MG**. The mammalian exercise pressor reflex in health and disease. Exp Physiol 2006;**91**(1):89–102.

94 **Alum M, Smirk FH**. Observations in man upon blood pressure raising reflex arising from the voluntary muscles. J Physiol 1937;**89**:372–83.

95 **Hayes SG, Kindig AE, Kaufman MP**. A comparison between the effect of static contraction and tendon stretch on the discharge of group III and IV muscle afferents. J Appl Physiol 2005;**99**:1891–96.

96 **Kaufman MP, Forster HV**. Reflexes controlling circulatory, ventilatory and airway responses to exercise. In: Rowell LB, Shepherd JT (eds) Handbook of Physiology, Exercise: Regulation and Integration of Multiple Systems. American Physiological Society: Bethesda, MD, USA; 1996.

97 **Williamson JW, Mitchell JH, Olesen HL, Raven PB, Secher NH.** Reflex increase in blood pressure induced by leg compression in man. J Physiol 1994;**475**:351–57.

98 **Stebbins CL, Ortiz-Acevedo A.** The exercise pressor reflex is attenuated by intrathecal oxytocin. Am J Physiol 1994;**267**:R909–15.

99 **Person RJ.** Somatic and vagal afferent convergence on solitary tract neurons in cat: electrophysiological characteristics. Neuroscience 1989;**30**:283–95

100 **Hunsperger RW.** Affective reaction from electric stimulation of brain stem in cats. Helv Physiol Pharmacol Acta 1956;**14**:70–92.

101 **Carrive P, Bandler R.** Control of extracranial and hindlimb blood flow by the midbrain periaqueductal grey of the cat. Exp Brain Res 1991a;**84**:599–606.

102 **McGaraughty S, Far D, Heinricher MM.** Lesions of the periaqueductal gray disrupt input to the rostral ventromedial medulla following microinjections of morphine into the medial or basolateral nuclei of the amygdala. Brain Res 2004;**1009**:223–27.

103 **Schenberg LC, Povoa RM, Costa AL, Caldellas AV, Tufik S, Bittencourt AS.** Functional specializations within the tectum defense systems of the rat. Neurosci Biobehav Rev 2005;**29**:1279–98.

104 **Johnson PL, Lightman SL, Lowry CA.** A functional subset of serotonergic neurones in the rat ventrolateral periaqueductal gray implicated in the inhibition of sympathoexcitation and panic. Ann NY Acad Sci 2004;**1018**:58–64.

105 **Finnegan TF, Chen SR, Pan HL.** Effect of the {mu} opioid on excitatory and inhibitory synaptic inputs to periaqueductal gray-projecting neurones in the amygdala. J Pharmacol Expl Ther 2005;**312**:441–48.

106 **Arnsten AFT, Goldman-Rakic PS.** Noise stress impairs prefrontal cortical cognitive function in monkeys: evidence for a hyperdopaminergic mechanism. Arch Gen Psychiatr 1998;**55**:362–68.

107 **Mobbs D, Marchant JL, Hassabis D et al.** From threat to fear: the neural organization of defensive fear systems in humans. J Neurosci 2009;**29**(39):12236–43.

108 **Critchley HD, Melmed RN, Featherstone E, Mathias CJ, Dolan RJ.** Volitional control of autonomic arousal: a functional magnetic resonance study. Neuroimage 2002;**16**(4):909–19.

Chapter 2

Baroreceptor activation therapy

A surgical approach to the treatment of hypertension

Peter W. de Leeuw and Abraham A. Kroon

Key points

1 The sympathetic nervous system plays an important role in blood pressure regulation. In patients with hypertension, notably in those resistant to drug treatment, the system is of pathogenetic significance.

2 Modulation of baroreceptor function may reduce sympathetic outflow to the heart and blood vessels, thereby inducing a fall in blood pressure.

3 Devices have been developed which, after implantation in the area of the carotid sinus, allow delivery of electrical energy locally; such stimulation of the baroreceptor area produces a sustained fall in pressure.

4 Device-based treatment of hypertension does not have major adverse effects and is well tolerated.

5 Although patients have initially been stimulated bilaterally, one-sided stimulation (preferably on the right side) appears to be sufficient for a good clinical response.

Introduction

Hypertension is a common disorder affecting approximately 1 billion people worldwide (1). It is a leading cause of cardiovascular morbidity and mortality. Stroke, myocardial infarction, and heart failure, as well as hypertensive kidney disease, are among the most frequent complications accounting for considerable disability and societal costs. The occurrence of such atherothrombotic complications is accelerated in the presence of other risk factors (hyperlipidaemia, smoking, etc.).

Hypertension sometimes is related to specific abnormalities such as renal artery stenosis or overproduction of aldosterone (primary hyperaldosteronism) or catecholamines (feochromocytoma). Whenever this is the case, the clinician will try to eliminate the causative factor. In most patients, however, no underlying cause can be found and the hypertension is classified as primary or essential. In all likelihood, both genetic and environmental factors are involved in the pressure rise of these patients.

Pathophysiological aspects of essential hypertension

Haemodynamically, blood pressure is characterized by a static and a dynamic component. The static component is determined mainly by cardiac output (CO) and total peripheral vascular resistance (TPR). The dynamic part is largely dependent upon vascular stiffness. Although a rise in CO may be responsible for an increased blood pressure, hypertension will not persist if TPR does not rise either. The typical profile of a younger hypertensive patient would be a normal or perhaps slightly elevated CO with an increased vascular resistance. At later ages, CO will be reduced and resistance further increased (2).

For more than a century, clinicians have believed that exaggerated salt consumption would lead to volume excess and, hence, elevated blood pressure. However, it is now known that only part of the population is sensitive to the effects of sodium and even then there is insufficient evidence that hypertension will develop as a consequence of volume retention per se. Studies have shown that plasma volume and, to a lesser extent, extracellular volume are inversely related to the height of blood pressure, which could be interpreted as an attempt of the body to lower its volume to compensate for the pressure rise. Along the same line of reasoning one could see the progressive fall in the levels of circulating renin as hypertension progresses, as an adaptive phenomenon (2).

Among the mechanisms that may cause a rise in blood pressure, an over-active autonomic nervous system ranks high. Indeed, many observations in hypertensives are in line with the possibility of adrenergic overdrive, such as a tendency in some individuals to display exaggerated heart rate responses to a variety of stimuli. In addition, high levels of plasma catecholamines and renin have been found in subgroups of mainly young hypertensives. More sophisticated techniques, such as muscle sympathetic nerve activity (MSNA) recordings, have confirmed greater adrenergic activity in hypertensives than in normotensives, and in both groups this activity tends to increase with age (3). It should be noted, however, that MSNA only detects sympathetic activity in a special nerve (usually the peroneal nerve) and this does not necessarily reflect overall sympathetic activity. Even more intriguing are the findings obtained from measurements of total and regional noradrenaline spillover. In as much as spillover of noradrenaline into the plasma is a marker of sympathetic outflow, this technique allows assessment of overall sympathetic activity in the body or just in a specific organ if one samples blood that is draining from that particular organ, e.g. the kidney. Small studies in normotensives have shown an overall correlation between MSNA and renal noradrenaline spillover (4), which suggests that MSNA may, indeed, also be a marker for sympathetic activity at other places than the leg. More specifically, it appears that both cardiac and renal sympathetic activity are increased in younger patients with primary hypertension and usually normal in older ones (5).

Under normal circumstances, the capacity of the body to counteract a rise in pressure is substantial. According to Guyton and co-workers, hypertension can only persist in the long run when the ability of the kidneys to excrete water and salt is impaired (6). In other words, if the kidneys, for whatever reason, fail to appropriately excrete a certain salt load, blood pressure will go up; otherwise pressure-natriuresis in the kidney will get rid of the excess of total body sodium and restore pressure to its initial level. Interestingly, the autonomic system also has a role in counteracting pressure rises and it does so through the baroreceptor system.

Baroreceptor function in hypertension

The role of the baroreceptor system in the regulation of blood pressure has been known for more than 150 years (7). In essence, the purpose of the baroreceptor system is to buffer both upward and downward excursions of blood pressure. The baroreceptors are located in the aortic arch, as well as at the carotid sinus level. They are not really responding to the pressure itself but rather to stretch of the vascular wall; so, they are more like mechanoreceptors than like baroreceptors. From the receptor area both myelinated A-fibres and unmyelinated C-fibres run into the central nervous system through the IXth (glossopharyngeal) and Xth (vagal) cranial nerves. More stretch of the carotid vascular wall or, for that matter, a rise in arterial pressure causes increased firing of the afferents, which will stimulate the cardiovascular control centre to lower sympathetic discharge and to enhance parasympathetic (vagal) tone. The opposite occurs when blood pressure falls. Given this mechanism, it is not surprising that bilateral dissection of the carotid nerves is associated with hypertension and tachycardia (8).

There is debate about the precise role of the baroreceptors ever since Guyton and colleagues proposed that the baroreflex system is not important for the long-term regulation of blood pressure but serves to regulate moment-to-moment variations in pressure (9). However, this view has been challenged by others who argued that Guyton and co-workers misinterpreted their own data and that baroreceptors do play a role in the long-term stabilization of pressure (10).

If baroreceptors are so important in counteracting hypertension, one may ask the question why they do not restore pressure once high blood pressure develops. The answer lies in the so-called resetting phenomenon, which means that the set point of the system gradually moves upwards when the receptors are chronically exposed to a higher pressure. In addition, Bristow and colleagues were the first to show that the baroreceptor system in patients with hypertension is not only reset, but also less sensitive (11). These investigators measured baroreceptor sensitivity from the relationship between changes in systolic blood pressure and those in the intervals between successive heartbeats after the administration of vasoconstrictor substances. It seems, therefore, that the baroreflex system more or less passively follows the development of hypertension.

Can dysfunction of the baroreceptor system cause hypertension? Data obtained in experimental animals suggest it can. Indeed, selective denervation of baroreceptors significantly increases blood pressure for several days (8). Moreover, in humans, hypertension may develop following neck surgery or radiotherapy in the carotid area (12). Interestingly, though, this form of hypertension is quite labile, which means that there are substantial upward as well as downward swings in blood pressure. Admittedly, this is a bit different from the situation in 'ordinary' hypertension where variability is more modest. Nevertheless, the observation that deafferentation of the carotid baroreceptors raises pressure justifies the hypothesis that stimulation of these structures may lower the pressure. In fact, these considerations have led to the development of devices with which it became possible to electrically stimulate the baroreceptor area in the intact human being.

Electrical stimulation of the baroreflex

Early experiments in animals

Bilgutay and colleagues who designed a device, which they called the baropacer, have done pioneering work in the field of baroreceptor activation therapy (13). Their instrument consisted of a compact implantable unit with two stainless steel electrodes that were attached directly to the baroreceptor area and sutured in the wall of the carotid arteries. When they stimulated the baroreceptors for 2 hours they were able to produce a substantial drop in blood pressure (13, 14). A few years later, Neistadt and Schwartz obtained similar results in dogs with experimentally induced hypertension when they applied a so-called radiofrequency (RF) stimulator that was attached to the carotid sinus nerve (15). Both devices stimulated the carotid baroreceptors bilaterally. However, it turned out that unilateral stimulation was effective as well, as shown by Griffith and Schwartz (16). These investigators used a pacemaker device with a bipolar electrode that was attached directly to the carotid sinus nerve and which reduced blood pressure irrespective of whether the contralateral sinus nerve was sectioned or not. Since then, several other groups have confirmed that animals subjected to carotid sinus nerve stimulation respond with a drop in pressure (17–21). In general, blood pressure quickly returned upon discontinuation of the stimulation. From these experiments one may conclude that stimulation of the carotid baroreceptor or carotid sinus nerve can, indeed, lower blood pressure, at least in experimental animals. The available data also show that it does not really matter what type of device is used, which site is stimulated, and what the prevailing level of pressure before the stimulation is, even though responses seem somewhat greater under hypertensive conditions.

Early experiments in humans

Carlsten and colleagues were the first to report on the effects of direct carotid sinus stimulation in humans (22). In five patients with neck cancer who required dissection of the carotid sinus region, they applied brief periods of electrical stimulation using a bipolar electrode. The experiment caused a prompt fall in mean blood pressure, pulse amplitude, and heart rate. Bilgutay and Lillehei, who had previously reported on their results in experimental animals, followed two patients who were treated with an electronic implantable stimulator for a period of up to 1 year (23). Although they used different devices in these patients, both of them exhibited significant reductions in blood pressure. The long-term results were somewhat equivocal though, as in one patient, blood pressure remained reduced, while in the other, it tended to rise again. Also, in the study of Schwartz and co-workers, results were not uniform (24). In 'only' eight of eleven patients whom they had treated for a variable period of time, they noticed a sustained fall in blood pressure of 30 to 100 mmHg systolic and of 24 to 80 mmHg diastolic. In two patients only marginal changes in pressure occurred and one patient died shortly after device implantation. Since then a large number of studies have confirmed the efficacy of baropacing, not only in the treatment of hypertension but also in the management of patients with coronary insufficiency (25). Unfortunately, though, these were all observational studies and case histories. No randomized controlled trials with the devices were carried out at the time. Undoubtedly, this lack of trials, together with the increasing availability of effective anti-hypertensive drugs that were well tolerated, has hampered the further introduction of such an invasive procedure as the baroreceptor activation therapy.

Recent developments

Since the beginning of this century, new devices with improved technology have been developed. This has resulted in the Rheos ™ Baroreflex Hypertension Therapy ™ System (Fig. 2.1) as a new prototype of a modern class of baropacing instruments. This is an

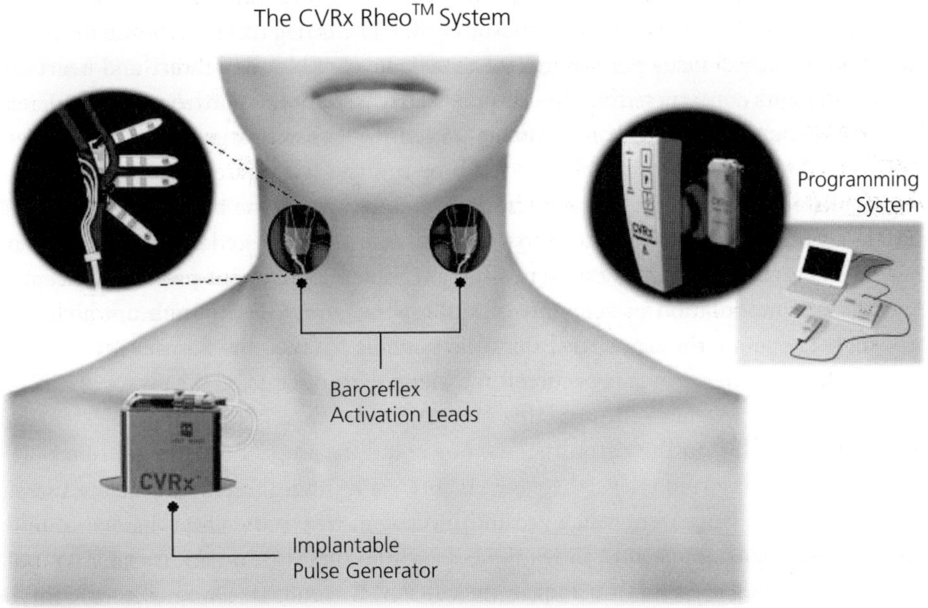

Fig. 2.1 Photograph of the Rheos System (32).

Reproduced from Expert review of medical devices, 5, Scheffers IJ, Kroon AA, Tordoir JH, de Leeuw PW., Rheos Baroreflex Hypertension Therapy System to treat resistant hypertension, p. 33–39, Copyright (2008), with permission from Informa.

open-loop system with electrodes that are attached surgically to both carotid arteries at close proximity to the bifurcation. Except for the two electrode leads, the device consists of an implantable pulse generator and an external programmer. The latter makes it possible to independently control the delivery of the activation energy for the left and right lead. It allows the programming of start and stop times, ramp function, dose settings, burst settings, pulse amplitude, pulse width, and pulse frequency separately for the left and right lead. This Rheos System has been extensively tested in experimental dogs by Lohmeier's group (26). Using a variety of hypertension models, including obesity-induced and angiotensin-dependent hypertension, the investigators were able to show that baropacing effectively reduced blood pressure over a prolonged period of time. Subsequently, the device was ready for evaluation in humans.

Acute effects of the Rheos System in humans

Schmidli and co-workers were the first to report that the device actually worked in humans (27). In 11 patients with a mean age of 70 years who needed elective carotid surgery, they placed a single-use electrode on the carotid sinus wall at the level of the origin of the internal carotid artery. This site was chosen because it was thought to have the greatest density of baroreceptors. Care was taken not put undue pressure on the artery and to hold the electrode in place. As the authors describe, the electrode was allowed to 'ride' on the vessel wall and to follow the pulsatile movements of this wall. Baseline blood pressure of the patients was 146 ± 30 mmHg systolic and 66 ± 17 mmHg diastolic, while their heart rate averaged 72 ± 7 beats per minute. At a stable level of blood pressure and heart rate, the investigators constructed a dose–response curve by applying incrementally increasing electrical currents (1-volt increments). Each level of activation was continued for 1 minute. With this approach, both blood pressure and heart rate fell significantly in a voltage-dependent way. On average, the maximal fall in systolic blood pressure was 23 mmHg and that in diastolic pressure 16 mmHg. Heart rate slowed down by 7 beats per minute. All these changes were statistically significant and provided proof of concept for device-based modulation of sympathetic outflow in humans. Although not absolutely proven, these data strongly suggest that it is possible to 'fool' the baroreceptor system. Importantly, no adverse events occurred and all patients completed the protocol successfully. Due to the peculiar setting of this investigation, it was not possible to extensively study multiple sites on the carotid sinus, nor could the impact of site differences (left versus right) be assessed. Nevertheless, it is interesting that the maximal reductions in systolic blood pressure were much greater in those in whom the carotid sinus could be easily identified, as opposed to the patients in whom this was not the case (31 versus 5 mmHg). This indicated that for long-term efficacy, it would be essential to identify as clearly as possible the point of maximal responsiveness. Since this was an acute study, the electrodes were removed again after the test. Therefore, from these initial results no inferences could be made about the sustainability of the effects in case of long-term stimulation.

Chronic effects of the Rheos System in humans

Following the acute study, long-term studies were set up to evaluate whether the baropacing system would be able to produce a sustained effect in hypertensive patients. The first of these was the so-called DEBuT-HT (Device-Based Therapy in Hypertension) trial (28). This was a multicentre, prospective, non-randomized feasibility study, which assessed the safety and efficacy of the Rheos System over a period of 3 months in treatment-resistant hypertensive patients. After the 3 months, patients could consent to an extended follow-up phase. The study was performed in patients over 21 years of age, whose blood pressure remained above ≥160/90 mmHg, despite treatment with at least three anti-hypertensive agents, including a diuretic. The protocol demanded that medications were kept constant for 2 months before entry and during the first 3 months of therapy, except when medically necessary. Exclusions included baroreflex failure, significant orthostatic hypotension, cardiac arrhythmias, chronic atrial fibrillation, clinically significant cardiac valvular disease or hypertension secondary to a treatable cause, carotid artery atherosclerosis with >50% stenosis, as determined by ultrasonography, prior implant or radiation in the carotid sinus region, currently implanted electrical medical devices, dialysis, and pregnancy or contemplated pregnancy. To allow for undisturbed tissue healing, the device was not activated until 1 month after implant. Thereafter, at each follow-up visit, therapy was individualized with the programmer to produce an optimal blood pressure reduction. A total of 45 patients with an average age of 54 years were enrolled into the trial. Baseline blood pressure, defined as the pressure 1 month after the implant just before the device would be activated, was 179 ± 29 mmHg systolic and 105 ± 22 mmHg diastolic and heart rate 80 ± 13 beats per minute. As illustrated in Fig. 2.2, stimulation produced a significant fall in blood pressure at 3 months. Although to a lesser degree, heart rate fell significantly as well. The median number of anti-hypertensive drugs was five at the start of the study and remained at that number. In the patients who consented to continued monitoring, efficacy was sustained over a follow-up period of 1 year and even after several years there were no signs of loss of efficacy (29). On the contrary, it appeared possible in many patients to reduce the number of medications. Although the study was uncontrolled, the changes in pressure could be compared to those in a concurrent group of resistant patients who refused participation in the trial. This comparison revealed far greater falls in pressure than in the patients in whom medical treatment was intensified.

Not surprisingly, in the early phase of the implantation procedures, adverse events were relatively common. One fatal procedure-related event occurred 6 days after implant due to angioneurotic oedema, before device activation. Although the cause could not be established, a drug reaction was suspected. Other procedure-related complications included: infection, peri-operative stroke with minimal residual effects, and tongue paresis, most likely due to intra-operative injury to the hypoglossal nerve. The only device-related adverse event was movement of the implantable pulse generator, resulting in the need for further surgery to reposition the implantable pulse generator (28). Overall, however, the safety profile of the device proved to be acceptable.

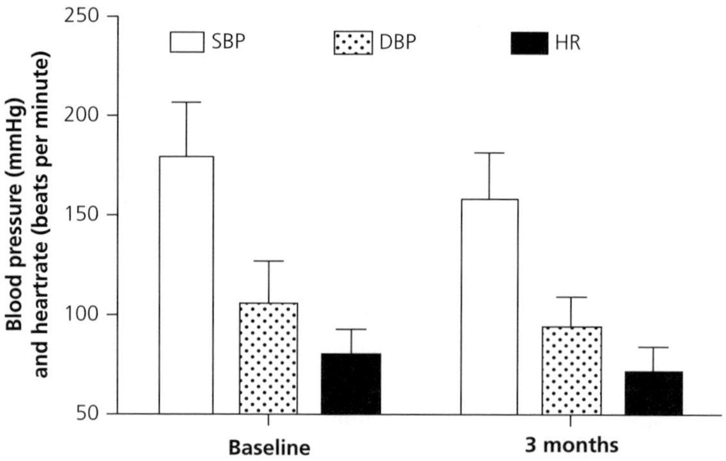

Fig. 2.2 Changes in blood pressure and heart rate after three months of BAT in the DEBuT-trial. At 3 months all values were significantly lower than at baseline ($p < 0.001$ for all).

Source data from Journal of the American College of Cardiology, 56, Scheffers IJ, Kroon AA, Schmidli J, Jordan J, Tordoir JJ, Mohaupt MG, et al., Novel baroreflex activation therapy in resistant hypertension: results of a European multi-center feasibility study., p. 1254–1258, Copyright (2010), with permission from Elsevier.

Notwithstanding its impressive results, DEBuT-HT was an observational study and caution is needed in the interpretation of the data that it generated. There was, thus, a need for a randomized controlled trial to compare stimulation with non-stimulation. This resulted in the Rheos Pivotal Trial (NCT00442286), which was a randomized, double-blind, parallel-design clinical trial designed to assess the efficacy and safety of the Rheos System in 265 patients with resistant hypertension (Fig. 2.3). Patients who gave their informed consent were randomized in a 2:1 ratio to either immediate activation (i.e. 1 month after the implant, group A) of the device or delayed activation (7 months after the implant, group B). Thus, the second, smaller group could be considered as a sham-operated or placebo group in this respect.

The primary outcome variables were efficacy and safety at 7 months after the operation when group A had received baroreceptor activation therapy (BAT) in the preceding 6 months and group B had had only medical treatment but with the baropacing system *in situ* during the same time period (30). After the 6-month assessment, the baropacer was switched on in patients from group B as well and 6 months later all measurements were repeated. This study clearly showed the necessity of doing proper randomized trials with a 'sham-group' in order to establish the true effect of devices such as the present one. Indeed, blood pressure fell not only in group A after 6 months of stimulation, but it did also in group B, yielding responder rates (primary endpoint) of 54 and 46%, respectively. This difference was not statistically significant. Even though the decrement in pressure was numerically greater in group A (16 vs. 9 mmHg), this was not significantly different either. However, the proportion of patients who reached the goal pressure of 140 mmHg

IMPLANT (month–1)	Blinded evaluation period (month 0–12)	Long-term follow-up
Group A (n = 181)	Device ON (continously)	Device ON
Group B (n = 84)	Device OFF (month 0–6) Device ON (month 7–12)	Device ON

Fig. 2.3 Design of the pivotal trial.
Source data from J Am Coll Cardiol, 58, Bisognano JD, Bakris G, Nadim MK, Sanchez L, Kroon AA, Schafer J, et al., Baroreflex activation therapy lowers blood pressure in patients with resistant hypertension: results from the double-blind, randomized, placebo-controlled rheos pivotal trial, p. 765–773, Copyright (2011), with permission from Elsevier.

or below systolic (a secondary endpoint) was greater in group A (42 vs. 24%; $p < 0.005$). This suggests that the device is, indeed, effective but the power of enhanced supervision per se should not be discarded, as the results from group B illustrate. Interestingly, at 12 months, when all patients had BAT, a sustained efficacy could be demonstrated with an equal change in pressure from baseline in both groups. As far as safety is concerned, the profile of adverse events was related primarily to the hypertension itself and to the operative procedure and not so much to the device or BAT (30).

Altogether, the Pivotal trial has taught us that BAT is a relatively safe mode of treatment that can lower blood pressure in patients who would otherwise be resistant to medical treatment. Nevertheless, it is essential to carefully select the patient for this procedure and to ascertain that everything has been done to lower the pressure in a non-invasive way.

Baroreceptor activation therapy and target organ damage

Obviously, time has been too short to establish whether BAT leads to a reduction in major cardiovascular complications, such as stroke or myocardial infarction. This would require a large, prospective trial, but given the invasive nature and costs of the procedure it is not likely that such a trial will be initiated shortly. On the other hand, one could evaluate target organ damage as a proxy for hard endpoints. So far, data are available for the heart and the kidney only.

In a subset of 34 patients who participated in the DEBuT and United States trials of the Rheos System, a standard echocardiogram was obtained before implant and after 3 and 12 months of active therapy (31). At baseline, patients had normal systolic function (ejection fraction: 65 ± 5%), but left ventricular (LV) size, as measured by LV mass index, was abnormal in the majority of patients. After 1 year of active therapy, LV mass index had fallen from 139 ± 35 to 108 ± 34 g/m^2 ($p < 0.01$) and midwall fractional shortening had increased ($p < 0.01$) at month 12, as compared to pre-implant. BAT increased left ventricular outflow tract diameter and arterial compliance. However, no significant correlation was observed between changes in systolic BP and LV mass index. Thus, BAT not only reduces BP, but also induces reverse cardiac remodelling in patients with drug-resistant hypertension.

More recently, some data with respect to renal function have become available. These show that 6 months after starting BAT, serum creatinine had risen significantly and estimated glomerular filtration rate (eGFR) had fallen. Although changes were small and probably not so relevant from a clinical point of view, they should be taken seriously. Further analyses revealed that the drop in blood pressure was the main determinant of the changes in serum creatinine and eGFR. It is likely, therefore, that the renal effects of BAT are haemodynamically determined. Whether the changes represent a true impairment of renal function or merely reflect normalization of a previously hyper-filtrating kidney needs to be established in more refined studies.

Future developments

Now that BAT has proven to be an effective and safe procedure, future research has to focus on improvements and simplification of the system. One development has already begun and that is the simplification of the device. The Barostim neo™ is a second-generation device with only one stimulation electrode, allowing for unilateral implantation and stimulation. Preliminary data with this new device show that it is as effective and safe as its predecessor. Apparently, unilateral stimulation suffices to achieve the desired effect. In a few patients in whom the technique of renal denervation failed, the Barostim neo™ still was able to reduce pressure to the same extent as in those without prior renal denervation. Future research must be directed towards finding the optimal spot to stimulate and to explore whether external stimulation is possible, i.e. without the need to operate. One can also think about developing closed-loop systems in which a pressure sensor is integrated in the device so that stimulation settings can be adapted to the prevailing level of blood pressure.

Conclusions

Over the past 50 years several attempts have been made to treat hypertension by means of baroreceptor stimulation. While these attempts failed initially, we have witnessed over the last 10 years a tremendous progress with the development of new devices that can be controlled much more easily and that have shown to be effective and safe. While surgery is still needed, the most recent system requires implantation at only one site so that perioperative morbidity can be minimized. Given the substantial drops in blood pressure that one can see even with prolonged stimulation, baroreceptor activation therapy may become the treatment of choice in patients with otherwise resistant hypertension and in those who cannot tolerate medication.

References

1 **Kearney PM, Whelton M, Reynolds K, Muntner P, Whelton PK, He J**. Global burden of hypertension: analysis of worldwide data. Lancet 2005;**365**:217–23.

2 **Birkenhäger WH, De Leeuw PW, Schalekamp MADH**. Control Mechanisms in Essential Hypertension. Amsterdam: Elsevier Biomedical Press; 1982.

3 **Yamada Y, Miyajima E, Tochikubo O, Matsukawa T, Ishii M**. Age-related changes in muscle sympathetic nerve activity in essential hypertension. Hypertension 1989;**13**:870–77.

4 **Wallin BG, Thompson JM, Jennings GL, Esler MD**. Renal noradrenaline spillover correlates with muscle sympathetic activity in humans. J Physiol 1996;**491**:881–87.

5 **Esler M, Lambert G, Jennings G**. Regional norepinephrine turnover in human hypertension. Clin Exp Hypertens A 1989;**11**:75–89.

6 **Guyton AC, Hall JE, Coleman TG, Manning Jr**. RD, Norman Jr RA. The dominant role of the kidneys in long-term arterial pressure regulation in normal and hypertensive states. In: Laragh JH, Brenner BM (eds) Hypertension. Pathophysiology, Diagnosis, and Management. New York: Raven Press; 1995:1311–26.

7 **Cooper A**. Guy's Hospital Report. In: Heymans C, Neil E (eds) Reflexogenic Areas of the Cardiovascular System. London: J&A Churchill; 1858:457.

8 **Korner P**. Essential Hypertension and its Causes. Neural and Non-Neural Mechanisms. New York: Oxford University Press; 2007.

9 **Guyton A**. Arterial pressure and hypertension. Philadelphia: WB Saunders Company; 1980.

10 **Sleight P**. Nonpharmacological treatments for hypertension. J Hypertension 2012;**30**:1516–17.

11 **Bristow JD, Honour AJ, Pickering GW, Sleight P, Smyth HS**. Diminished baroreflex sensitivity in high blood pressure. Circulation 1969;**39**:48–54.

12 **Heusser K, Tank J, Luft FC, Jordan J**. Baroreflex failure. Hypertension 2005;**45**:834–39.

13 **Bilgutay AM, Wingrove RC, Simmons RL, Dahlstrom IJ, Lillehei CW**. A new concept in the treatment of hypertension utilizing an implantable electronic device: 'Baropacer'. Trans Am Soc Artif Intern Organs 1964;**10**:387–95.

14 **Bilgutay AM, Lillehei CW**. Treatment of hypertension with an implantable electronic device. Jama 1965;**191**:649–53.

15 **Neistadt A, Schwartz SI**. Effects of electrical stimulation of the carotid sinus nerve in reversal of experimentally induced hypertension. Surgery 1967;**61**:923–31.

16 **Griffith LS, Schwartz SI**. Reversal of renal hypertension by electrical stimulation of the carotid sinus nerve. Surgery 1964;**56**:232–39.

17 **Agishi T, Temples J, Peirce EC, 2nd**. Electrical stimulation of the carotid sinus nerve as an experimental treatment of hypertension. J Surg Res 1969;**9**:305–09.

18 **Neufeld HN, Goor D, Nathan D, Fischler H, Yerushalmi S**. Stimulation of the carotid baroreceptors using a radio-frequency method. Israel J Med Sci 1965;**1**:630–32.

19 **Myers GH, Parsonnet V, Holcomb W, Zucker IR, Lewin G**. An experimental radio-frequency carotid-sinus pacemaker. Med Res Eng 1968;**7**:13–16.

20 **Michaelis LL, Gilmore JP**. Renal effects of electrical stimulation of the carotid sinus nerve. Surgery 1969;**65**:797–801.

21 **Resnicoff SA, Harris JP, Hampsey JP, Schwartz SI**. Effects of sinus nerve stimulation on arterial resistance and flow patterns of specific vascular beds. Surgery 1969;**66**:755–61.

22 **Carlsten A, Folkow B, Grimby G, Hamberger CA, Thulesius O**. Cardiovascular effects of direct stimulation of the carotid sinus nerve in man. Acta Physiol Scand 1958;**44**:138–45.

23 **Bilgutay AM, Lillehei CW**. Surgical treatment of hypertension with reference to baropacing. Am J Cardiol 1966;**17**:663–67.

24 **Schwartz SI, Griffith LS, Neistadt A, Hagfors N**. Chronic carotid sinus nerve stimulation in the treatment of essential hypertension. Am J Surg 1967;**114**:5–15.

25 **Scheffers IJ, Kroon AA, de Leeuw PW**. Carotid baroreflex activation: past, present, and future. Curr Hypertens Rep 2010;**12**:61–6.

26 **Lohmeier TE, Iliescu R**. Chronic lowering of blood pressure by carotid baroreflex activation: mechanisms and potential for hypertension therapy. Hypertension 2011;**57**:880–86.

27 **Schmidli J, Savolainen H, Eckstein F et al.** Acute device-based blood pressure reduction: electrical activation of the carotid baroreflex in patients undergoing elective carotid surgery. Vascular 2007;**15**:63–69.

28 **Scheffers IJ, Kroon AA, Schmidli J et al.** Novel baroreflex activation therapy in resistant hypertension: results of a European multi-center feasibility study. J Am Coll Cardiol 2010;**56**:1254–58.

29 **Krum H, Schlaich M, Sobotka P, Scheffers I, Kroon AA, de Leeuw PW**. Novel procedure- and device-based strategies in the management of systemic hypertension. Eur Heart J 2011;**32**:537–44.

30 **Bisognano JD, Bakris G, Nadim MK et al.** Baroreflex activation therapy lowers blood pressure in patients with resistant hypertension: results from the double-blind, randomized, placebo-controlled Rheos pivotal trial. J Am Coll Cardiol 2011;**58**:765–73.

31 **Bisognano JD, Kaufman CL, Bach DS, Lovett EG, de Leeuw P**. Improved cardiac structure and function with chronic treatment using an implantable device in resistant hypertension: results from European and United States trials of the Rheos System. J Am Coll Cardiol 2011;**57**:1787–88.

32 **Scheffers IJ, Kroon AA, Tordoir JH, de Leeuw PW**. Rheos Baroreflex Hypertension Therapy System to treat resistant hypertension. Exp Rev Med Dev 2008;**5**:33–39.

Chapter 3

Deep-brain stimulation and blood pressure disorders

Alexander L. Green, Erlick A. C. Pereira, and Jonathan A. Hyam

Key points

1. Deep-brain stimulation (DBS) is an established treatment for neurological disorders and has a low morbidity profile.
2. DBS can increase or decrease arterial blood pressure in humans.
3. Varying location of electrode within the neural networks conferring blood pressure alters its effect on blood pressure.
4. The periaqueductal grey (PAG) mediates the 'flight or fight' reaction and opioid and non-opioid analgesia.
5. PAG stimulation in humans has been found to increase or decrease blood pressure by up to 16 mmHg and alter heart rate, baroreceptor sensitivity, heart rate variability, and muscle sympathetic nerve activity.

Introduction

Deep-brain stimulation (DBS) is a technique where fine electrodes are surgically implanted into areas of the human brain in order to alter function (1). Although the technique was first used in an experimental context to treat psychiatric disorders and pain in the 1950s (2), its use became popularized in the late 1980s and 1990s in the treatment of tremor and Parkinson's disease (PD) (3). To date, over 50,000 people worldwide have been treated with DBS and it continues to grow both in terms of numbers of patients treated per condition, as well as a growing number of indications. The more common indications include PD, dystonia (a movement disorder involving abnormal muscle contractions), tremor, pain, epilepsy, depression, obsessive–compulsive disorder, and Tourette's syndrome (1). Indeed, many of these indications now have randomized trial evidence proving their efficacy. As DBS is practised by a growing number of surgeons, there has been a search for more indications, largely due to the fact that it is known that the brain influences virtually every system in the body. The control of the autonomic nervous system is an obvious corollary, as it can be seen in Chapter 2 that the nervous system has a significant top-down influence on cardiovascular control. As the reader will see later in this chapter, there is good evidence that control of the cardiovascular system (CVS), including blood pressure (BP) and other aspects of autonomic control, are possible, but first it is useful to describe the technique of DBS.

The technique of deep-brain stimulation

Needless to say, as with any surgical technique, there are many permutations on the technique of DBS. The basic principle is that the patient has their brain scanned whilst held in a *base ring* that is attached to a *localizer* (Fig. 3.1A). The localizer consists of a number of rods or *fiducials* that are detected on the scan. As some are vertical and some diagonal, it is possible to calculate any point in 3D space, depending on where the rods are on any given horizontal slice. Simple Cartesian coordinates are taken from this and used to target the electrodes. Stereotaxy has its origins (at least in animals) in the nineteenth century but since Spiegel and Wycis first combined a frame with positive contrast ventriculography to localize intracerebral structures in the 1940s (4), there are now a multitude of different

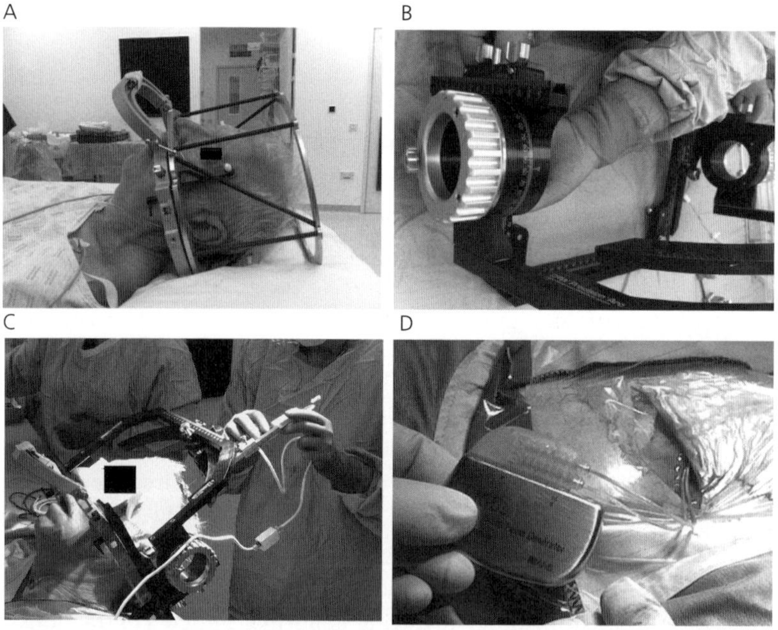

Fig. 3.1 The stereotactic procedure for implantation of deep brain electrodes. (A) Patient with base ring and localizer attached to head. (B) The stereotactic frame assembled with coordinates entered. (C) Frame applied to patient to guide electrode insertion. (D) Implantable pulse generator to be placed in the infraclavicular area.

types. Whilst some surgeons prefer magnetic resonance (MR) compatible frames, such as the Leksell® frame, others feel that this leads to image distortion (5) and that accuracy is better using a computed tomography (CT) scan during the procedure, in order to obtain the coordinates relative to the patient. This CT scan is then fused electronically to a pre-existing MR scan of the patients' brain. The surgeon selects the target(s) according to the condition (e.g. subthalamic nucleus (STN) or globus pallidus interna (GPi) for PD, peri-aqueductal grey (PAG), or sensory thalamus for pain, etc.) and the software gives a coordinate that, when put into the stereotactic frame (attached to the base ring in theatre rather than the localizer), will guide the electrode to target (Fig. 3.1B, C). Some targets, such as the STN, are easily visible on MR, whereas others, such as the motor or sensory thalamic nuclei, have to be calculated 'blind' by using coordinates relative to known landmarks, such as the mid-commissural point. This obviously leads to a certain inaccuracy and some surgeons operate on patients whilst awake in order to observe the clinical effect of stimulating at a particular point, and adjust the target as necessary. In addition (or instead of), some surgeons use microelectrode recording techniques to characterize the target—and structures on its approach—neurophysiologically, to determine the best position. Whichever technique is chosen (and some use visual targeting alone), the basic principle is to drill either a 2.7 mm twist drill hole or a 14 mm burr hole and use the frame to guide the electrode to target. The electrode is fixed to the skull and connected, via an extension lead, to an implantable pulse generator (like a pacemaker that provides the battery power and means to change the parameters, such as voltage and frequency). The pulse generator is placed in a sub-cutaneous pocket, usually in the chest wall (Fig. 3.1D).

Brain stimulation and blood pressure

It is widely established that the medulla contains the major nuclei that control heart rate, blood pressure, and respiration. Information from the peripheral arterial and cardiopulmonary baroreceptors and chemoreceptors passes, via the glossopharyngeal and vagus nerves, to the caudal nucleus of the tractus solitarius (NTS) (6). From here, impulses are transmitted to the nucleus ambiguus (NA), the dorsal motor nucleus of the vagus nerve (DMNX), and then to the rostral and caudal ventrolateral medulla (RVLM/CVLM) (7, 8). The parasympathetic system is activated by the NA and DMNX, which contain parasympathetic preganglionic neurones that alter contractility of the heart and heart rate via the vagus. The sympathetic system is activated by the CVLM, whose neurones synapse on the sympathetic preganglionic intermediate lateral (IML) neurones that innervate blood vessels and the adrenal medulla and, via catecholamine release, alter the basal tone of blood vessels (9, 10). Although this is an over-simplification and there is considerable interaction between these autonomic medullary centres, this mechanism is essentially a reflex to maintain cardiovascular homeostasis.

In 1953, Kabat showed that PAG stimulation can alter blood pressure (11). Later, in 1956, Hunsperger described the 'defence' reaction in the rat (12). This is an integrated response that is associated with survival in the wild. For example, if escape from danger is *possible*, the response involves a 'fight or flight' reaction that includes raised blood pressure and heart rate, non-opioid mediated analgesia, and emotional effects such as fear (13, 14, 15). Conversely, if escape is *not possible* and it is safer to remain undetected, the reaction consists of lowered blood pressure, opioid-mediated analgesia, and a 'withdrawal reaction', as well as fear (16, 17). Other components of the defence reaction include vocalization, pupillary changes, micturition, and changes in skeletal blood flow (18). It was soon established that the PAG is an important area involved in the defence reaction. Furthermore, the columns of the PAG are functionally distinct and opposite; activation of the dorsomedial and dorsolateral columns evokes the 'fight or flight' response and activation of the lateral and ventrolateral columns produces the passive coping responses (14, 19). This was perhaps the first evidence that the role of the PAG in autonomic control is as a 'higher' centre to influence the cardiovascular system in times of environmental stress, such as during an attack or an emotional situation or pain. Evidence for an anatomical substrate for this 'higher' control is abundant. For example, serotonergic and adrenergic sympathetic pathways project onto the rostroventromedial medulla (20, 21), the rostroventrolateral medulla, locus coeruleus (22), and pontobulbar reticular formation (23), amongst others. PAG neurones also project to cardiac vagal preganglionic neurones in the nucleus ambiguus, dorsal motor vagal nucleus, and the nucleus of the tractus solitarius (22).

As described the PAG also has reciprocal connections with a number of higher centres. Many of these centres are involved in cardiovascular regulation. Of particular note is the hypothalamus, as nearly all its nuclei influence blood pressure and heart rate. Many of the descending connections from the hypothalamus pass through, and are influenced by, PAG. For example, the hypotensive response elicited by lateral hypothalamus stimulation can be attenuated by lidocaine injection into PAG (24). Stimulation of the paraventricular nucleus (PVN) of the hypothalamus causes hypertension by inhibiting sympathetic output (25). This nucleus receives afferents from other hypothalamic nuclei, amygdala, insular and prefrontal cortex, as well as lower nuclei, such as VLM and NTS. In return, it sends efferents to VLM, NTS, DMNX, and the IML. The PAG has reciprocal connections with both PVN and LHN. In addition, the PAG has direct reciprocal connections with amygdala, prefrontal cortex, and insular cortex (26, 27). As with PAG connections to lower centres, these 'higher' connections also exhibit specificity with particular columns of the PAG. Thus, the role of PAG in autonomic regulation is probably as an 'integrator' of emotional/higher influence on cardiovascular control, similar to its role in pain control.

Why the PAG is important—using the opportunity of DBS

Deep-brain stimulation of the *human* PAG has been used for many years for the treatment of severe, refractory neuropathic pain (28, 29, 30). Given the known role of the PAG in autonomic function in humans, it is a logical step to ask if human PAG stimulation alters blood pressure or any other autonomic parameters. In fact, in North and Levy's textbook of *Neurosurgical Management of Pain* in 1997, Young and Rinaldi described changes in blood pressure observed intraoperatively when electrodes were placed in the PAG (31).

They found these changes useful as a marker that the electrode was in the correct position. Given these observations, we decided to look at these effects in a methodical way.

First, if we take BP, in a study of 15 chronic neuropathic pain patients (a total of 17 electrodes) we have demonstrated that acute stimulation of the PAG at either 10 or 50Hz leads to significant alterations in BP (32). Mean reduction of systolic BP was 14.2 ± 3.6 mmHg in seven patients with electrodes in the ventral PAG and mean increase was 16.73 ± 5.9 mmHg in six patients with dorsal electrodes. Four electrodes had no effect. These results are shown in Fig. 3.2.

There are two important points to make regarding these data. First, the BP changes were not associated with changes in visual analogue scores of pain, i.e. there was not likely to be an analgesic confound. Second, BP changes were in normotensive subjects and only in the acute setting, so although possible, they do not prove that DBS can be used to treat hypertension.

What are the mechanisms of the BP changes?

The two most powerful mediators of BP, both sympathetically controlled, are peripheral vasoconstriction (which increases BP) and cardiac contractility. In our studies, we found that, although diastolic BP (DBP) alters significantly with stimulation, it does not alter to the same degree as systolic BP (SBP). The pulse pressure (PP = SBP – DBP) is therefore increased with increasing BP. Increased PP, however, may be due to increased stroke volume, so with many variables, it is difficult to be sure of the mechanisms of increasing BP without directly measuring the various components. In addition to the changes in PP, there are analogous increases in dP/dt, i.e. how fast the BP rises with time. This, again, may be due to increased cardiac contractility (33), but there could also be a component related to total peripheral resistance (which in turn can affect PP). Reduction of BP is associated with similar changes, i.e. decreased PP and dP/dt. There were no changes in heart rate, suggesting lack of a vagal mechanism. A recent report (in which the authors are involved) has demonstrated, using Doppler flowmetry of the brachial artery, that a reduction in arterial blood pressure was associated with a reduced total peripheral resistance and an increased mean brachial blood flow (34). These are preliminary data and need to be replicated in a number of patients before they become robust. However, it is direct studies such as this that will shine some light on the mechanisms by which PAG stimulation alters BP. Other studies that will be useful are those looking directly at cardiac stroke volume and contractility using echo-cardiography.

What are the underlying central nervous system mechanisms?

As with the underlying causes of BP changes, the best way of determining whether changes in the output of the CNS leading to BP change are sympathetically or parasympathetically mediated, is by direct measurement. One way of measuring sympathetic nerve activity is to measure it directly from peripheral autonomic nerves, a technique called 'microneurography' or measurement of muscle sympathetic nerve activity (MSNA) (35). Studies in our laboratory showed a decrease or increase in MSNA burst frequency, amplitude, and baroreflex sensitivity, depending on whether ventral or dorsal PAG was stimulated (36).

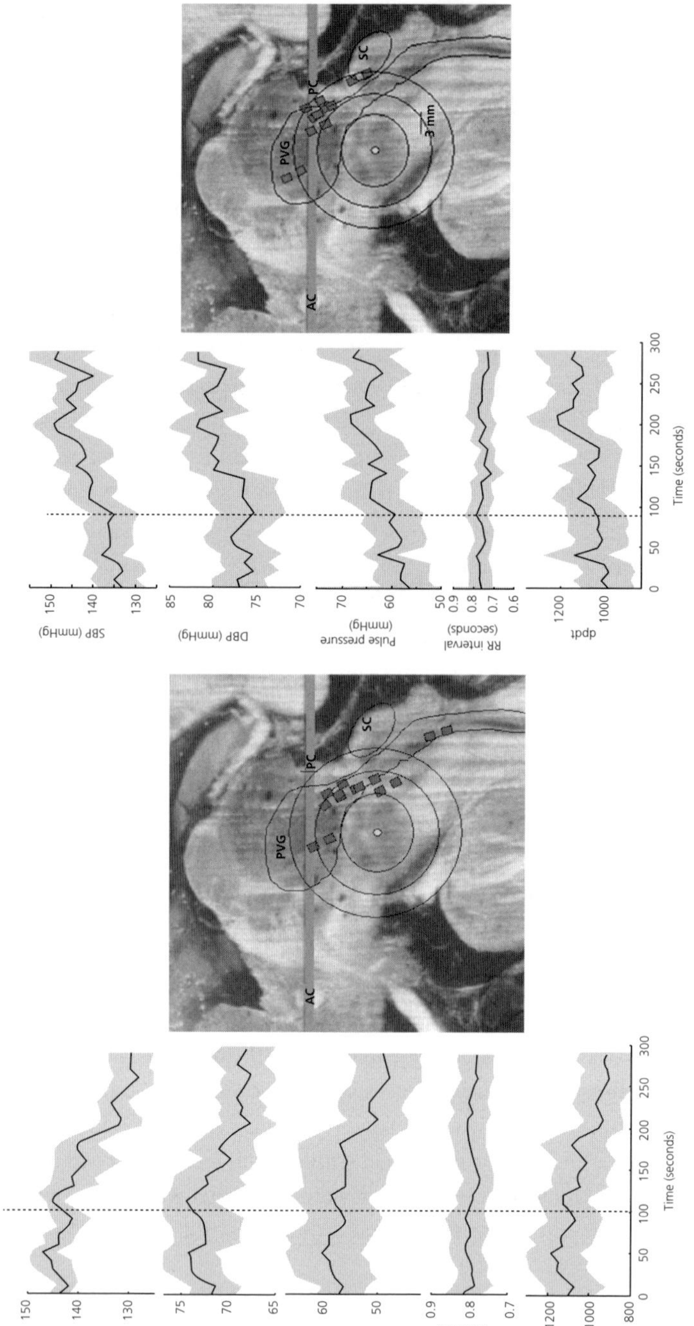

Fig. 3.2 Mean changes in cardiovascular variables with stimulation points indicated in the central schematics. Ventral squares (left hand group) represent the contacts of the DBS electrodes that when stimulated reduced BP and associated variables, except RR interval. The dorsal (right hand group of squares indicate points that increased BP (right-hand side). Grey areas = standard error of the mean, vertical lines = start of stimulation, spot = centre of red nucleus (for orientation), SC = superior colliculus, PVG = periventricular grey area, AC = anterior colliculus, PC = posterior colliculus. (See Plate 2.)

However, another less direct method (and less reliable) is to look at heart rate variability (HRV) or blood pressure variability (BPV). By breaking down the continuous signal into spectral frequencies using a technique called *power spectral analysis*, we can infer relative degrees of sympathetic/parasympathetic change (37). For example, the low frequency peak (called Meyer's wave, at around 0.1 Hz) is said to be related to sympathetic activity (38). Detection of the parasympathetic component using HRV or BPV is more controversial but the ratio of low:high frequency is generally held to be more useful. In our studies, we found that BP changes were associated with changes in the low-frequency component of BPV (32) indicating that there are changes in sympathetic activity, although without direct measurements it is hard to be sure.

Dorsal versus ventral electrodes

As Carrive and Bandler and others have shown (14), in the animal it is important which longitudinal column of the PAG is stimulated as to whether there is a hypertensive or hypotensive response. Indeed the same appears to be the case in humans. Without histology it is not possible to determine whether an electrode is definitively in a ventral or dorsal column as the spatial resolution of MR is not accurate enough. However, when the most ventral versus the most dorsal electrodes were divided into two groups, on average the ventral electrodes reduced mean arterial BP (ABP), whereas the most dorsal increased it (32). Therefore, it would appear that the animal experiments over the past 80 years are translatable into humans!

What is the likelihood that DBS will be used to treat BP related conditions?

The main problem with this concept is that DBS has a risk attached to it. The risk of intracranial haemorrhage visible on a post-operative scan may be as high as 5%, although the risk of symptomatic haemorrhage is nearer 2% and the risk of permanent neurological deficit probably closer to 1 in 200 (39). However, it is likely that this risk would be higher in patients with severe hypertension. Hypertension is generally asymptomatic until it leads to stroke or myocardial infarction, so DBS would be purely a prophylactic therapy. If the risk of electrode implantation or manipulating deep-brain areas were reduced, this concept may become closer to reality. However, we know that DBS can render a hypertensive patient normotensive, both in the short- and long-term (40, 41). In addition, this antihypertensive effect has been demonstrated to be independent of pain relief and not associated with any side-effects (41). A more likely candidate, at least in the near future, is the treatment of postural or 'orthostatic' hypotension. Postural hypotension is a significant clinical problem that affects a large number of people, particularly the elderly (42) and in extreme cases, has even led some clinicians to implant sub-cutaneous norepinephrine pumps (43). If we are able to increase BP by stimulating dorsal PVG/PAG, are we able to affect postural responses of BP? Ascending projections of barosensitive adrenergic cells in the rostroventrolateral medulla project to PAG (44). There is evidence that the PAG projects to preganglionic cardiac vagal neurones in the nucleus ambiguus and chemical

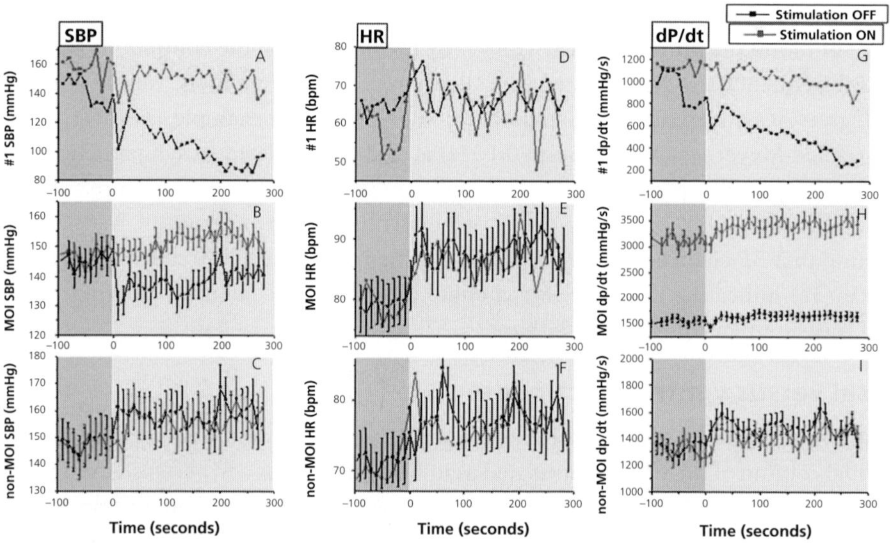

Fig. 3.3 Modulation of BP responses to standing. (A) in a group of five asymptomatic patients undergoing DBS for pain, the usual reduction in BP on standing (black line) is reversed with PAG stimulation (red line). Grey area = patient sitting, white area = patient standing. (B) An individual patient with postural hypotension. Stimulation not only reversed the BP changes on standing but also successfully treated the clinical condition. (See Plate 3.)

stimulation of the PAG inhibits baroreflex vagal bradycardia in rats (45). We have previously shown that human postural BP responses can be influenced using DBS (46). In this study it was demonstrated that stimulation can completely reverse any reduction in BP associated with standing, even treating a symptomatic patient effectively (Fig. 3.3).

These findings were not associated with changes in heart rate (HR) per se, but there were significant changes in HR variability consistent with increasing sympathetic activity. So what is the mechanism of reduced BP reduction with standing? In young and middle-aged healthy subjects, baroreflex sensitivity decreases on standing (47, 48). In autonomic neuropathy, such as that of diabetes, it has been shown that it is lower in the supine position and there is less reduction on standing than in normal subjects (49). In our study, we demonstrated that stimulation significantly raises sensitivity in the sitting position and reduces the magnitude of reduction on standing. This suggests that the reversal of postural changes in blood pressure is associated with increased baroreflex sensitivity.

Other brain areas and other systems involved in autonomic control

It is beyond the scope of this chapter to discuss every brain area and every part of the autonomic nervous system that may be influenced with stimulation (for review, see (50)).

However, descriptions of a few recent examples will give an idea of the potential scope. As described, the medulla oblongata is an area very rich and powerful in autonomic control but it has to be considered as part of a large system with influence from many areas (Fig. 3.4). The medulla itself, using existing DBS techniques, is not a very inviting area for any neurosurgeon! It is a long way from the surface of the brain and packed with many

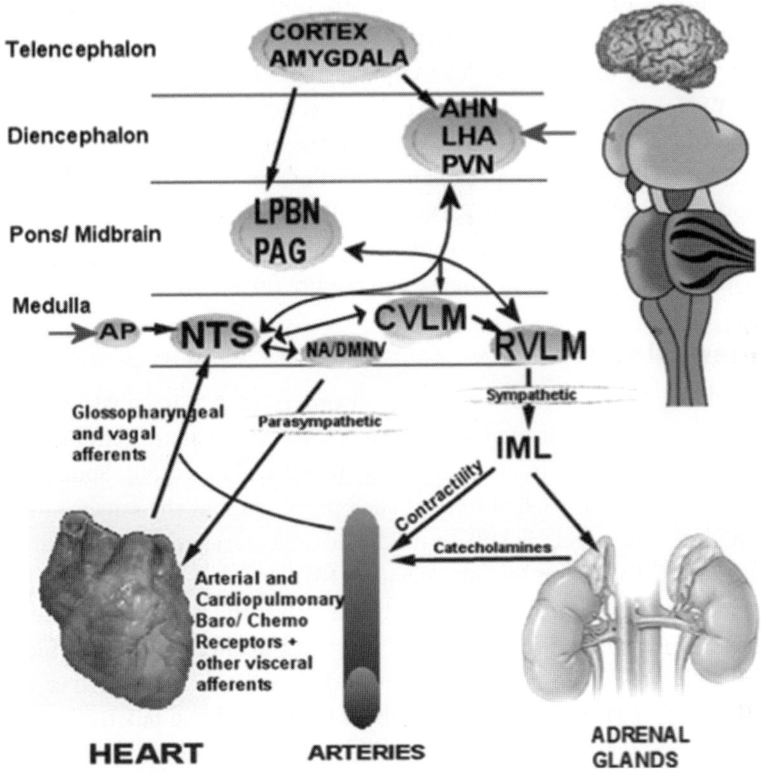

Fig. 3.4 Neural control of the cardiovascular system. The medulla contains areas rich in cells that are involved in the baroreceptor reflex and represents the termination of inputs from end-organs, such as the heart and arterial smooth muscle. These areas, in turn, are influenced by higher areas up to the telencephalon. Abbreviations: AHN, anterior hypothalamic nucleus; LHA, lateral hypothalamic nucleus; PVN, paraventricular nucleus of the hypothalamus; LPBN, lateral parabrachial nucleus; PAG, periaqueductal grey; NTS, nucleus of the tractus solitarius; CVLM, caudal ventrolateral medulla; RVLM, rostral ventrolateral medulla; NA, nucleus ambiguus, DMNV, dorsal motor nucleus of the vagus; AP, area postrema; and IML, intermediolateral cell column.

Reproduced from Experimental Physiology, 93, Green, A. L. and Paterson, D. J., Identification of neurocircuitry controlling cardiovascular function in humans using functional neurosurgery: implications for exercise control, p. 1022–1028, Copyright (2008), with permission from John Wiley & Sons Ltd.

Original figure adapted from Basic and Clinical Neurocardiology, Edited by J. Andrew Armour and Jeffrey L. Ardell, from J. Michael Wyss, Scott H. Carlson, and Suzanne Oparil: The Pathogenesis of Hypertension, ch.13, Copyright (2004), with permission from Oxford University Press.

nuclei that are important in sustaining life. Therefore, we have to use the knowledge gained from areas that we currently stimulate, as follows.

The respiratory system

Airway calibre, secretion, blood flow, and microvascular permeability are all under the control of the autonomic nervous system (51). Whilst the medulla is known to be important in breathing control, supramedullary centres have been implicated using functional imaging techniques (52, 53, 54). Bronchoconstriction is known to be important in the pathogenesis of asthma and other respiratory diseases and it is well known that bronchoconstriction is under the influence of the parasympathetic *airway-related preganglionic neurones* (AVPNs) (55. These, in turn, have connections to brain areas, including PAG, that are used in DBS for pain (56, 57). We have recently demonstrated that stimulation of both PAG and STN improves peak expiratory flow rate (PEFR) up to 14% in patients undergoing DBS for either pain or Parkinson's disease, respectively (58). These findings demonstrate that DBS may be used to alter lung function, although whether this effect is useful in patients with respiratory disease will require further investigation (59).

Gastrointesinal system

Much research in gastrointestinal dysmotility disorders, such as irritable bowel syndrome, has revealed aberrant visceral afferent reflex arcs with neuronal projections via the dorsal columns and spinothalamic tracts to the ventrobasal thalamus (60). Spinal cord stimulation has, therefore, been trialled to treat such problems, but the sensory thalamus is a further intuitive brain target for DBS to modulate the enteric nervous system and relieve intractable visceral discomfort (see also Chapter 10).

Another important avenue of translational research is the hypothalamic control of satiety and investigation of the ventromedial ('satiety') and lateral hypothalamic ('feeding') nuclei as sites for DBS in the control of eating and, therefore, anorexia nervosa and obesity, respectively (61, 62). The nucleus accumbens is an additional putative brain target for obesity control with substantial animal evidence for its role in reward processing that may translate into controlling dietary preferences.

DBS for functional gastrointestinal disorders and obesity is yet to reach patients, but provides an exciting potential neurosurgical alternative to gastric stimulation and bariatric gastric surgery.

Urinary system

Central nervous system control of the bladder is poorly understood, but it is known that stretch receptors in the bladder wall activate afferents that eventually terminate in the midbrain PAG. These neurones in turn project to the pontine micturition centre, which projects to preganglionic sacral neurones that activate the smooth muscle of the bladder wall (see (63) for review). Integrity of these areas is essential for normal bladder control (64). Another important area is the orbitofrontal cortex (OFC) that projects to parts of the

PAG that contain bladder afferents (65). Disrupting the OFC in rats causes dysfunction of micturition in rats (64) and conscious voiding effort in humans activates the OFC (66). Bladder function has been investigated in the context of other areas such as subthalamic nucleus (STN) stimulation in Parkinson's disease (PD) (67). Bladder function is often deranged in PD but Herzog et al. showed that STN stimulation improves bladder capacity and, as shown using positron emission tomography (PET), that the PAG is activated at the same time. Thus, it may be a reduction of dopaminergic projections to PAG that result in the initial bladder dysfunction in these patients. Evidence to support this hypothesis is that gamma aminobutyric acid (GABA) levels usually decrease in the PAG during the micturition reflex but in 'Parkinsonian' rats treated with the dopamine-depleting 6-OHDA lesion in the substantia nigra pars compacta, GABA actually increases (68).Taken together, these various findings would suggest that there are brain areas in humans that could be stimulated in order to improve bladder function per se, as recently demonstrated by our group in rodents and humans (69).

Pedunculopontine nucleus region

Whilst the classic targets for treatment of PD include STN and GPi, a relatively 'new' nucleus is the pedunculopontine nucleus (PPN) region. Following the demonstration that PPN stimulation improves gait and axial stability in non-human primates (70), it has subsequently been shown to provide positive clinical benefit in PD patients with axial instability and 'on' gait freezing, i.e. not in the periods when the medication is wearing off and the patient is slowing down prior to their next dose (71, 72, 73). The PPN region is in an area of the brainstem rich in autonomic nuclei, such as the locus coeruleus that stimulates noradrenaline in stress and anxiety states (74) and the parabrachial nucleus that has a role in thermoregulation and respiration (75). The PPN itself is a nucleus that is known to be important in sleep and indeed stimulating areas in the vicinity of the PPN has been shown to cause a shift from sleep to the waking state in animals (76). There is also evidence that it may be involved in the startle response or the sudden galvanization of an organism (including humans) into action (77). Thus stimulation of the PPN either through direct stimulation or stimulation of the surrounding structures may provide insights into potential mechanisms of autonomic control or indeed future therapeutic strategies. A recent example of this is the demonstration that PPN stimulation in PD patients leads to a reduction in magnitude of the blood pressure fall associated with head up tilt.

Conclusions

Gotoh et al. (78) provided a demonstration of an elegant system that could control beat-to-beat blood pressure in the rat using brainstem stimulation, feedback from peripheral arterial pressure monitoring, and an intervening microprocessor. Thus we know that it is possible to control autonomic factors using central nervous system stimulation. Given the various reports on the autonomic effects of DBS, it is a logical conclusion that in the future, brain manipulation by one means or another may be possible in order to treat a wide range of conditions, including those affecting the cardiovascular, respiratory, or urinary systems. The largest barrier to using DBS, as it stands, is the risk associated with it. This is justifiable in the case of advanced neurological diseases, such as PD or dystonia, that severely limit the individuals' activities of daily living and involve symptoms that significantly impair quality of life. In the case of hypertension, which is often asymptomatic, one needs to either justify the risk or provide brain stimulation/manipulation with lower risk. Whilst not possible at the moment, a number of promising techniques and advances, such as nanotechnology, may eventually provide the answers. For example, nanowires can be threaded through tiny arteries deep into the brain via peripheral blood vessels and have been shown to be able to record electrical activity on the parenchymal side of tiny vessels (79). It is only a matter of time before technologies such as these can be used to stimulate brain areas that are risky and difficult to get to using contemporary means and autonomic functions can be altered using 'DBS'.

References

1 **Pereira EA, Green A, Nandi D, Aziz T**. Deep brain stimulation: indications and evidence. Exp Rev Med Dev 2007;**4**(5):591–603.

2 **Heath RG**. Electrical self-stimulation of the brain in man. Am J Psychiatr 1963;**120**:571–77.

3 **Benabid AL, Pollak P, Seigneuret E, Hoffmann D, Gay E, Perret J**. Chronic VIM thalamic stimulation in Parkinson's disease, essential tremor and extra-pyramidal dyskinesias. Acta Neurochir Suppl (Wien) 1993;**58**:39–44.

4 **Spiegel EA, Wycis H, Marker M et al**. Stereoencephalotomy. Proc Soc Exp Biol Med 1948;**69**(1):175–77.

5 **Sumanaweera TS, Glover G, Hemler P et al**. MR geometric distortion correction for improved frame-based stereotaxic target localization accuracy. Magn Reson Med 1995;**34**(1):106–13.

6 **Sumal KK, Blessing W, Joh T, Reis D, Pickel V**. Synaptic interaction of vagal afferents and catecholaminergic neurons in the rat nucleus tractus solitarius. Brain Res 1983;**277**(1):31–40.

7 **Hancock MB**. Evidence for direct projections from the nucleus of the solitary tract onto medullary adrenaline cells. J Comp Neurol 1988;**276**(3):460–67.

8 **Aicher SA, Saravay RH, Cravo S et al**. Monosynaptic projections from the nucleus tractus solitarii to C1 adrenergic neurons in the rostral ventrolateral medulla: comparison with input from the caudal ventrolateral medulla. Journal of Comparative Neurology 1996;**373**(1):62–75.

9 **Malhotra V, Kachroo A, Sapru H**. Role of alpha 1-adrenergic receptors in the intermediolateral column in mediating the pressor responses elicited by the stimulation of ventrolateral medullary pressor area. Brain Res 1993;**626**(1–2):278–86.

10 **Smith JE, Jansen A, Gilbey M, Loewy A**. CNS cell groups projecting to sympathetic outflow of tail artery: neural circuits involved in heat loss in the rat. Brain Res 1998;**786**(1–2):153–64.

11 **Kabat H, Magoun HW, Ranson SW**. Electrical stimulation of points in the forebrain and midbrain. The resultant alteration in blood pressure. Arch Neurol Psych 1935;**34**:931–55.

12 **Hunsperger RW**. Role of substantia grisea centralis mesencephali in electrically-induced rage reactions. Progress in Neurobiologyl 1956;(2):289–94.

13 **Carrive P, Bandler R**. Control of extracranial and hindlimb blood flow by the midbrain periaqueductal grey of the cat. Exp Brain Res 1991;**84**(3):599–606.

14 **Carrive P, Bandler R**. Viscerotopic organization of neurons subserving hypotensive reactions within the midbrain periaqueductal grey: a correlative functional and anatomical study. Brain Res 1991;**541**(2):206–15.

15 **McGaraughty S, Farr D, Heinricher M.** Lesions of the periaqueductal gray disrupt input to the rostral ventromedial medulla following microinjections of morphine into the medial or basolateral nuclei of the amygdala. Brain Res 2004;**1009**(1–2):223–27.

16 **Johnson PL, Lightman S, Lowry C.** A functional subset of serotonergic neurons in the rat ventrolateral periaqueductal gray implicated in the inhibition of sympathoexcitation and panic. Ann N Y Acad Sci 2004;**1018**:58–64.

17 **Finnegan TF, Chen S, Pan H.** Effect of the {mu} opioid on excitatory and inhibitory synaptic inputs to periaqueductal gray-projecting neurons in the amygdala. J Pharmacol Exp Ther 2005;**312**(2):441–48.

18 **Schenberg LC, Povoa R, Costa A, Caldellas A, Tufik S, Bittencourt A.** Functional specializations within the tectum defense systems of the rat. Neurosci Biobehav Rev 2005;**29**(8):1279–98.

19 **Bittencourt AS, Carobrez A, Zamprogno L, Tufik S, Schenberg L.** Organization of single components of defensive behaviors within distinct columns of periaqueductal gray matter of the rat: role of N-methyl-D-aspartic acid glutamate receptors. Neuroscience 2004;**125**(1):71–89.

20 **Cameron AA, Khan I, Westlund K, Willis W.** The efferent projections of the periaqueductal gray in the rat: a Phaseolus vulgaris-leucoagglutinin study. II. Descending projections. J Comp Neurol 1995;**351**(4):585–601.

21 **Farkas E, Jansen A, Loewy A.** Periaqueductal gray matter input to cardiac-related sympathetic premotor neurons. Brain Res 1998;**792**(2):179–92.

22 **Farkas E, Jansen A, Loewy A.** Periaqueductal gray matter projection to vagal preganglionic neurons and the nucleus tractus solitarius. Brain Res 1997;**764**(1–2):257–61.

23 **Odeh F, Antal M.** The projections of the midbrain periaqueductal grey to the pons and medulla oblongata in rats. Eur J Neurosci 2001;**14**(8):1275–86.

24 **Pajolla GP, Tavares R, Pelosi G, Correa F.** Involvement of the periaqueductal gray in the hypotensive response evoked by L-glutamate microinjection in the lateral hypothalamus of unanesthetized rats. Autonom Neurosci 2005;**122**(1–2):84–93.

25 **Martin DS, Egland M, Barnes L, Vogel E.** Adrenergic nerves mediate the venoconstrictor response to PVN stimulation. Brain Res 2006;**1076**(1):93–100.

26 **Rizvi TA, Ennis M, Behbehani M, Shipley M.** Connections between the central nucleus of the amygdala and the midbrain periaqueductal gray: topography and reciprocity. J Comput Neurol1991;**303**(1):121–31.

27 **Bandler R, Keay K, Floyd N, Price J.** Central circuits mediating patterned autonomic activity during active vs. passive emotional coping. Brain Res Bull 2000;**53**(1):95–104.

28 **Hosobuchi Y.** Subcortical electrical stimulation for control of intractable pain in humans. Report of 122 cases (1970–1984). J Neurosurgery 1986;**64**(4):543–53.

29 **Richardson DE, Akil H.** Long term results of periventricular gray self-stimulation. Neurosurgery 1977;**1**(2):199–202.

30 **Owen SL, Green A, Stein J, Aziz T.** Deep brain stimulation for the alleviation of post-stroke neuropathic pain. Pain 2006;**120**(1–2):202–06.

31 **Young RF, Rinaldi P.** Brain stimulation in Neurosurgical Management of Pain eds: North R, Levy R New York, Springer 1997.

32 **Green AL, Wang S, Owen S et al.** Deep brain stimulation can regulate arterial blood pressure in awake humans. Neuroreport 2005;**16**(16):1741–45.

33 **Germano G, Pecchioli V, Germano U et al.** Un parametre additionnel de fonction ventriculaire gauche derive du profil oscillometrique arteriel. Archives des Maladies du Coeur et des Vaisseaux 1998;**91**(8):947–50.

34 **Carter HH, Dawson E, Cable N et al.** 'Deep brain stimulation of the periaqueductal grey induces vasodilation in humans. Hypertension 2011;**57**(5):e24–25.

35 **Victor RG, Seals D, Mark A.** Differential control of heart rate and sympathetic nerve activity during dynamic exercise. Insight from intraneural recordings in humans. J Clin Invest 1987;**79**(2):508–16.

36 **Sverrisdottir YB, Green A, Aziz T et al.** Differentiated baroreflex modulation of sympathetic nerve activity during deep brain stimulation in humans. Hypertension 2014;**63**(5):1000–10.

37 **Pagani M, Lombardi F, Guzzetti S et al.** Power spectral analysis of heart rate and arterial pressure variabilities as a marker of sympatho-vagal interaction in man and conscious dog. Circ Res 1986;**59**(2):178–93.

38 **Pagani M, Montano N, Porta A et al.** Relationship between spectral components of cardiovascular variabilities and direct measures of muscle sympathetic nerve activity in humans. Circulation 1997;**95**(6):1441–48.

39 **Park JH, Chung S, Lee C, Jeon S.** Analysis of hemorrhagic risk factors during deep brain stimulation surgery for movement disorders: comparison of the circumferential paired and multiple electrode insertion methods. Acta Neurochirurgica (Wien) 2011;**153**(8):1573–78.

40 **Pereira EA, Wang S, Paterson D, Stein J, Aziz T, Green A.** Sustained reduction of hypertension by deep brain stimulation. J Clin Neurosci **17**(1):124–27.

41 **Patel NK, Javed S, Khan S et al.** Deep brain stimulation relieves refractory hypertension. Neurology 2011;**76**(4):405–407.

42 **Rutan GH, Hermanson B, Bild D, Kittner S, LaBaw F, Tell G.** Orthostatic hypotension in older adults. The Cardiovascular Health Study. CHS Collaborative Research Group. Hypertension 1992;**19**(6 Pt 1):508–19.

43 **Oldenburg O, Mitchell A, Nurnberger J et al.** Ambulatory norepinephrine treatment of severe autonomic orthostatic hypotension. J Am Coll Cardiol 2001;**37**(1):219–23.

44 **Haselton JR, Guyenet P.** Ascending collaterals of medullary barosensitive neurons and C1 cells in rats. Am J Physiol 1990;**258**(4 Pt 2):R1051–63.

45 **Inui K, Nosaka S.** Target site of inhibition mediated by midbrain periaqueductal gray matter of baroreflex vagal bradycardia. J Neurophysiol 1993;**70**(6):2205–14.

46 **Green AL, Wang S, Owen S, Paterson D, Stein J, Aziz T.** Controlling the heart via the brain: a potential new therapy for orthostatic hypotension. Neurosurgery 2006;**58**(6):1176–83; discussion 1176–83.

47 **Bahjaoui-Bouhaddi M, Henriet MT, Cappelle S, Dumoulin G, Regnard J.** Active standing and passive tilting similarly reduce the slope of spontaneous baroreflex in healthy subjects. Phys Res 1998;**47**(4):227–35.

48 **Cooper VL, Hainsworth R.** Carotid baroreceptor reflexes in humans during orthostatic stress. Exp Physiol 2001;**86**(5):677–81.

49 **Zhang Y, Critchley L, Tam Y, Tomlinson B.** Short-term postural reflexes in diabetic patients with autonomic dysfunction. Diabetologia 2004;**47**(2):304–11.

50 **Hyam JA, Kringelbach M, Silburn P, Aziz T, Green A.** The autonomic effects of deep brain stimulation–a therapeutic opportunity. Nat Rev Neurol;2012: **8**(7):391–400.

51 **Barnes PJ.** Neural control of airway function: new perspectives. Mol Asp Med 1990;**11**(5):351–423.

52 **Evans KC, Shea S, Saykin A.** Functional MRI localisation of central nervous system regions associated with volitional inspiration in humans. J Physiol 1999;**520 Pt 2**:383–92.

53 **Corfield DR, Fink GR, Ramsay SC, Murphy K, Harty HR, Watson JD, Adams L, Frackowiak RS, Guz A.** Evidence for limbic system activation during CO_2-stimulated breathing in man. J Physiol 1995;**488**(1):77–84.

54 **Quanjer PH, Lebowitz M, Gregg I, Miller M, Pedersen O.** Peak expiratory flow: conclusions and recommendations of a Working Party of the European Respiratory Society. Eur Resp J Suppl 1997;**24**:2S–8S.

55 **Barnes PJ**. Is asthma a nervous disease? The Parker B. Francis Lectureship. Chest 1995;**107**(3 Suppl.):119S–25S.

56 **Hadziefendic S, Haxhiu M**. CNS innervation of vagal preganglionic neurons controlling peripheral airways: a transneuronal labeling study using pseudorabies virus. J Autonom Nerv Syst 1999;**76**(2–3):135–45.

57 **Haxhiu MA, Jansen A, Cherniack N, Loewy A**. CNS innervation of airway-related parasympathetic preganglionic neurons: a transneuronal labeling study using pseudorabies virus. Brain Research 1993;**618**(1):115–34.

58 **Hyam JA, Brittain J, Paterson D, Davies R, Aziz T, Green A**. Controlling the lungs via the brain: a novel neurosurgical method to improve lung function in humans. Neurosurgery 2012;**70**(2):469–77; discussion 477–68.

59 **Hyam JA, Aziz T, Green A**. Control of the lungs via the human brain using neurosurgery. Prog Brain Res 2014;**209**:341–66.

60 **Krames ES, Foreman RD**. Spinal cord stimulation modulates visceral nociception and hyperalgesia via the spinothalamic tracts and postsynaptic dorsal column pathways: a literature review and hypothesis. Neuromodulation 2007;**10**:224–37.

61 **Torres N, Chabardes S, Benabid A**. Rationale for hypothalamus-deep brain stimulation in food intake disorders, obesity. Adv Tech Standards Neurosurg 2011;**36**:17–30.

62 **Halpern CH, Wolf J, Bale T et al**. Deep brain stimulation in the treatment of obesity. J Neurosurg 2008;**109**(4):625–34.

63 **Holstege G**. Micturition and the soul. J Comp Neurol 2005;**493**(1):15–20.

64 **Matsumoto S, Hanai T, Yoshioka N, Shimizu N, Sugiyama T, Uemura H**. Medial prefrontal cortex lesions inhibit reflex micturition in anethetized rats. Neurosci Res 2006;**54**(1):66–70.

65 **An X, Bandler R, Ongur D, Price JL**. Prefrontal cortical projections to longitudinal columns in the midbrain periaqueductal gray in macaque monkeys. J Comp Neurol 1998;**401**(4):455–79.

66 **Griffiths D, Derbyshire S, Stenger A, Resnick N**. Brain control of normal and overactive bladder. J Urol 2005;**174**(5):1862–67.

67 **Herzog J, Weiss P, Assmus A et al**. Subthalamic stimulation modulates cortical control of urinary bladder in Parkinson's disease. Brain 2006;**129**(Pt 12):3366–75.

68 **Kitta T, Matsumoto M, Tanaka H, Mitsui T, Yoshioka M, Nonomura K**. GABAergic mechanism mediated via D receptors in the rat periaqueductal gray participates in the micturition reflex: an in vivo microdialysis study. Eur J Neurosci 2008;**27**(12):3216–25.

69 **Green AL, Stone E, Sitsapesan H et al**. 'Switching off micturition using deep brain stimulation at midbrain sites. Ann Neurol 2012;**72**(1):144–47.

70 **Jenkinson N, Nandi D, Aziz T, Stein J**. Pedunculopontine nucleus: a new target for deep brain stimulation for akinesia. Neuroreport 2005;**16**(17):1875–76.

71 **Plaha P, Gill S**. Bilateral deep brain stimulation of the pedunculopontine nucleus for Parkinson's disease. Neuroreport 2005;**16**(17):1883–87.

72 **Pereira EA, Muthusamy K, De Pennington N, Joint C, Aziz T**. Deep brain stimulation of the pedunculopontine nucleus in Parkinson's disease. Preliminary experience at Oxford. Br J Neurosurg 2008;**22(Suppl. 1)**:S41–4.

73 **azzone P, Lozano A, Stanzione P et al**. Implantation of human pedunculopontine nucleus: a safe and clinically relevant target in Parkinson's disease. Neuroreport 2005;**16**(17):1877–81.

74 **Itoi K, Sugimoto N**. The brainstem noradrenergic systems in stress, anxiety and depression. J Neuroendocrinol 2010;**22**(5):355–61.

75 **Morschel M, Dutschmann M**. Pontine respiratory activity involved in inspiratory/expiratory phase transition. Philos Trans R Soc Lond 2009;**364**(1529):2517–26.

76 **Moruzzi G, Magoun H**. Brain stem reticular formation and activation of the EEG. 1949. J Neuropsychiatr Clin Neurosci 1995;**7**(2):251–67.

77 **Reese NB, Garcia-Rill E, Skinner R**. The pedunculopontine nucleus–auditory input, arousal and pathophysiology. Progr Neurobiol 1995;**47**(2):105–33.

78 **Gotoh TM, Tanaka K, Morita H**. Controlling arterial blood pressure using a computer-brain interface. Neuroreport 2005;**16**(4):343–47.

79 **Llinas RR, W. K., Nakao M, Hunter I, Anquetil PA**. Neuro-vascular central nervous recording/stimulating system: Using nanotechnology probes. J Nanoparticle Res 2005;**7**:111–27.

Chapter 4

Lateral medullary decompression for essential hypertension

Peter J. Jannetta and Kenneth F. Casey

Key points

1 Essential (primary) hypertension is driven by sympathetic hyperactivity.
2 Neurogenic hypertension results from perturbations in the brainstem vasomotor control loop.
3 Excitatory afferents, including from the vagal nerve, activate sympathetic hyperactivity.
4 Pulsatile blood vessels can drive sympathetic activity when in contact with the retroolivary region of the medulla.
5 Microvascular decompression of the pulsatile blood vessels can relieve neurogenic hypertension.

Introduction

Normal regulation of a pulsatile blood pressure is essential to the proper functioning of the human organism. Blood pressure control involves a variety of sites in the body, but the brainstem is an integral site for the feedback and control of blood pressure. Extra-cranial and extra-neural input reaches this region via the blood, cerebrospinal fluid, and neural pathways from peripheral receptors. Over-activity of one of these input loops causes a response in the blood pressure levels. Our current therapy for essential hypertension fails to address the cause in one-third of the people so afflicted. We offer a partial solution to this conundrum.

The autonomic nervous system (ANS), by virtue of its two divisions, parasympathetic and sympathetic, plays an enormous role in homeostasis throughout the body. The regulation of metabolic activities, heat production, and peripheral vascular system, as well as a component of cardiac output and blood pressure regulation, have all been well established in literature (1). When this balance is disrupted, the end effect is hypertension. We will look at some of the experimental and clinical data that examine what are the consequences of this imbalance. Many papers have looked at hypertension-driven damage, such as left ventricular hypertrophy and vascular damage, as well as blood pressure effects on the eyes, kidneys, and brain, as evidence of the secondary effects of hypertension. These effects are seen to occur even in the face of controlled hypertension. The overall effect of medical control is to slow the progression of damage in the target organs. The dysregulation of the energy expenditure and the caloric outputs demonstrate that this process can produce metabolic, haemodynamic, and finally neurohormonal excess that can be demonstrated to correlate with rapid thermogenesis and the occurrence of weight gain disproportionately in the fat stores. This is the postulated mechanism for the occurrence of obesity, related to hypertension.

There is interest in the genetics' field to identify a phenotype that may predispose to raised blood pressure. There have been no solid results as yet. This interest extends to the production of the inflammatory and other cytokines seen to accompany hypertension. Some authors have suggested that inflammatory states exist either as a primary or secondary response to this sympathetic augmentation, and that secondary cellular changes occur but do not result in clinical detectable loss of cells, but rather metabolic uncoupling in some instances and metabolic over-activity in others. This constellation of features serves to underscore the challenge in the treatment of hypertension.

The more pressing question is what lies at the tipping point to cause the imbalance in the normal control systems, i.e. the ANS?

The key to unlocking this cascade of damage is to identify the weak link in the feedback chain.

Why do we need arterial blood pressure anyway?

It has been postulated throughout the recorded history of medicine that the pulse represents signs of life itself. Certainly in Eastern medicine there is ascribed diagnostic value to the pulse. The practitioners of this ancient art refer to the five elements of pulse diagnosis and, coupled with tongue diagnosis, use both to reach an accurate picture of the state of health of the patient. The pulse is used to confirm the impression of the primary process. It is not a diagnostic tool per se, but should be coordinated with the other findings of traditional diagnosis. The pulse diagnosis is used to follow the effects of the treatment as well, but the science of pulse diagnosis postulates there is a chronicity and a pulsatility that are really at the heart of that diagnostic endeavour. As such, when one looks at the blood pressure as a disease process, mainly hypertension, we need to evaluate whether the hypertension relates to the maximum pressure exerted, i.e. the systolic pressure, or whether we are looking at the pulsatility changes that occur, i.e. a combination of the heart rate with the pressure, or are we looking at the force exerted on the system continuously, i.e. the mean arterial pressure? We have known since the time of the early Middle Ages that pulsatile blood flow is important for overall perfusion. The work done in the early days of extracorporeal bypass showed that non-pulsatile delivery of blood was quite different, physiologically and functionally, from pulsatile flow. The importance of pulsatility for pathologic changes in the microcirculation has been well documented (2–4). This despite the fact that blood was adequate in delivering oxygen for exchange in the tissues as well as clearing substances, such as CO_2, lactate, and other by-products in either manner of flow. Pulsatility explains the normal flow patterns seen in the coronary circulation, despite the countering pressure of the muscle wall contractions (5). One of the early discoveries in this area made reference to the fact that the absence of pulsatile blood flow leads to vasomotor instability that was not seen in subjects with pulsatile blood flow (6). In addition, a substantial amount of research documents the importance of pulsatile blood flow in capillary circulation and the importance of the pulsatile blood flow in maintaining the appropriate nature of flow within the capillaries relative to the sheer layers and alignment of the blood cells. These researchers also demonstrated that kidney function is improved in the presence of pulsatile blood flow, both as to the output of urine and its composition (7–9). However, these authors did not look at anything more than the pulsatility (as contrasted with the pulse pressure). Nonetheless, Page demonstrated that renin release is affected by an alteration in the pulse pressure, rather than a decrease in the mean arterial pressure (10). It is also well described by Hanes (11), and then subsequently Neil (12), that the pulsatile blood pressure is important in the origin of vascular tone through its action on the various stretch receptors. Some of their work speculated, as did Wilkins and Taylor (13), that the effect of the non-pulsatile systems pushing the initial pulse wave of the blood through the vascular tree could indeed stimulate the stretch receptors more proximally; however, they could not maintain this tone evenly or throughout the system. The pulsatile systems of perfusion performed much better in this regard. This raises the question of whether a difference between the central pulsatility and the peripheral pulsatility results in a disorder of vasomotor tone and this disorder subsequently then leads to alterations in tone and function, such as is seen in vascular wall composition in hypertension. Pulsatile blood flow is also important for haemodynamics across the capillary wall in the interstitial spaces, and a series of experimental work demonstrated the changes in blood tissue, tissue hypoxia, metabolic acidosis, capillary pressure, and ultimately blood clotting when comparing pulsatile versus non-pulsatile blood flow. Many of these authors asked the question whether the pulsatile blood flow or the pressure itself was the issue. McMaster and Parsons (14) looked at movement of dye and demonstrated that the change in the calibre of the vessel may in fact affect some of these exchanges. McDonald (15) pursued that by measuring the volume changes in vessels and its effect on interstitial pressure, but tied these observations to interstitial fluid and lymph production or flow, rather than vasomotor tone in these capillary areas. Haley and Creech looked at the concept of whether pulse pressure itself was important as to its effects on oxygen consumption in the brain and cerebral vessel resistance. They were able to show that decreasing the pulse pressure utilizing non-pulsatile perfusion reduced oxygen consumption in the brain, but did not change cerebrovascular reactivity in their model (16). They also showed that other metabolism, and the blood flow itself, remained unchanged, suggesting that the cells were reacting to the differences in pulse pressure, not perfusion or exchange. This was shown to be the same for the production of cerebrospinal fluid as well. Thus, taken together (and utilizing some of the large body of work in comparative anatomy and physiology), these data document that the changes in pressures, both for mean arterial pressure and pulse pressure, are of less consequence then the pulsatility. Indeed, a comparison of the aquatic circulatory system and that of the land primates demonstrates the importance of an increasing pulsatility within the circulatory system. This body of work would indicate that in the mammalian primate a number of cellular and extracellular processes are quite dependent on pulsatility, rather than mean arterial pressure. Thus it will come as no surprise that a good deal of research has shown that there are interrelated homeostatic mechanisms that regulate various aspects of the mean arterial pressure, pulse pressure, and pulsatility. The question that we pose in this chapter is: does neurogenic hypertension represent a subgroup of patients in whom this derangement in control occurs due to external forces on these control systems?

Essential hypertension, which accounts for some 95% of people with hypertension, is present throughout the world. Various studies have concluded that approximately 2 billion people are estimated to have hypertension and as many as one-third of those patients have persistent hypertension in the face of appropriate medical care and in the absence of secondary causes for hypertension (conditions that affect the kidneys, heart, endocrine system, and arteries). Hypertension is a modifiable risk factor for coronary heart disease, stroke, kidney failure, and eye-related hypertensive disorders, among others. The costs of this disease process, both direct and indirect, have been estimated to be as high as 80–90 billion US dollars. This is despite the fact that population estimates suggest that well over three-quarters of the patients with hypertension are aware that they have hypertension and are taking the medications, but up to one-third continue to have inadequately controlled blood pressure (16). The prevalence of hypertension is relatively evenly spread among the various nations of the world, but the Carnes' group have demonstrated a range of 60–70% among the Polish population and 3–5% in rural India (17). Other critics have written that data collected in rural areas are suspect, but what appears to be generally agreed upon is that high blood pressure in the young is increasing and that this is seen in as many of 10–15% of adolescent groups worldwide. Certainly the question has been raised as to whether this is linked to a change in weight, but the observation that prevalence is increasing despite these concerns is pervasive (18). Henry and Caselle in 1969 raised the provocative question as to the interaction of psychosocial factors on the prevalence or increase in essential hypertension and its control. They postulated that 'difficulties of adaptation . . . and the status of ambiguity . . . may result in years of repeated arousal of the vascular autonomic hormonal functions due to the organized perception of certain events as threatening'. They concluded that repeated arousal of the defence alarm system may, in fact, drive hypertension (19). The hypothalamic–pituitary–adrenocortical (HPA) axis is recruited by the organism in response to real or perceived threats to homeostasis ('stress'). The system is maintained by the hypothalamic cells of the paraventricular nucleus (PVN). Excitation of these neurons is mediated by several sources: direct (and perhaps indirect) inputs from brainstem neurons regulating autonomic tone/arousal; circumventricular organs monitoring blood and cerebrospinal fluid (CSF) constituents; and local-circuit neurons within the hypothalamus and basal forebrain. Kona pulled together a rather wide-ranging account of the various arguments related to the pathogenesis of essential hypertension in which he skilfully wove together the material from societal, psychosocial, dietary, and central systems. Following the undeniable impacts of his work is the effect of those various related spheres of influence on the neural system, specifically the neural regulatory system of hypertension. So, little doubt remains that the brain is deeply involved in the pathogenesis of arterial hypertension. Research over several decades has demonstrated the interplay at various points throughout the system, but the bulk of the direction of that research has led to specifically the concept that the interplay between sympathetic neural system and the imbalance of the feedback loop resulted in more hormonal alterations to the normal control of blood pressure, resulting in elevated blood pressure.

In the early 1960s, several authors began to look at the issue of neurally generated hypertension and sought to elucidate its pathogenesis. Initial animal work was quite promising and provided evidence that the adrenergic neural systems were certainly well within the mix for both the control of, and abnormal maintenance of, elevated blood pressure. Oparil and co-workers demonstrated that both the development and maintenance of arterial hypertension involved the adrenergic systems in 1968 (20). This opened the lines of enquiry to the topic.

Normal blood pressure has been described as being multifactorial and multifocal in origin and its maintenance. The onset of hypertension invites us to look at where the processes are effected. Grassi (21) summarized this approach succinctly: first, angiotensin II stimulation; second, alterations in plasma osmolarity; third, effects of hypoxia and altered respiratory drive on chemoreceptor groups; fourth, vascular cytokine inflammatory effects; fifth, peripheral stimulation from renal and baroreceptors input. One could also look at hypertension as the interplay of these sites, wherein the reciprocal pathways generate an imbalance, tipping the system toward higher pulsatility and dysfunctional pressures. This could include anatomical alterations in the system. A new concept in neurological circles is that of the connectome. This refers to the network of anatomical and thus functional pathways through which various neurones and astrocytes interact. The importance of this concept applies to systems that apparently work in parallel. The parasympathetic system and the sympathetic system generally maintain a balance of outputs to maintain homeostasis in any appropriate system. Each system is constantly active, and if the sympathetic system is activated in a 'flight or fight' mode, the parasympathetic responses are designed to tone down the excesses of that activity. The origin of the tonic activity in the sympathetic arm of the autonomic nervous system is key to maintaining the balance, even under general anaesthesia. These tonically active cells are predominantly in the cardio-accelerator and vasomotor systems of the SNS. While specific sets of cells appear to be grouped for muscle-directed preganglionic tasks, others are directed to the vasoconstrictor system; both act in concert at the central information 'nodes' in reciprocal connections with the rostral central nervous system.

One mechanism of looking at the hypertensive pattern is that the normal flow of signals originates in the reciprocal loop between the area postrema, nucleus tractus solitaries

(NTS), and rostral ventrolateral medulla (RVLM) (22). These three centres are, in turn, interconnected to the circumventricular organs (CVO). A great deal of experimental work suggests that certain CVO, namely the paraventricular nucleus, the organ of the lamina terminalis, and the subfornicial organ, all act on the NTS. However, only the efferents from the area postrema have significant fibre tracts. The parventricular nucleus was postulated in 1980 to be an efferent system that by responding to its visceral and hormonal components in the circulating fluids, in turn activated the 'vasopressinergic' projections to the brainstem centres and periphery (23). Zoccal (24) has suggested that this system can be affected by alterations in the respiratory cycle. Chronic hypoxia, such as is seen in sleep apnoea, produces alterations in angiotensin II and coupling with the respiratory excitatory drive. This results in sympathetic hyperactivity. At the PVN, angiotensin II is produced in response to the aforementioned stimuli. In addition, neural activation coming from the periphery via the vagus and glossopharyngeal nerves can stimulate a response in the PVN (25). This system then directly innervates the RVLM. The sympathetic premotor sites are thought to be the neurones that drive the hyperactivity (26). The area postrema and rostral ventral medullary nucleus receive direct input from the vagus. Both inputs produce an increase in ANG II, which is a prohypertensive compound. ANG II and its counterbalance system ACE2 are found ubiquitously in animal brain models. The role of the central renin–angiotensin system (RAS) in the elevation of sympathetic hyperactivity is well accepted. These substances exert a vasopressor effect on the region of the brainstem that includes the nucleus tractus solitariius.

A brief review of the circumventricular organs (CVO) include the three most closely identified with the control of blood pressure: the organum vasculosum of the lamina terminalis, the subfornicial organ, and the area postrema. The remaining sites of CVO are the median eminence, pineal gland, posterior pituitary gland, and the subcommissural area. A review of the literature surrounding the role of these three CVO in blood pressure control includes data from lesion studies, stimulation studies, and chemical interventions.

Lesions in the anterior ventricular region (OVLT or AV3V) have been shown to blunt the effect of angiotensin II induced pressure changes, as well as alter water homeostasis. However, lesions in the AV3V region do not blunt the effect of an electrolytic lesion in the NTS, which are known to cause sustained hypertension. The combination lesions are interesting. NTS-lesioned animals that experience an AV3V lesion show less sympathetic adrenal activity. Interestingly, there was also activation of the immune system, specifically T-cells and leukocyte cellular adherence, which is a by-product of the effect on the nucleus tractus solitarius dysfunction. The OVLT is composed of two types of cells: tanycytes (specialized ependymal cells) and other glial cells. The former are more numerous and make extensive contact with the non-fenestrated capillaries found here.

Considering the area postrema, we have another site of interest as it lies relatively close to the nucleus tractus solitarius. The area postrema lies close to the vagal triangle, separated by a thin funiculus, and is composed of specialized ependymal cells and tanycytes. Ependymal and tanycytes can participate in transport of neurochemicals into and out of the cerebrospinal fluid from its cells or adjacent neurones, glia, or vessels. Ependyma and tanycytes may also participate in chemoreception. A recent study has indicated the existence of prolactin-binding sites specific to the area postrema. This hormone is an integral part of the osmoregulatory system. Of particular interest, however, for the area postrema, is that, of the different circumventricular organs, and especially the three most closely involved in blood pressure regulation, this is the only one that receives efferents directly from the vagus. Each of the others, the OVLT, SFO, and PVN, receives afferents from the nucleus tractus solitarius and differ in their other efferents. Only the area of postrema has reciprocal innervation with the nucleus tractus solitarius as well as the dorsal motor nucleus of the vagus (27). Wheeler proposed that the experimental information could suggest that hyperactivity in the vagus from cross-compression, effects reciprocal innervation in the nucleus tractus solitarius via the area of postrema, as well as directly in the rostral medulla, as demonstrated earlier by Fagius (31). This activity could well drive various observations seen in the inflammatory systems, the cytokine systems, and the neuroadrenergic or sympathetic augmentation seen in hypertension.

The sympathetic system in neurogenic hypertension

Building on the work of several decades of animal experimentation, researchers began to look more closely at how the sympathetic nervous system might be involved in control for blood pressure. Experiments looking at the amounts of plasma catecholamines were largely frustrating as the evidence was inconclusive. It took the development, as is often the case, of newer techniques to evaluate the impact of the system activation on humans. Two major areas in that regard were the development and use of radio-labelled neurotransmitters, which were then both supplemented and finally supplanted by microneurographic recording of sympathetic nerve traffic. Microneurography became a viable technique based on the work done in the Department of Physiology at Uppsala in the mid-1960s (28). The researchers there, who were looking at the activity of the muscle systems, and particularly the fusimotor system, developed and perfected the technique of inserting a needle into a human nerve and amplifying a recording of the normal amount of sympathetic traffic. This was building on previous work done by those authors.

Briefly, recordings can be made from single and myelinated fibres, both efferents and afferents. Microneurography is done using a 200-micrometer diameter electrode that has a non-insulated tip. As in other clinical neurophysiologic situations, amplification of the signal to improve a signal-to-noise ratio, coupled with bandpass filters, provides the output called the neurogram. Some of the original work done by Hagbarth and Valbo from Uppsala included looking at the sympathetic nerve traffic as it related to the pulse and respiratory activities. This early work documented the inverse relationship between blood pressure and sympathetic nerve traffic in the muscles, i.e. when blood pressure decreased, sympathetic nerve activity increased and the converse was also true. Macefield and co-workers were able to demonstrate the firing frequency at rest and its change during various provocations in their 2002 paper (29). Indirectly, this allowed them the evaluation of baroreceptor activity and utilizing this nerve traffic data to determine the amount of released neurotransmitter (norepinephrine) during these variations. The group also found that looking at sympathetic nerve traffic in the patients with essential hypertension revealed more bursts in these patients at rest and this was seen in a large group of adults with hypertension. So, more sympathetic nerve traffic resulted in more norepinephrine in the system. Mancia subsequently reported (30) that patients in cardiac failure had increased sympathetic nerve traffic, but baroreflex modulation was still intact. At the time, one of the prevailing theories was that baroreceptor reflex activity was decreased in cardiac failure and hypertension. An essential feature of the concept that neurogenic hypertension may have its aetiology in vascular cross-compression starts with the work by Fabias (31) when he demonstrated (on himself) that the temporary deafferentation in the glossopharyngeal vagal nerve complex resulted in an increase in sympathetic nerve traffic and hypertension, and that cardiac rhythmicity was also affected. This change in sympathetic nerve activity may have happened indirectly through the changes in the baroreceptor reflex activity. One of the issues raised by this experimental group was that when sensory stimuli were delivered to the deafferented nerve group, there were arousal bursts much the same as was raised earlier in the concept of increased arousal defence mechanisms. In the non-anaesthetized nerve arm the responses were not seen, suggesting that this activity is normally suppressed by baseline neural traffic. This led to the conclusion that the deafferentation uncovered a tonic response in the sympathetic system. Conceptually, this can be related to the underlying response seen after disinhibition in the injured spinal cord. The remarkable body of work that originated from the initial group at Uppsala and its components is intriguing as it sets the stage for refining understanding of the sympathetic nervous system in human hypertension. Floras' (32) group was able to show that sympathetic activation and nerve traffic parallels the magnitude of the blood pressure elevation in patients with mild and moderate hypertension. Additionally, Grassi cited other studies that are important because they show a high correlation in both moderate and severe essential hypertension between the sympathetic nerve traffic and both the mean arterial pressure and, to a lesser extent, the heart rate. By contrast, the patients with secondary hypertension showed very little sympathetic nerve traffic, despite elevated heart rate and elevated blood pressure (33). Grassi makes the point that sympathetic hyperactivity appears to be unique to the central vasomotor portion of the system, rather than the entire system, as no sympathetic hyperactivity was seen in the neurones involved in skin circulation, which is also under sympathetic control via the thermoregulatory system. Other groups as well as Grassi's had concluded that measuring plasma catecholamines was not going to be a reliable marker for sympathetic nerve activity, but could be utilized in focal experiments, such as venous drainage in the arm and the like, with some degree of correlation. Nonetheless, this does not appear to be a useful technique to investigate in a human subject. At the current time, few data exist about the evaluation of this neurotransmitter and its spillover in the central nervous system, either by means of using tritiated markers in brain imaging or in measurement of the CSF levels. This may well be an area for evaluation in the future. Preliminary work by

Eide in 1979 (34) demonstrated an elevation of cerebrospinal fluid norepinephrine in the relation to diastolic blood pressure was seen in primary hypertension, but not in patients with secondary hypertension. In 1984, Cudeddu (35) looked at cerebrospinal fluid norepinephrine levels and found them to be markedly different between hypertension and normotensive patients, and that this could be affected by the administration of clonidine, despite the fact that the clonidine had no effect on the blood pressure or plasma norepinephrine levels. Grassi raised the question as to the point of the feedback, in which the central system was affected. He queried whether it was activity secondary to the renin–angiotensin system elevation observed in patients with essential hypertension or hypothalamic sympathetic nervous activity mediated to other central systems in response to the abnormal feedback loop plus or minus the effect of external stimuli and perhaps sodium intake. Several of the papers at this time also alluded to the fact that sympathetic hyperactivity resulted in a phenomenon termed 'insulin resistance' by triggering alternations in plasma insulin levels as measured by insulin resistance in skeletal muscles (36, 37). A group looked at the central sympathetic activity using microneurography. They looked at a group of patients utilizing both MRI and neurography contemporaneously. They found that patients with neurovascular compression had significantly greater sympathetic activity than patients that did not. However, given the patients with higher pulse pressures, the activity was still higher than patients who had either normal pressure or mild pressure elevations (37, 38). In the clinical setting, microneurography is an alternate way to measure sympathetic nerve cells; however, it can be somewhat cumbersome and is technically demanding. An additional way to quantitate sympathetic/parasympathetic activity is the low- to high-power frequency ratios from the electrocardiogram. These are obtained utilizing standard parameters (39) and involve sampling electrocardiogram for the R-wave fiducial. A commercially available algorithm is utilized to transform the fiducial data as a power equation. Low frequency is defined as 0.05 to 0.15 Hz and high frequency 0.15 to 0.4 Hz. The low-frequency component is sympathetic activity, whereas the high-frequency component represents the parasympathetic activity. This ratio is an indicator of the sympathetic and vagal balance in the normal setting. This technique is based on the concept of heart rate variability analysis as a measure of autonomic nervous system function. While there are three types of method, frequency domain analysis has been suggested as most well-correlated with measurement of sympathetic balance (40). The time domain method utilizes primarily the standard deviation between the normal beats. Thayer (41) looked at a time domain variability during sitting, standing, and different stressors. Utilizing the Pearson correlations with the standard deviation of the square root, they found a high correlation between the normal time domain, as well as the spectral domain, of the low-frequency/high-frequency ratio and this was found to be useful both in evaluation of normal patients and patients with activity and stressors throughout the period of evaluation. One criticism of the aforementioned method is that heart rate analysis may have some element of chaos; however, Eckberg (42) did not find this to be a valid criticism. The experimental data support that vagal stimulation, vagal mechanical change, and sectioning the vagus, all result in reproducible changes in the high-frequency variant. Initially, the low-frequency variant was considered suspect; however, its correlation with microneurography has raised the level of acceptance of this component of the ratio. Several papers demonstrate that the low-frequency component is well correlated with microneurography. It also is correlated with norepinephrine spillover as an invasive measure of cardiac sympathetic activity. Nonetheless, even in later stages of hypertension, the ratio continues to represent the effect of the autonomic nervous system on the heart. In fact, Notarius suggested that the diminishing spectral analysis of the low-frequency component is the most accurate representation of the sympathetic state, rather than the trend in that setting (43).

Is there an inflammatory role in the origin or maintenance of neurogenic hypertension?

In the past 2 or 3 years there has been an explosion of interest in the concept of the primary or secondary role of inflammation in neurogenic hypertension. As we have shown from the previous data, the sympathetic nervous system is activated prior to the onset of hypertension. This was also seen in the animal model for hypertension, i.e. the spontaneous hypertensive rat, in which sympathetic hyperactivity precedes the onset of hypertension (44). Several authors have raised the question of whether an inflammatory state precedes, and/or is driven by, effects in circumventricular organs in which activation of the inflammatory tree produces secondary over-expression of various hormone systems or enzyme systems, with subsequent altered regulation of the receptor groups. One could then envision the situation in which hypertension could be produced by alterations in the T-cell system causing so-called inflammation-related hypertension, alterations in the angiotensin II renin system (so-called chemical hypertension), and alterations in the peripheral system (so-called secondary hypertension).

Youn and their group at Beonsel in Korea demonstrated that the T-cell population from patients with hypertension show an increased role for pro-inflammatory CD8 T-cells, which are a cytotoxic group of cells, and that they also were related to an increase in certain types of chemokines in that this T-cell chemokine was seen in the proximal and distal tubules of these patients. There is considerable evidence in humans that inflammation and secondary hypertension are important in specialized cases such as pulmonary hypertension and seen also in pre-eclampsia. However, until the recent paper by Youn, human data was lacking. (45)With sympathetic hyperactivity in the brainstem, several areas have been investigated as to their responses. The nucleus tractus solitarius, which has reciprocal innervation with the rostral ventral medullary area, has been a particular target of investigators. Of interest, they have seen elevation of certain enzymes and down-regulation of others. One of the more intriguing ones is the molecule alone as junctional adhesion molecule 1, which was first noted to be up-regulated in the spontaneous hypertensive rat. When this was placed in the normotensive rat via gene transfer technique, blood pressure was seen to elevate in the normotensive rat model. The conclusion of several authors then was that the elevation of this enzyme was correlated with hypertension and the question that arises is whether the hypertension is driven by sympathetic hyperactivity relative to the expression of the gene or secondary arterial distention (which elevates JAM-1 production). Junctional adhesion molecule-1 (JAM1) is part of the family of the JAM proteins. The JAM proteins were described in 1998 as proteins predominantly expressed in endothelial and epithelial intercellular junctions, suggesting that this protein and the family of proteins, subsequently described as JAM-1, JAM-2 and JAM-3, have a primary role in cell–cell interactions. These cell–cell interactions appear to help both reseal tight junctions and change barrier function in vascular endothelium. JAM-1, which is associated with a great deal of inflammation, appeared to be important in regulating a set point for arterial pressure in the nucleus tractus solitaries. These pro-inflammatory molecules are expressed in the nucleus tractus solitaries, and secondary vascular inflammation and infiltration occur, which may affect the ability of the cells to carry on their normal feedback function (46) There are some conflicting results that point to brainstem intermittent hypoxia, which elevates these systems as well (47). In addition, there have been a number of papers that have looked at mitochondrial dysfunction and secondary impairment of vasomotor tone and its potential relationship to oxides produced in the rostral ventral medulla in response to blood flow changes, which were possibly direct or related to alterations in the angiotensin-converting enzyme system.

The grey matter angiotensin system is an important component of homeostasis in the brain in terms of vasomotor control and the electrolyte balance. This system includes the angiotensinogen, angiotensin-converting enzymes, and the renin system and then the secondary receptors for those systems. The angiotensin system has been noted to have several subgroups and angiotensin II and its receptor groups appear to be an integral component of altering baroreflex sensitivity in the presence of increased sympathetic tone. Indeed, Fang showed that angiotensin-converting enzyme type II over-expression would make angiotensin type II into a peptide of angiotensin (1–7), which is a much more potent peptide. Angiotensin (1–7) increases the bradycardiac component, promotes vasodilatation, and has an anti-hypertensive effect; therefore, over-expression of this agent could potentially reverse hypertension (48). While angiotensin-converting enzyme type II is found in the heart and other locations throughout the body, it is also found in the brain, especially in the area of the subfornicial organ. Interestingly, the subfornicial organ and other components of the circumventricular organs are also involved in regulation of blood pressure and volume homeostasis through their basic activities of sampling blood and CSF. They are also affected by oxidative impairment of mitochondrial electron chain and the oxygen radicals produced as a consequence of that. The subfornicial organ, in turn, affects the area of the NTS in the brainstem.

Neurogenic hypertension—where is it broken?

In the early 1980s, a good deal of experimental work came together from correlative anatomic studies to suggest that the rostral medulla oblongata on the central lateral surface is a part of the vasomotor regulatory system. This was deduced from electrolytic lesions and focal electrical stimulation that produced inverse results, namely the lesion produced a drop in blood pressure and stimulation an increase in blood pressure. In addition, Amendt's work (48), demonstrating that projections from this area into the interomediolateral cell column were also activated, was consistent with this being the end of the sympathetic outflow tract in vasomotor control. The sympathetic system is thought to have its origin in the lateral hypothalamic nuclei and then involves integration, at the level of the nucleus tractus solitariius, then, via reciprocal innervation between the NTS and rostral lateral ventral medullary area, the projections proceed to the anteromedial lateral cell column. A good deal of the animal work shows that these ventrolateral medullary relay neurones are part of the hypothalamic response described previously as a defence response. An excellent study by Dampney (49) found that there was a very focal area in the midst of the ventrolateral cells in which micro-injections produced a clearcut response of a pressor nature that was not seen in the sites surrounding this area, which they entitled the ventrolateral pressor area. Afferents to this area included cells found in nucleus tractus solitarius and its pathways and the nucleus parabrachialis in the pons. These input cells also were localized to a very concise area. This was in concordance with the work from several other investigators (50). In the lab model, Dampney showed that the pressor response from electrical stimulation came from this group of ventrolateral cells and demonstrated increased sympathetic discharge, as well as peripheral effects. Criticism of the stimulation model has been that cells at a distance that have dendrites in the area of stimulation could be affected and so this observation, while important, is certainly not conclusive. However, several investigators looked at the fact that sympathetic preganglionic neurones activated muscle vasoconstrictor activity, as well as peripheral vasoconstrictor sites. The sympathetic vasomotor pathways received input from specific supraspinal sources, and one of the notable facts of these supraspinal sources is the maintenance of tonic activity. Investigators attempting to determine the mechanism for this tonic activity, as well as its implications, have looked at brain networks between the nucleus tractus solitarius, the ventrolateral medullary group, and the parabrachial nucleus. This was based on the observation that the interomediolateral cell column, termed the final pathway of sympathetic activation, has projections that come from the rostral ventral medullary area, caudal nuclei, the A5 cell group, the paraventricular thalamic nucleus, the lateral hypothalamic area, and the central grey area of the brain (51, 52). In the animal model, the cell groups within this area had been defined by their response to clinical standing and had been termed the A1 neuro-adrenergic neurones and the C1 adrenergic neurones. These neurones are grouped about the rostral ventral area of the medulla in close proximity to the inferior olive and lateral to it, as well as ventral to the nucleus tractus solitarius in the same region. Work that initially stimulated interest in this area suggested this area has been more responsible for blood pressure control. It originated with Dittmar (53), who, in doing a series of transections of the brainstem, demonstrated that transection of the rostral medulla at the level of the olive dropped the blood pressure and hence he termed this area the vasomotor centre. Subsequent investigators began to define this area more precisely utilizing a combination of cooling, micro-injections of antagonist and agonist agents, and tracer studies to identify the cell groups. Ross's lab (54) demonstrated the opposing effects of the excitatory amino acid glutamate and inhibitor amino acids of gamma aminobutyric acid. He then proceeded in a series of experiments to look for a tonic discharge that correlated with the activities for a so-called pacemaker property. Pacemaker properties are defined as neurones that generate a rhythmic pattern of discharge in response to intrinsic stimuli rather than depending on the synaptic, neurohormonal release of a modulator or after discharges to maintain firing status. There are some additional cellular electrophysiological properties that are well detailed. Sun and Guyenet, in 1985, were able to demonstrate that the cells in the retrofacial portion of nucleus paragigantocellularis lateralis represent a certain group of cells with spontaneous activity and spinal projections consistent with the concept of a vasomotor tonic projection system (55). However, one area in which the most exciting experiments exist is that of Suns' group, which demonstrated that the high frequency but low stimulation of the vagus produced activation in the cells in this region and produced a change in activity of the rostral brain cell medullary motor neurones, which resulted in uniform increase in their firing rates (56). These activities were able to be manipulated by blocking both excitatory and inhibitory pathways, confirming the findings of electrical stimulation. The concept that manipulation of the vagal input to this region could affect these pacemaker cells and increase sympathetic output is at the heart of the subsequent observation by Jannetta and Gendell, in which they postulated that neurogenic hypertension was related to vascular cross-compression of this site. Utilizing their double-balloon model, they were able to fulfil Koch's postulates in the primate (57). Their data correlated with that of Dampney and McAllen, wherein they showed in the animal model that two distinct regions in the medulla oblongata on the ventral surface produce excitation in the sympathetic nerves. There is a mixed area of cells that lie immediately lateral and posterior to the inferior olive. Stimulation here produces both central vasomotor and peripheral vasomotor effects, as are seen in response to the electrolytic lesioning, agonist and antagonist blockers' micro-injections (Fig. 4.1).

The concept that alterations in the activity of the vagal nerve can produce a change in the sympathetic nerve traffic is widely accepted. It may well be that as a potential therapeutic target, given the diverse nature of the area postrema, nucleus tractus solitarius, and RVLM area in their chemical nature, that simply reducing the driving input, mainly the sympathoexcitatory input, will allow the rest of the system to reset towards normal, thereby preventing both recurrence of blood pressure elevation, as well as secondary effects of hypertension on different organ systems, such as the left ventricular, peripheral vascular distention, and the kidneys. Whether this is accomplished by a direct means or indirectly by blunting the effect of the other three types of hypertension is currently not entirely clear in the human, but there are certainly suggestions that this could be the case, looking at the accumulative animal model data, largely from the spontaneous hypertensive rat data, considered an excellent model for human hypertension. In Jannetta's original model of the primate baboon, we had similar findings (57).

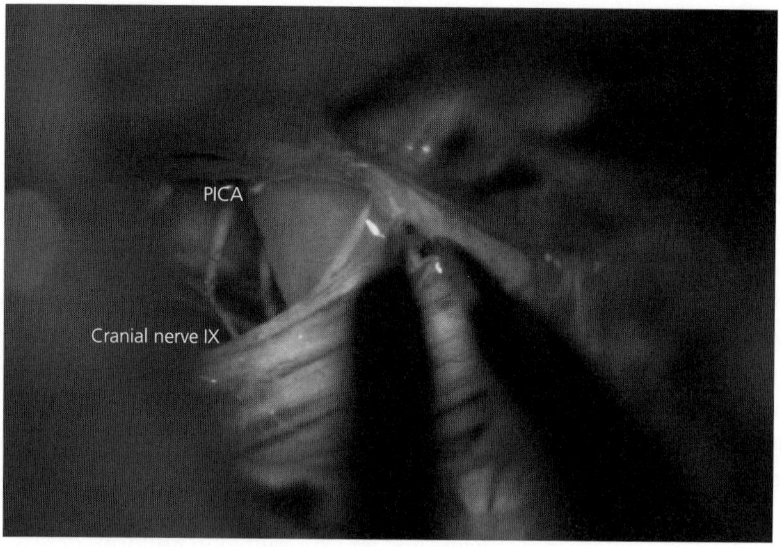

Fig. 4.1 The area encircled in front of the IXth and Xth cranial nerve entry zones contain the sympathoexcitatory cell groups for those nerves.

Neurogenic hypertension—the clinical phase

In the observation by Jannetta and Gendel that hypertension may be related to intracranial arterial pathology, namely neurovascular cross-compression (NVC), a genesis of an elaboration of the pathophysiology of hypertension was initiated (58). The hypothesis of vascular cross-compression rests upon the concept that arterial or venous pulsatile pressure on brainstem and cranial nerve structures can produce dysfunction. Jannetta initially made these observations and completed the first operative procedure in June 1966. It is well accepted that the aetiology of hemifacial spasm and its cure are due to neurovascular compression (NVC) and its relief. What we think is more intriguing about hemifacial spasm is the observation that there is nuclear hyperactivity that is a consequence of the chronic compression of the vulnerable portion of the cranial nerve. This central excitation explains a number of the clinical features of hemifacial spasm. Other disease processes, including trigeminal neuralgia, glossopharyngeal neuralgia, and other cranial nerve compression syndromes have evolved from this initial compilation of medical observations over the preceding 50 years of neurosurgery. We mention these other syndromes to reinforce the clinical evidence that vascular cross-compression can produce cranial nerve and brainstem dysfunction. Following the 1978 paper, Jannetta (56) extended their observations to 53 patients where cross-compression of the lateral medulla was seen in 51 of the 53 patients roentgengraphically. Vascular decompression was effective in 42 of the 51 patients; 32 of the 42 patients were relieved of their hypertension and 4 were improved. This led to the hypothesis that a subgroup of patients with essential hypertension could be treated by removing the pressure or the pulsatility against the brainstem in that location.

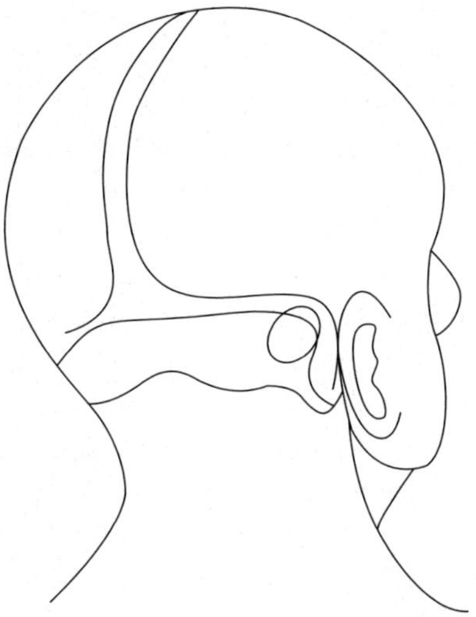

Fig. 4.2 Retromastoid craniectomy.

This has enabled additional groups to look at the concept of the origin of neurogenic control of blood pressure and the effect that decompression has on the carotid baroreceptor reflex travelling in cranial nerves IX and X (Fig. 4.2).

The output in the descending sympathetic neurones that go to both the heart and peripheral muscular systems, originate in the same area, as demonstrated by Sun and Gayette (57). Since the cardiac vagal efferents to the neurogenic vasomotor centre are C fibres, they may well be more susceptible to mechanical and pulsatile effects. In the normal physiologic model, the C fibres largely sense the degree of arterial and atrial calibre and, to a lesser extent, with other fibres respond to the systolic pressure and the left ventricular distention, which is an indirect measure of the diastolic pressure. In Jannetta's initial clinical observations, increased activity of the sympathetic nervous system affecting peripheral resistance was thought to be a part of essential arterial hypertension. What was not known was whether this was a by-product of sympathetic over-activity or was a primary affect, which then altered the feedback loop. Looking at the spontaneous hypertensive rat data compared to the normotensive animals, the atrial C fibre receptors are noticeably up-regulated in the spontaneously hypertensive rat. The decreased sensitivity of the left-sided cardiopulmonary vagal efferents may be related to changes in the fibres themselves or to a decrease in the sensitivity to the pulsatility or change in arterial wall size during the normal cardiac cycle. Cross-compression of the vagal efferents of IX and X may play a role in decreasing the brain's messaging traffic, rather than a change in affected fibres directly. This remains an area of additional research. As noted earlier in the discussion of the homeostatic features of arterial blood pressure(Why do we need Blood Pressure anyway), so too here, the effects on the root entry zone of the IXth and Xth cranial nerves in the region of the retroolivary sulcus do require a certain degree of pulsatility. This was nicely shown by Jannetta (55) in an animal model of primate hypertension. Jannetta et al.

discussed whether the pulsatility itself was the damaging agent or whether the pulsatility was stimulating the central nuclei, such as we saw earlier in the experiments that demonstrated that high-frequency low-amplitude stimulation of the vagal efferents resulted in excitation of the vasomotor system in the medulla. One part of the hypothesis put forth by Jannetta suggests that the sympathoexcitatory distribution in the vagus is asymmetrical. That is to say, the output through the NTS and RLVN on the left side exerts its major activity on the heart and vascular system above the diaphragm. The right side of the heart in its vagal and glossopharyngeal output, bears a greater effect on the subdiaphragmatic ANS system. Subsequently, the group at Erlangen (58) evaluated a series of patients and found that cross-compression of the ventrolateral medulla could be visualized on pre-operative imaging studies and that decompression of those patients resulted in salutary effects on the blood pressure. Interestingly, they referred to neurovascular compression as an example of a secondary form of compression wherein the aetiology is ascribed to a source outside the normal vasomotor control system, much the same as in kidney disease. In their group of patients, 7 of 8 patients were normotensive at 3 months after surgery; however, the patients still required anti-hypertensive medicines (58). The group at Hanover produced an interesting paper in which autopsy data from 34 patients with arterial hypertension were examined: 24 had essential hypertension, while 10 had a secondary cause. They also included a control group with normal pressure. After normalizing the patient's for sex and age range, they evaluated the pathology and histology from both a macrostructural and a microcellular perspective. They found that in all 24 cases with essential hypertension there was arterial cross-compression in the ventrolateral medulla in at least one location. They noted that there was also some compression on the right side and the typical offending vessel in either case was the posteroinferior cerebellar artery, the vertebral artery either alone or in conjunction with the posteroinferior cerebellar artery, and, least likely, the anteroinferior cerebellar artery. Interestingly, their diagram of the area of neurovascular compression coincides quite nicely with that of Sun for the motor and mixed areas from the animal model. Their light microscopic histology examinations, which included Mason trichrome and Kluver–Barrera staining, was performed looking for a wide variety of changes. No difference was seen in the cell types and nerve fibres in terms of pathological losses, including no evidence of demyelination (59).

Other authors have previously suggested that hypertension was one of the risk factors for the development of cranial nerve cross-compression syndromes. These pathology results raised the counter-argument that the elongation of the vessels and atherosclerotic changes may have come about as a consequence of neurovascular compression starting with these normal vessels. The importance of this is that the vessels do not need pathologic changes within the vessel wall, which in fact would alter the pulsatility, but rather they have a normal pulsatility and pulse pressure. Jannetta, building on observations by Dandy, reasoned the same for trigeminal neuralgia. Some researchers speculated that the pattern of compression, that is the points at its neurovascular cross-contact, were different in arterial hypertension cases as opposed to other cranial nerve syndromes. Specifically the volume of nerve tissue compressed was greater in the arterial hypertension group. This was reasoning from Sun's animal work on the volume of tissues involved in the retroolivary sulcus. An observational study reported that small vessels, from 0.3 to 2 mm, can cause neurovascular compression for the traditional cranial nerve syndromes, but that it required much larger vessels for arterial hypertension. Following that, a group made up by Schmitz from Berlin looked at a protocol to visualize this and found a low result of vascular cross-compression utilizing their criteria for the left RLVM compared to normotensive controls. They utilized 3D fast-imaging with steady-state precession and time of flight sequences to visualize vessels in proximity to these neurosensitive sites. It should be noted that in the paper by Kabota, when he was looking at combined hyper-dysfunction syndrome and vascular cross-compression syndrome, he noted that patients who had combined cross-compression had a much higher rate of having concomitant hypertension. This was significantly higher in patients with a single cross-compression and was also noted to be more elevated in the single decompression group based on population, although it was not statistically significantly different. The technique of microvascular decompression utilizes a retromastoid craniectomy (Fig. 4.2). The area detailed in Fig. 4.1 is approached from the dorsal aspect. Vessel decompression is accomplished by elevating the offending vessel(s) (posterior inferior cerebellar artery and vertebral artery) and placing a felt pad to reduce pulsatility against the nerves and brainstem (Figs 4.3 and 4.4).

The last several decades have seen an increase in various publications of a clinical nature relative to the concept of neurogenic hypertension and the fact of focal compression at the rostral ventral medullary area and its resolution produces relief (60). The possibilities for how neurogenic hypertension comes about would include the sympathetic firing rate, baroreflex down-regulation, and the renin–angiotensin system in the brain. An alteration in the norepinephrine uptake might be involved, as evidenced by the elevated

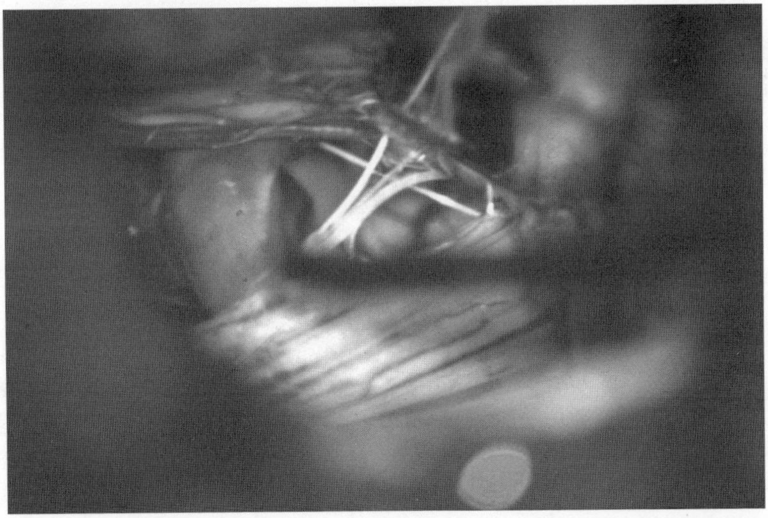

Fig. 4.3 Upper: the Posterior inferior cerebellar artery(PICA) is seen compressing the entry zone at the retroolivary sulcus. Lower: the instrument is elevating the vessel away from the brainstem.

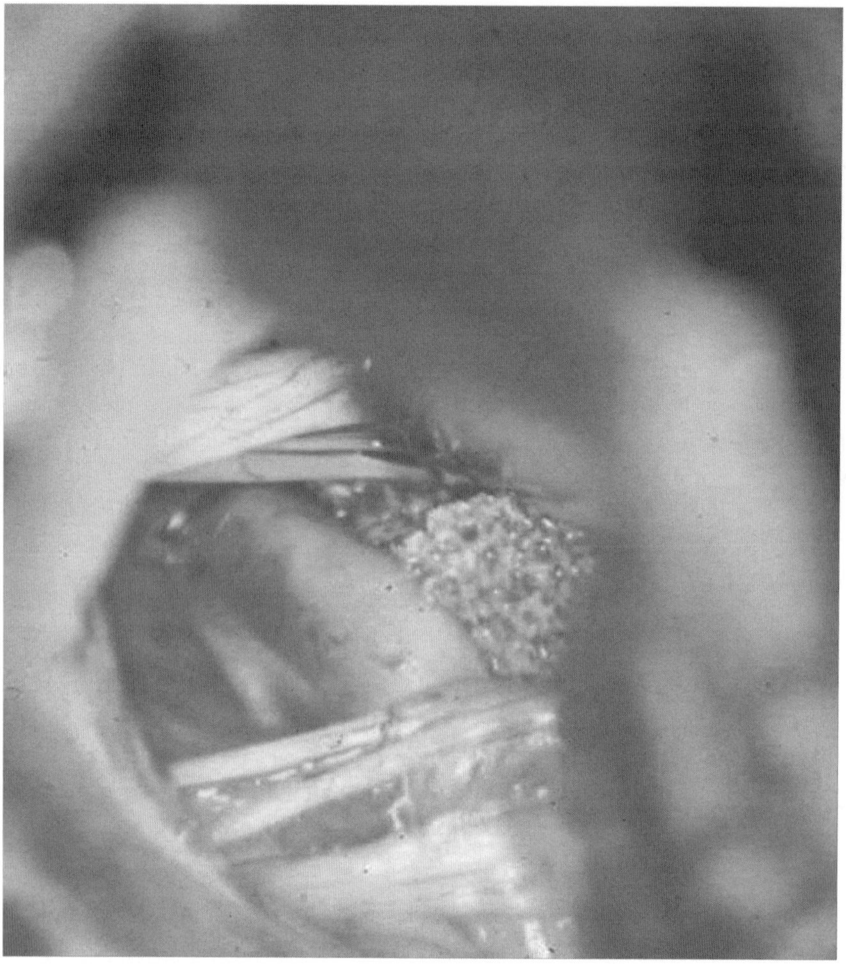

Fig. 4.4 Felt sponge is seen between the artery and brainstem.
Source data from Hypertension, 62, Youn JC, Yu HT, Lim BJ, Koh MJ, et al., Immunosenescent CD8+ T Cells and C-X-C Chemokine Receptor Type 3 Chemokines Are Increased in Human Hypertension, pp. 126–133, Copyright (2013), American Heart Association; Experimental Physiology, 95(5), Waki H, Gouraud SS, SS, Maeda M, and Paton JFR, Evidence of specific inflammatory condition in nucleus tractus solitarii of spontaneously hypertensive rats, pp. 595–600, Copyright (2010), John Wiley and Sons.

plasma catecholamines. This finding may be due, not to increased production, but rather decreased re-uptake. In humans this has been investigated by several groups, but most eloquently in the study in which spillover rates in various models was related to the onset of hypertension. The spillover rate is the concept referring to the infusion analysis of tritiated norepinephrine. With that, both systemic and regional areas can be evaluated so as to further understand and elucidate the sites that may be involved. In humans, altered re-uptake does not appear to have a genetic origin or an alteration in the transport chains, as eloquently demonstrated with some of the blocker agents. This was done by putting in nonsense gene substitutions by several different groups. The re-uptake also showed a reduced turnover in the heart and this was seen also in healthy controls, in which, when central sympathoinhibition was created with chemical means, there was an increased norepinephrine spillover. As with other papers, this work suggests that central sympathetic activity is at the heart of abnormal blood pressure regulation. The papers taken together would indicate that the hypothesis of alterations in the rostral medullary complex in the brainstem as the primary driving event, which could be in response to an external stimulus (compression). It also suggests this alteration is at the heart of many of the changes seen systemically, both centrally and peripherally, in hypertension.

Patients who form the roughly the one-third of individuals who have refractory hypertension may be screened for the sympathetic hyperactivity early in their course by obtaining measures of the plasma catecholamines, which, while non-specific for location, certainly suggest an overall elevation in the sympathetic tone. Although some observers have called in to question the usefulness of the spectral ratio of the heart, this also could be used as a preliminary screening test, thereby identifying a group of patients who would benefit from microneurography at two or three sites to look at sympathetic nerve traffic. An additional appropriate screening measure would then be to use a clonidine test administered orally or transdermally to identify the drop in central sympathetic traffic to suggest this subgroup of patients. Ultimately, if the patient has been on a long-term diuretic or dihydropyridine calcium channel blocker, there may be an increase in sympathetic outflow, which would be more resistant to the clonidine and looking at the asymmetric dimethylarginine levels, which is an indigenous nitric oxide sympathetic inhibitor could be determined as a plasma marker as well.

These markers could identify a subgroup of patients where no additional chemical therapies are likely to be appropriate, as well as providing a means of following the effects of an intervention. In patients in the original and subsequent surgical series, control of blood pressure is sometimes slow to occur. This would be expected with the multifocal nature of blood pressure alterations. In some cases blood pressure reductions did not occur, which would be consistent with the underlying theory in vascular cross-compression, namely, that ongoing cross-compression can and does cause alterations in facilitatory pathways, that may be difficult to reverse after long standing activation of the aberrant pathways.

Conclusions

The range of medical literature over the last 20 years clearly supports the neuroadrenergic hypothesis of hypertension. These various animal and human studies document both the nature of the central events, as well as the consequences in peripheral events, as to their contribution towards hypertension-related diseases. At the current time, it would appear that there is no specific genotype that links itself either in individual patient or patient subgroups to identify patients who might develop hypertension. The current therapeutic target then is the elevated sympathetic activity. Different therapeutic interventions may be aimed at reducing, while not eliminating, central sympathetic excitation either with chemicals or other means. The work done by subsequent groups raises the question of not IF the adrenergic theory of neurogenic hypertension is correct, but rather whether the peripheral effects are more dominant than the central effects. This may be an important question to answer in the future to effectively counter hypertension with appropriate therapy. As mentioned in the Introduction, some 30% of patients with hypertension are refractory and most estimates indicate that between 1 and 1.5 billion people in the world will be affected by hypertension, suggesting that there is a high degree of urgency to this quest. If the peripheral treatments currently in use are effective for two-thirds, one question that of course begs an answer is, why are the refractory patients refractory? The compression theory suggests that, much the same as in other vascular cross-compression states, the presence of cross-compression is not the only driving factor for an event. As seen in facial pain from cross compression, face pain can be caused by intrinsic damage to the nerves, such as in the case of multiple sclerosis, or extrinsic compression, such as from a tumour in addition or in place of vascular cross-compression. Thus, in the case of hypertension, central effects seen in the complex of the nucleus tractus solitarius, the area of postrema, and the rostral ventrolateral medulla at an earlier stage may explain those patients who respond to oral medications. However, even in the group of patients with oral medications, the peripheral effects of the disease, such as seen in the heart and kidneys, progress. The concept that alteration of this central sympathetic excitation could be halted through a more direct means raises the potential that the secondary scourges of hypertension could be reduced, or even eliminated, with appropriate surgical therapies.

References

1. Autonomic nervous system anatomy [home page Medscape reference] available at http://emedicine.medscape.com/article/ 1922943/overview. accessed October 2014
2. **Ogata T, Ida Y, Nonoyama A, Takida J, Sasaki H, cited by Close GH**. Extracorporal maintenance of circulation and respiration. Physiol Rev 1960;**40**:826–919.
3. **Close GH Jr**. Extracorporal maintenance of circulation and respiration. Physiol Rev 1960;**40**:826–919.
4. **Hooker DR**. Study of isolated kidney: the influence of pulse pressure on renal function. Am J Physiol 1910;**27**:24–44.
5. **Goto N, Van Bavel E, Giezeman MJM, Spaan JA**. Vasodilatory effect of pulsatile pressure on coronary resistance vessels. Circ Res 1996;**79**:1039–45.
6. **Taylor KM, Bain WH, Russell M, Brannan JJ, Morton IJ**. Peripheral vascular resistance in angiotensin-II levels during pulsatile and non-pulsatile cardiopulmonary bypass. Thorax 1979;**34**:594–98.
7. **Judson WE, Rausch NH**. Effects of acute reduction of renal artery blood pressure on renal hemodynamics and excretion of electrolytes in water. J Lab Clin Med 1957;**50**:923.
8. **Senning A, Andres J, Bornstein P, Norberg B, Andersen MN**. Renal function during extracorporal circulation at high and low flow rates: experimental studies in dogs. Ann Surg1960;**151**:63–70.
9. **Kohlstaedt KG, Page IH**. Liberation of renin by perfusion of kidneys following reduction of pulse pressure. J Exper Med 1940;**73**:201–16.

10. **Hamans C**. Reflexogenic areas of cardiovascular system. Perspect Biol Med 1960;**3**:409–17.
11. **Neil E**, Afferent impulse activity in cardiovascular receptor fibers. Physiol Rev 1960;**40**(suppl. 4):201–208.
12. **Wilkens H, Regelson W, Hoffmeister FS**. The physiologic importance of pulsatile bloodflow. NEJM 1962;**267**(9):443–46.
13. **McMaster PD, Parsons R**. Physiologic conditions existing in connective tissue: interstitial spread of viral dyes. J Exper Med. 1949;**69**:247–64.
14. **McDonald BA**. Lateral pulsatile expansion of arteries. J Physiol 1953;**119**:280.
15. **Halley MM, Reentsma K, Creech O**. Cerebral blood flow, metabolism and brain volume in extracorporal circulation. J Thoracic Surg 1958;**36**:506–18.
16. **Kearney PM, Whelton M, Reynolds K, Whelton TK, Jiang H**. World wide prevalence of hypertension: a systematic review. J Hypertension 2004;**22**(1):11–19.
17. **Bartosh SM, Aronson AJ**. Childhood hypertension: an update on etiology, diagnosis and treatment. Ped Klin NA. 1999;**46**(2):235–52.
18. **Wolf-Maier K, Cooper RS, Kramer H et**.al. Hypertension: a systemic review. J Hypertension. 2004;**43**:10–17.
19. **Kearney PM, Whelton M, Reynolds K, Whelton TK, Jiang H**. World wide prevalence of hypertension: a systemic review. J Hypertension 2004;**22**(1):11–19.
20. **Henry AP, Cassel JC**. Psychosocial factors in essential hypertension: recent epidemiologic and animal experimental evidence. Am J Epid 1969;**90**:191–200.
21. **Opario S, Zaman MA, Calhoun DA**. Pathogenesis of hypertension 2003. Ann Intern Med. **139**(9):761–76.
22. **Grassi G, Seraballe G, Fosca Quarti-Trevano**. The neurogenic hypothesis in hypertension: current evidence. Exp Physiol 2009;**95**:581–86.
23. **Frerrario CM, Averill DD**. Do primary dysfunctions in the neural control of arterial pressure contribute to hypertension? Major pathogenic factors in hypertension. Supplement 1 Hypertension 1991;**18**(3):i38–51.
24. **Swanson LW, Sawchenko PE**. Paraventricular Nucleus: The Site for the Integration of Neuroendocrine and Autonomic Mechanisms. Neuroendocrinology 1980;**31**(6):410–17.
25. **Zoccal DB, Paton JF, Machado BH**. Do Changes in the Coupling Between Respiratory and Sympathetic Activities Contribute to Neurogenic Hypertension? Clin Exp Pharmacol Physiol 2009; 36:1188–96.
26. **Sawchenko PE, Brown ER, Chan RKW**. The Paraventricular Nucleus of the Hypothalamus in the Functional Neural Anatomy of Visceromotor Responses to Stress, Progress in Brain 1966; **107**:201–22.
27. **Osborn JW, Fink GD, Sved AF, Toney GM, Raizada MK**. Circulating Angiotensin-II and Dietary Salt: Converging Signals from Neurogenic Hypertension, Current Hypertension Reports 2007; **9**(3):228–35.
28. **Johnson AK**. Circumventricular Organs and Their Role in Visceral Functions, www.acucentre.com.au/neuro01/centreg/creg14.pdf
29. **Fagius J, Wallin BG, Sundlof G, Nerhed C, Englesson S**. Sympathetic Outflow in Man after Anesthesia of Glossopharyngeal and Vagus Nerves. Brain 1985;**108**:423–38.
30. **Valbo AB, Hagbarth KE, Wallin BG**. Microneurography: How the Technique Developed and Its Role in the Investigation of the Sympathetic Nervous System J Appl Physiol 2004;**96**:1262–69.
31. **Macefield VG, Elam M, Wallin BG**. Filing Properties of Single Post Ganglionic Sympathetic Neurons. Autonon Neurosci 2002;**95**:146–59.

32. **Mancia G, Mark AL**. Arterial Baroreflexes in Humans. Dean: Shepherd JT, Abboud FM, eds. Handbook of Physiologic, section 2: The Cardiovascular System. Bethesda, Maryland. Am Physiol Soc 1983; 755–93.
33. **Floras JS, Harah K**. Symphatoneuro and Hemodynamic Characteristics of Young Subjects with Mild Essential Hypertension. J Hypertens 1993 June;**11**(6):647–55.
34. **Mancia G, Ferrari A, Gregorini L, Parati G, Promodosi G**. Blood Pressure and Heart Rate Variabilities in Normotensive and Hypertensive Human Beings. Circ Res 1983;**53**:96–104.
35. **Eibe I, Kolloch R, DeQuattro V, Miano L, Dugger R, VanderMeulen J**. Raised Cerebrospinal Fluid Norepinephrine in Some Patients with Primary Hypertension. Hypertension. 1979, May–June;**1** (3):255–60.
36. **Cubeddu LX**. Clonidine Reduces Elevated Cerebrospinal Fluid Catecholamine Levels in Patients with Essential Hypertension. Lif Sci 1984;**35**:1365.
37. **Defronzo RA, Ferrannini B**. Insulin Resistance: A Multifaceted Syndrome Responsible for NIDDM, Obesity, Hypertension, Dyslipidemia and Atherosclerotic Cardiovascular Disease in Diabetes Care, care.diabetesjournals.org/content/14/3/173.abstract.
38. **Ferrannini B, Buzzigoli G, Bonadonna R, Giorico MA, Oleggini M, Graziadei L**. Insulin Resistance in Essential Hypertension. NEJM 1987;**317**:350–57.
39. **Swif PA, Meaney JF, Graham LN, Stoker JB, Mackintosh AF, Mary David A**. Relationship of Neurovascular Compression to Central Sympathetic Discharge in Essential Hypertension. J. Am Coll Cardiol. 2004;**43**(8):1453–58.
40. **Lombardi F, Sandrone G, Pruner S**. Heart Rate Variability as an Index of Sympathovagal Action after Acute Myocardial Infarction. Am J Cardiol 1987;**60**:1239–45.
41. **Ori Z, Monir G, Weiss J, Sayhouni X, Singer DH**. Heart Rate Variability. Frequency Domain Analysis. Cardiol Clin 1992;**10**(3):499–537.
42. **Eckberg DL**. Symphathovagal Balance, A Critical Appraisal. Circulation. 1997;**96**:3224–32.
43. **Notarius CF, Floras JS**. Limitations of the use of Spectral Analysis of Heart Rate Variability for the Estimation of Cardiac Sympathetic Activity in Heart Failure. Europace 2001;**3**(1):29–38.
44. **Youn JC, Yu HT, Lim BJ, Koh MJ, Lee J, Chang DY, Choi YS, Lee SH, Kang SM, Jang Y, Yoo OJ, Shin EC, Park S**. Immunosenescent CD8+ T cells and C-X-C chemokine receptor type 3 chemokines are increased in human hypertension. Hypertension 2013 Jul; **62**(1):126–33. doi: 10.1161/HYPERTENSIONAHA.113.00689. Epub 2013 May 28.
45. **Waki H, Gouraud SS, Maeda M, Paton JF**. Evidence of specific inflammatory condition in nucleus tractus solitarii of spontaneously hypertensive rats.Exp Physiol. 2010 May; **95**(5):595–600. doi: 10.1113/expphysiol.2009.047324. Epub 2009 Nov 18.
46. **Paton JF, Waki H**. Is Neurogenic Hypertension Related to Vascular Information in the Brainstem? Neurosci Behav Rev 2009; **33**(2):89–94.
47. **Fang Y, Xia H, Cai Y, Halabi CM, Becker LK, Santos RA, et al**. Brain Selective Overexpression of Human Angiotensin-Converting Enzyme Type II Attenuates Neurogenic Hypertension. Circ Res 2010;**106**(2):373–82.
48. **Amendt K, Czachurski J, Dembowski K, Seller H**. Neurones Within the Chemo Sensitive Area on the Ventral Surface of the Brainstem Which Project to the Anteromediolateral Column. Pfluqers Arch 1978;**375**(3):289–92.
49. **Dampney RA, Goodchild AK, Robertson LG, Montgomery W**. Role of Ventrolateral Medulla in Vasomotor Regulation: A Correlative Anatomical and Physiologic Study. Brain Res 1982;**249**:223–35.
50. **Dampney RA**. Brainstem Mechanisms in the Control of Blood Pressure. Clin Exp Hypertension 1981;**3**:379–91.
51. **Ross CA, Ruggiero DA, Park VH, Joh TH, Sved AF, Fernandez-Pardal AF, et al**. Tonic Vasomotor Control by the Rostral Ventrolateral Medulla: Affect of Electrical or Chemical Stimulation on

the Area Containing C1 Adrenalin Neurons on Arterial and Pressure Heart Rate in Plasma Catecholamine in Vasopresin, J Neurosci 1984;**4**:474–94.

52. **Sun MK, Young BS, Hackett JT, Guyenet PG**. Reticulospinal Pacemaker Neurons of the Rat Rostral Ventrolateral Medulla, Repetitive Symphatoexcitatory Function: An Intracellular Study In Vitro. Brain Res 1988;**442**:229–39.
53. **Sun MK, Guyenet PG**. Arterial Baroreceptor in Vagal Inputs to the Symphatoexcitatory Neurons in the Rat Medulla. Am J Physiol 1987;**252**:R699–09.
54. **Janetta PJ, Segal R, Wolfson SK, Dujovny M, Semba A, Cook ED**. Neurogenic Hypertension: Etiology and Surgical Treatment. Observations in Experimental Non-Human Primate Model. Ann Surg 1985;**202**(2):253–61.
55. **Janetta PJ, Segal R, Wolfson SK**. Neurogenic Hypertension: Etiology and Surgical Treatment. 1. Observations in 53 patients. Ann Surg 1985;**201**(3):291–98.
56. **Brown DO, Guyent PG**. Electrophysiologic Study of Cardiovascular Neurons in the Rostral Ventrolateral Medulla. Circ Res 1985;**56**:359–69.
57. **Geiger H, Naraghi R, Schobel HP, Frank H, Stervel RB, Fahlbush R**. Decrease of Blood Pressure by Ventrolateral Medullary Decompression in Essential Hypertension. Lancet 1998;**352**(9126):446–48.
58. **Naraghi R, Daab MR, Walter GF, Kleinberg B**. Arterial Hypertension and Neurovascular Compression at the Ventrolateral Medulla, A Comparative Microanatomical and Pathological Study. J Neurosurg 1992;**77**:103–12.
59. **Morimoto S**. Decrease in Blood Pressure and Sympathetic Nerve Activity by Microvascular Decompression of the Rostral Ventral Medulla in Essential Hypertension. Stroke 1999;**30**:17-7–17-10.
60. **Sindou M**. Is there a place for microsurgical vascular decompression of the brainstem for apparent essential blood hypertension? a review. http://www.ncbi.nlm.nih.gov/pubmed/25411145 Adv Tech Stand Neurosurg. 2015;**42**:69–76. doi: 10.1007/978-3-319-09066-5_4.

Chapter 5

Device-based approaches to target renal sympathetic nerves for hypertension

Markus Schlaich and Murray Esler

Key points

1. Over-active sympathetic nerves contribute to the development of hypertension.
2. Sodium retention, release of renin, and vasoconstriction are the main mediators of the rise in BP caused by stimulation of renal sympathetic nerves.
3. Therapeutic targeting of the sympathetic nervous system at various levels has been tested using direct surgical approaches, deep-brain stimulation, device-aided regulation of breathing, baroreflex stimulation, and, most recently, catheter-based renal denervation.
4. While several clinical studies have demonstrated that catheter-based renal denervation is generally safe and commonly associated with a significant and sustained reduction in blood pressure, the latest most rigorous trial failed to demonstrate an effect beyond that of a sham control, although it is questionable whether renal denervation has actually been achieved in this trial.
5. Further prospective and properly designed trials are warranted to ultimately delineate the future role of renal denervation for treatment of hypertension and other conditions characterized by sympathetic overactivity.

Introduction

Sympathetic nervous system (SNS) activation is a common feature of arterial hypertension and has been demonstrated to contribute to the development and progression of the hypertensive state. The use of surgical procedures and, to a lesser extent, devices, has a long history in the management of hypertension. Indeed, surgery has been the preferred treatment modality in some forms of secondary hypertension for decades. Furthermore, surgical section of the sympathetic chain and splanchnic nerves was commonly used before effective pharmacologic treatment of hypertension was available. Faced with the failure of conventional pharmacological treatment of hypertension, devices and surgical procedures are being increasingly evaluated. The wider 'device revolution' in cardiovascular medicine has now come to hypertension with the testing of a device to lower blood pressure by guiding respiration, direct electrical stimulation of brain regions influencing blood pressure, the re-evaluation of a device to stimulate the arterial baroreceptors, surgical neurovascular depression of the brainstem to overcome presumed vascular compression of bulbar regions controlling sympathetic outflow and blood pressure, and development and testing of catheter-based approaches using radiofrequency energy for ablation of renal nerves.

Here we briefly review the anatomy and physiology of the renal nerves and their involvement in hypertension and other relevant disease states, the available clinical data on safety and efficacy of renal nerve ablation, discuss other potential implications, and introduce some of the new devices currently under investigation for renal denervation (RDN).

Therapeutic targeting of sympathetic nerves: a brief historical overview

While the first identifiable description of the anatomy of the sympathetic nervous system by Thomas Willis dates back to 1664, it was not until 1727 that the neural control of blood vessel calibre became apparent as a physiological concept through the work of du Petit, who demonstrated conjunctival vessel dilatation after section of cervical sympathetic nerves (1). More than a century later, Stelling in 1840 suggested that the vasomotor fibres were sympathetic nerves originating in the central nervous system and supplying the peripheral blood vessels. In 1852, Claude Bernard and others observed dilatation of blood vessels by sectioning sympathetic nerves and a rise in blood pressure upon electrical stimulation of the cut nerves, thereby identifying these as 'pressor nerves' (2). However, it was not until 1932 that Adrian described actual sympathetic discharges from direct recordings of electrical impulses in both pre- and post-ganglionic sympathetic fibres of cats and rabbits (3). Von Euler in 1946 then identified noradrenaline as the major neurotransmitter of sympathetic nerves (4). In the early decades of the twentieth century, Cannon (5) popularized the concept of the 'fight and flight' response to stress through his research on sympathetic nerves.

Accordingly, prior to the availability of effective pharmacologic drug therapy, surgical RDN was applied since the early 1920s and 1930s with thoraco-lumbar splanchnicectomy being the most commonly used form of surgical sympathectomy. It has been reported that the average survival time of patients in the malignant phase of hypertension at the time was only 8 months. Although the results of sympathectomy in hypertension were not subjected to rigorous scientific analysis, a relatively high rate of long-term improvement of hypertension was reported. Sympathectomy at the time was performed in either one or two stages and required a prolonged hospital stay (2 to 4 weeks) with a long recovery period (1 to 2 months). In a large population study, including 1266 hypertensive patients who underwent splanchnicectomy and 467 hypertensive control subjects treated by low-salt diet only, the 5-year mortality rates were 19% and 54%, respectively. Forty-five per cent of those who survived the surgery had significantly lower blood pressure afterwards, and the anti-hypertensive effect lasted 10 years or more (6). Another large observational study of more than 2000 patients, 1506 of whom underwent splanchnicectomy, demonstrated a satisfactory blood pressure response in about half of the patients who underwent splanchnicectomy (6). Interestingly, sympathectomy rendered blood pressure more sensitive to anti-hypertensive drugs, allowing a reduction in the number and doses of administered drugs. While surgical sympathectomy was effective in lowering blood pressure and improve outcomes in many cases it carried severe post-operative complications: prolonged hospitalization, orthostatic hypotension, syncope, incontinence (both urinary and faecal), and difficulties in walking. As a consequence, and due to the advent of effective pharmacological anti-hypertensive therapies, surgical sympathectomy for the treatment of hypertension was soon abandoned.

Role of the sympathetic nervous system in cardiovascular and metabolic control

Experimental and humans studies from the past three decades not only confirmed the critical role of the SNS in hypertension (7–10), but also provided conclusive evidence for a role of an over-active SNS in the pathophysiology of a variety of other clinically relevant conditions, such as insulin resistance (11), congestive heart failure, renal disease (12), and others.

Renal efferent and afferent nerves lie within the adventitia of the renal arteries and form a network that constitutes a significant control system for the physiological regulation of blood pressure and renal function, as summarized by Bertog et al. (13) (Fig. 5.1).

The efferent renal sympathetic nerves originate from the intermediolateral column of the spinal cord from T8 to L1. Nerves carrying fibres that project to the kidney are derived from the celiac plexus and its subdivisions (7). The kidney, including the renal vasculature, the tubules, the juxtaglomerular cells (14), and the renal pelvic wall (15), all have a rich supply of efferent sympathetic nerves. The release of noradrenaline from renal sympathetic nerve terminals has three major consequences: (i) it stimulates β_1-adrenoceptors on juxtaglomerular granular cells to release renin, thereby increasing activity of the renin–angiotensin–aldosterone system; (ii) it decreases urinary sodium and water excretion via enhanced tubular reabsorption (16); and (iii) it reduces renal blood flow and glomerular filtration rate via constriction of the renal vasculature (17).

The kidneys also have abundant afferent sensory innervation, with sensory nerve fibres projecting from the kidney to the central nervous system via the dorsal root ganglia. The cell bodies of the afferent renal nerves are located in ipsilateral dorsal root ganglia predominantly from T12 to L3. In contrast to the widespread distribution of the efferent

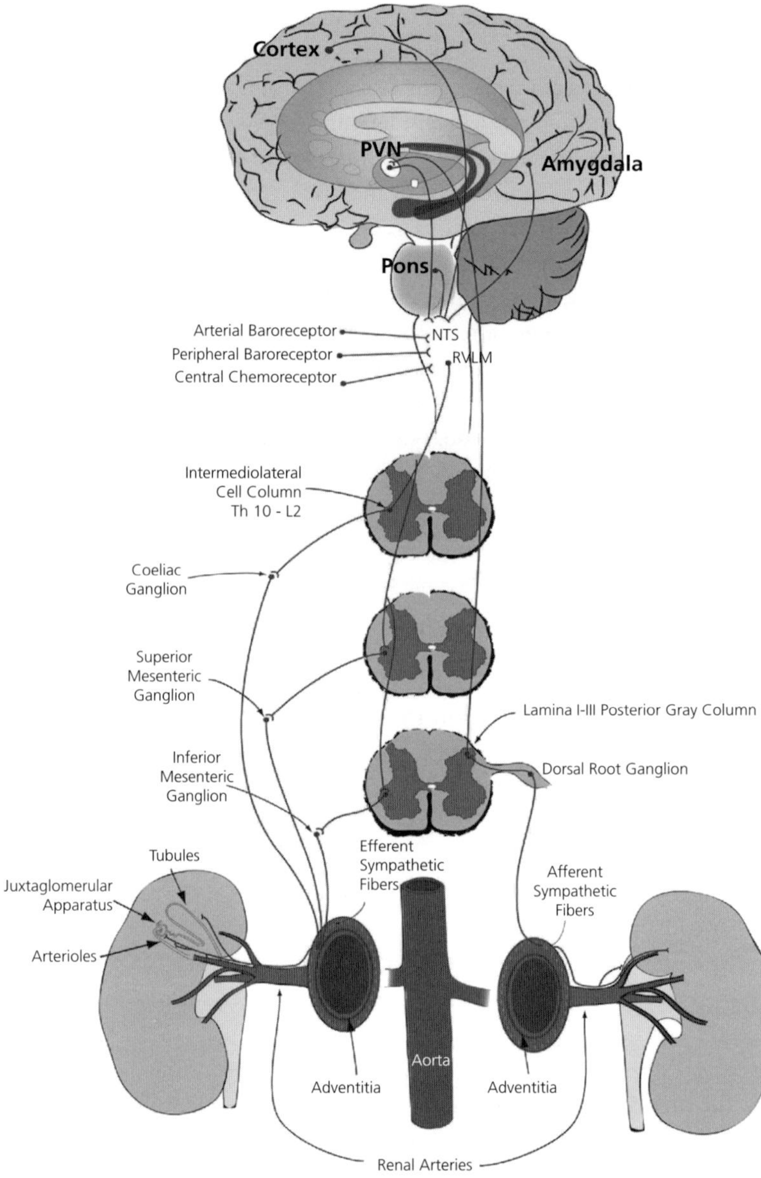

Fig. 5.1 Schematic of the anatomy of the sympathetic nervous system (for details see text). NTS = solitary tract nucleus; PVN = paraventricular nucleus; RVLM = rostral ventrolateral medulla.

Reproduced from JACC Cardiovasc Interv., **5** (3), Bertog SC, Sobotka PA, Sievert H., Renal denervation for hypertension., p. 249–58, Copyright (2012), with permission from Elsevier.

sympathetic nerve fibres in the kidney, the major locations of the afferent renal sensory nerves are in the renal pelvic area. The pelvic pressure is a major determinant of afferent renal nerve activity and increments in urine flow rate increase the firing rate of renal afferent fibres. This in turn results in a decrease in efferent renal sympathetic nerve activity and an increase in urinary sodium excretion, a renorenal reflex response. An increase in efferent renal nerve activity modulates afferent renal activity by the release of norepinephrine, which activates α_1-adrenoceptors (ARs) and α_2-ARs on renal sensory nerves (15).

The specific role of renal sympathetic nerve activity in hypertension

While the pathogenesis of essential hypertension is multi-factorial, sympathetic nervous system activation has been established as a major contributor to the development of hypertension. Based on direct recordings of muscle sympathetic nerve activity and measurement of the release of noradrenaline from organs critically involved in circulatory control, such as the kidney and the heart, it is now well established that arterial hypertension is commonly neurogenic, the blood pressure rise being initiated and sustained by increased sympathetic activity (9, 18). The increase in the number of sympathetic bursts to the skeletal muscle circulation has been related directly to the degree of blood pressure elevation (19).

Studies employing radiotracer dilution methodology to measure overflow of norepinephrine (NE) from the kidneys to plasma have provided unequivocal evidence for increased renal norepinephrine spillover rates in patients with essential hypertension (9, 20). Furthermore, elevated NE spillover from the heart is also often present and is commensurate with the typical haemodynamic profile seen in hypertensive patients (21, 22). Importantly, sympathetic activation is commonly present in subjects with borderline hypertension and even in normotensive individuals with a strong genetic predisposition to develop hypertension, indicative of a causal role of sympathetic activation in blood pressure elevation (23).

The consequences of increased sympathetic outflow to the kidneys, perhaps most important in this context, include volume retention via tubular sodium reabsorption (16), reduced renal blood flow through neurally mediated vasoconstriction (17, 24), and release of renin from the juxtaglomerular apparatus (25), all of which can contribute to blood pressure elevation, both acutely and in the long term. Accordingly, targeting the sympathetic nervous system appears to be a logical therapeutic approach for the treatment of hypertension.

Recent surgical and device-based approaches to target SNS overactivity

Surgical intracranial neurovascular depression

Studies in experimental animals have identified regions in the medulla oblongata, which, when stimulated, increase sympathetic nervous outflow and blood pressure. The clinical counterpart of this is the suggestion that human hypertension commonly is due to compression of the medulla by tortuous arteries, principally the posterior inferior cerebellar artery (26). Surgery has been devised to eliminate this vascular compression of the brainstem, and claims have been made for substantial consequential blood pressure lowering (26, 27), but this is problematic in that adequately controlled clinical trials have not yet been performed (see Chapter 4).

Devices for regulating breathing

There is now considerable data to support the hypothesis that chronic reduction of respiratory rate lowers blood pressure. This blood pressure lowering appears to be via stimulation of a number of cardiovascular reflexes, including slowly adapting pulmonary stretch receptors. In doing so, a slower breathing rate increases baroreceptor sensitivity. Reductions in nocturnal respiratory rate may also attenuate, or even prevent, apnoeic episodes associated with central sleep apnoea or Cheyne–Stokes breathing. Reduction in respiratory rate and increase in baroreceptor sensitivity leads to vasodilatation in a number of relevant vascular beds, including skeletal muscle, splanchnic and renal beds. There is clearly overlap between reduced breathing frequency and relaxation exercises to aid stress minimization. Mental relaxation has been associated with inhibition of stress-induced arteriolar vasoconstriction, which in turn leads to hypertrophy and increased stiffness within the arteriolar wall of resistance vessels.

A number of commercial entities have developed home breathing programmes to reduce respiratory rate to <10 breaths/min. The RESPeRATE device (InterCure, Lod, Israel) utilizes a musical pattern through earphones to slow breathing via a relatively prolonged expiration. This device also records the patient's actual achieved inspiratory and expiratory rates for later analysis. A number of randomized controlled trials (using Walkman-type devices without controlled breathing musical patterns as control) have shown that these programmes can result in both short-term and sustained reductions in systemic blood pressure values.

What is unclear is the degree of continued use of the device needed to maintain sustained blood pressure reductions. Furthermore, studies of the impact of withdrawal of this approach on blood pressure levels have not yet been performed. Nevertheless, controlled breathing appears to be a safe, non-invasive approach to influence blood pressure regulation, although the strong claims made for blood pressure lowering with such device-guided respiration (44) has been disputed (57), and to this point have not been substantiated in studies of rigorous design.

Deep-brain stimulation

Stimulating electrodes permanently placed in the brain are increasingly used in neurological disorders, such as Parkinsonism and chronic pain syndromes. Opportunistic advantage has been taken of this electrode placement in patients with comorbid hypertension, to stimulate also brain regions capable of lowering blood pressure (46, 54, 55). This can occur with the stimulation of CNS depressor regions, or electrical inhibition of pressor regions (see Chapter 3).

Stimulation of the arterial baroreceptor with an implantable device

In the presence of sustained elevation of blood pressure, the arterial baroreflex quickly resets. The set point for the reflex becomes the higher, prevailing blood pressure, so that there is no baroreflex drive operating to restore the pressure to normal levels. In experimental models of hypertension, however, activation of central baroreflex pathways by ongoing electrical stimulation of carotid sinus baroreceptor nerves reduces sympathetic outflow from the central nervous system and lowers blood pressure, an effect that persists for weeks without adaptation.

Accordingly, baroreflex stimulation devices have been developed for the treatment of patients with hypertension, and are currently undergoing clinical testing. The Rheos^{R} implantable carotid sinus stimulator (CVRx, Minneapolis, MN, USA) has been studied in patients with severe hypertension refractory to drug therapy (see Chapter 2).

Transcatheter renal nerve ablation

With the advances in technology and the availability of minimally invasive procedures, the concept of selective sympathectomy or, more specifically, renal denervation, was recently revisited and culminated in the development of catheter-based devices for renal denervation. The Symplicity Catheter System (Medtronic Ardian, Mountain View, CA, USA) was the first of its kind and specifically designed for endovascular radiofrequency ablation in the renal artery. With a guide catheter positioned in the renal artery via femoral artery access, the RF ablation catheter is advanced into the renal artery and connected to a radiofrequency generator. A series of 2-minute ablations are then delivered along each renal artery, distally to proximally, with longitudinal and rotational separation to achieve circumferential coverage of the renal artery, thereby targeting the renal nerves located in the adventitia of the vessel wall. Typically, 4–8 ablations are performed in each renal artery (28) (Fig. 5.2). The outcomes of Symplicity HTN-1 and HTN-2 studies in patients with resistant hypertension demonstrated the safety and efficacy of such an approach.

While histological data are unavailable from humans, a recent study performed in swine (29) investigating vascular histopathology at 6-months, demonstrated nerve fibrosis, replacement of nerve fascicles with fibrous connective tissue, and thickening of the epineurium and perineurium. In all treated vessels, fibrosis was found in 10 to 25% of the total media and underlying adventitia, whereas no significant smooth muscle hyperplasia or inflammatory components were evident. The results suggested that the healing process was complete. There was no renal arterial stenosis or thrombosis observed by angiography. No gross or microscopic abnormalities were observed.

Renal nerve ablation as treatment for drug-resistant hypertension

While over-activity of renal nerves is a feature of several clinically relevant conditions rendering renal denervation a potentially helpful therapeutic approach, at present, data from proper clinical trials is only available from patient cohorts with treatment resistant hypertension.

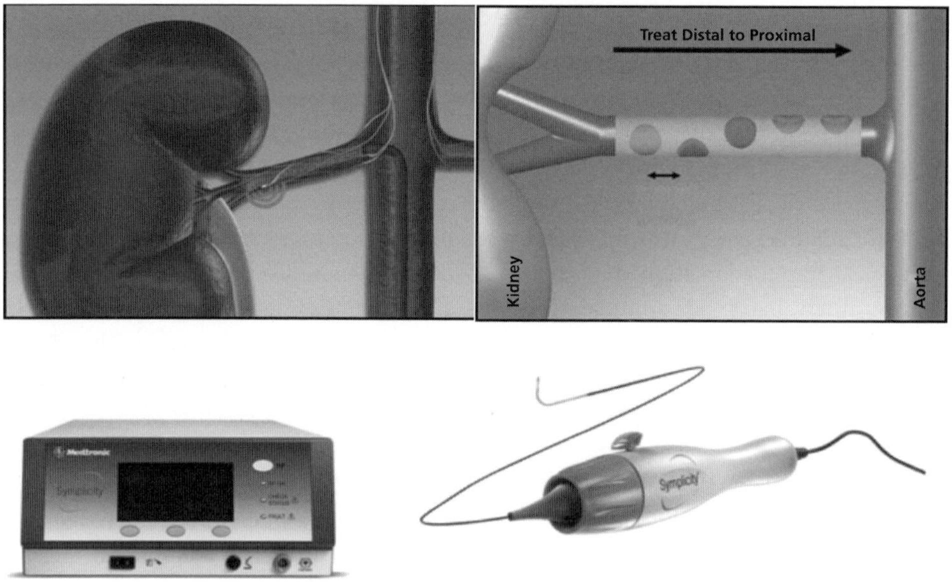

Fig. 5.2 Catheter-based renal denervation technology and treatment algorithm (for details see text).

Symplicity HTN-1 Symplicity HTN-1, an initial first-in-human experience, was a non-randomized study to evaluate the efficacy and safety of this approach in patients with treatment-resistant hypertension, defined as the failure of at least three anti-hypertensive drugs in adequate doses, typically including a diuretic, to reach target blood pressure levels. Altogether, 45 drug-resistant hypertensive patients with average baseline office blood pressure of 177/101 mmHg (SD 20/15 mmHg) and on 4.7 anti-hypertensive medications were recruited. Office blood pressure after RDN was reduced by −14/−10, −21/−10, −22/−11, −24/−11, and −27/−17 mmHg at 1, 3, 6, 9, and 12 months, respectively. The concurrent reduction in renal noradrenaline spillover by 47% assessed in a subgroup of 10 patients indicated that this procedure indeed targets the renal sympathetic nerves. Importantly, this BP decrease was recently reported to be maintained over 2 years (30) (Fig. 5.3). In this longer term follow-up study of 153 patients, baseline mean office BP was 176/98 ± 17/15 mmHg on an average of five anti-hypertensive drugs. Complication-free peri- and post-procedural follow-up was reported in 97% of patients (149 of 153), with one renal artery dissection and three femoral artery pseudo-aneurysms reported as minor adverse events. Post-procedure office BPs were reduced by 20/10, 24/11, 25/11, 23/11, 26/14, and 32/14 mmHg at 1, 3, 6, 12, 18, and 24 months, respectively. These data indicate that renal sympathetic denervation results in a substantial reduction in BP that is sustained out to ≥2 years of follow-up.

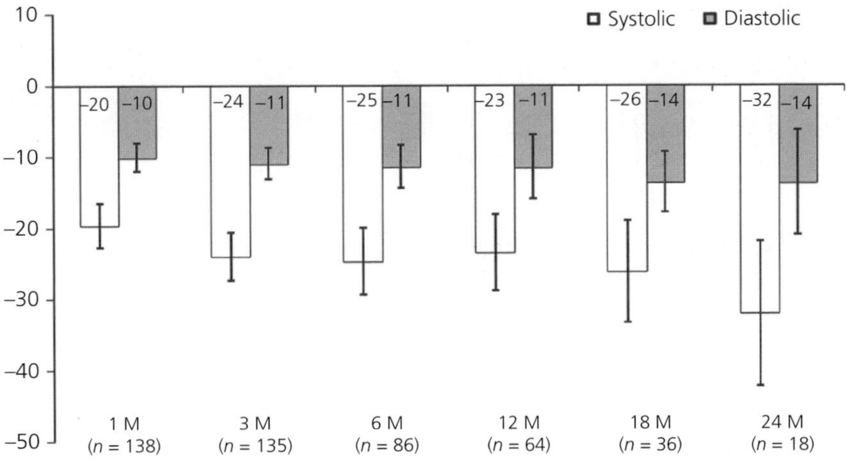

Fig. 5.3 Effects of RDN on blood pressure reduction in Symplicity HTN-1 with follow-up to 2 years.
Reproduced from Hypertension, 57 (5), Symplicity HTN1 Investigators, Catheter-based renal sympathetic denervation for resistant hypertension: durability of blood pressure reduction out to 24 months, p. 911–7, Copyright (2011), with permission from Wolters Kluwer Health.

Symplicity HTN-2 Following this first-in-human proof-of-concept and safety study, a randomized controlled clinical trial was initiated, which included a total of 106 patients from 24 centres in Australia and Europe. Inclusion criteria were similar to those of the initial safety and proof-of-concept trial with patients required to have a baseline systolic office BP ≥160 mmHg (≥150 mmHg for patients with type 2 diabetes) despite compliance with ≥3 anti-hypertensive medications. Patients were then randomized to either undergo renal nerve ablation treatment ($n = 52$) or to continue with conventional drug treatment as part of the control group ($n = 54$).

Both groups had similar baseline characteristics and anti-hypertensive regimen with the exception of estimated glomerular filtration rate (eGFR), which was lower in the active treatment group (77 ml/min vs. 86 ml/min; $p = 0.013$). Renal safety could be confirmed as demonstrated by unchanged mean eGFR both in the control and the treatment group at 6 months follow-up (31). Follow-up imaging of renal arteries 6 months after renal denervation did not reveal vascular damage. Of 49 patients who underwent renal denervation and were assessed at 6 months, 43 had renal imaging at 6 months (37 renal duplex imaging, 5 MRI, and 5 CT angiography). One patient had a possible progression of an underlying atherosclerotic lesion, without the need for intervention (65). In this context a case report indicates a possible association between RF ablation treatment and the occurrence of a renal artery stenosis (32).

In keeping with the results from Symplicity HTN-1, a significant difference in the primary endpoint of office blood pressure of 33/11 mmHg ($p < 0.001$ for both systolic and diastolic BP) was noted between the renal denervation group and the control group in the Symplicity HTN-2 trial (Fig. 5.4) (31). Home BP recordings confirmed the observed office

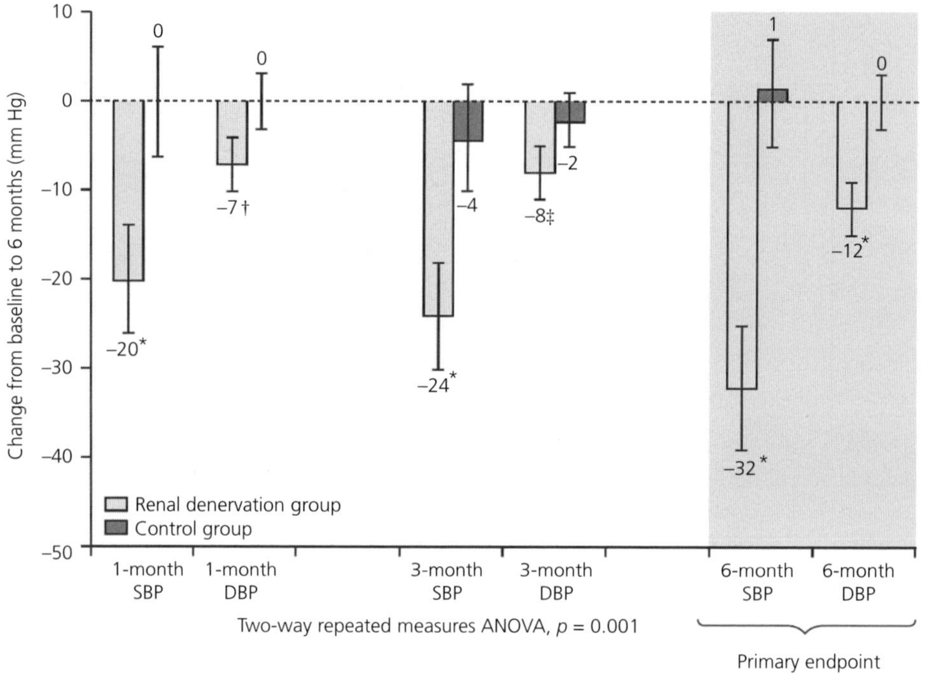

Fig. 5.4 Blood pressure reduction in Symplicity HTN-2 the treatment and control group up at 3- and 6-month follow-up.

Reproduced from The Lancet., 376 (9756), Esler MD, Krum H, Sobotka PA, Schlaich MP, Schmieder RE, Bohm M., Renal sympathetic denervation in patients with treatment-resistant hypertension (The Symplicity HTN-2 Trial): a randomised controlled trial, p. 1903–9, Copyright (2010), with permission from Elsevier.

BP changes with a reduction in home BP by 20/12 ± 17/11 mmHg in the renal denervation group and a rise of 2/0 ± 13/7 mmHg in the control group ($p < 0.001$). Blood pressure control defined as systolic BP <140 mmHg was achieved in 39% of patients in the denervation group and in 3% of patients in the control group. It is important to note that there is substantial variability with regards to the blood pressure effects and that the procedure failed to reduce blood pressure in ~16% of treated patients. Whether this may be related to the age of patients, duration of hypertension, established target organ damage, the number of ablation treatments, or other factors is currently unclear.

24-hour ambulatory blood pressure recordings were only available from 20 patients in the renal denervation group. While the average 24-hour ambulatory blood pressure at 6 months changed in parallel with office-based and home-based (20/12 mmHg; SD 17/11) blood pressure measurements, the magnitude of the blood pressure fall was less pronounced with a mean decrease of 11/7 mmHg (SD 15/11; $p = 0.006$ for systolic blood pressure change, $p = 0.014$ for diastolic blood pressure change) from baseline to 6 months. Averages did not change for 25 patients in the control group.

Data on the 1-year results of Symplicity HTN-2 have confirmed the safety of the approach and demonstrated sustained blood pressure effects (33). After the 6-month primary endpoint was met, renal denervation in control patients was permitted. One-year results on patients randomized to immediate renal denervation ($n = 47$) demonstrated a mean fall in office systolic blood pressure of −28.1 mmHg (95% confidence interval, −35.4 to −20.7; $p < 0.001$), which was similar to the 6-month fall of −31.7 mmHg (95% confidence interval, −38.3 to −25.0; $p = 0.16$ versus 6-month change), confirming durability of the BP effect at least until 1-year post-procedure. Furthermore, the mean systolic blood pressure of the crossover group 6 months after the control patients had undergone renal denervation procedure was also significantly lowered (from 190.0 ± 19.6 to 166.3 ± 24.7 mmHg; change: −23.7 ± 27.5; $p < 0.001$) (33).

While longer term follow-up data, up to 2 years, are now available from Symplicity-HTN-1 (64) and 1-year follow-up data from Symplicity HTN-2 (33), this may not yet be sufficient to ascertain the long-term safety and durability of the effect. Indeed, renal and heart transplant models indicate that renal sympathetic efferent nerves may regrow anatomically after injury, raising the possibility of finite time-limits in the physiologic effects of the procedure.

The absence of clinical findings of vessel pathology at 6 months in Symplicity HTN-2 makes it unlikely, albeit not impossible, that vessel pathology may develop either acutely or at longer term follow-up, as recently described in a case report (32). This needs to be addressed in future studies and ongoing long-term follow-up of treated patients.

Symplicity HTN-3 The latest and the largest clinical trial of catheter-based renal denervation, Symplicity HTN-3, has been reported very recently (34). This study was a rigorously designed randomized, blinded, sham-controlled trial. Patients in the control group underwent renal angiogram and a sham procedure. Patients' enrolment criteria were essentially the same as previous Symplicity trials. Patients had to be treated with at least three anti-hypertensive medications at maximally tolerated dose, including a diuretic. Stable medication regimens were to be implemented and had to be unchanged for at least 2 weeks prior to enrolment. Subsequently, patients needed to again fulfil the blood pressure criterion, which was systolic blood pressure ≥160 mmHg on the next visit. Automated 24-hour ambulatory blood pressure monitoring was performed to confirm an average 24-hour systolic blood pressure ≥135 mmHg to exclude patients' white-coat hypertension. Renal denervation was performed by means of Medtronic Symplicity Flex renal-denervation system, and, similar to previous studies, the safety and efficacy endpoints were assessed at 6-month follow-up. During the 6-month follow-up period, the regimen of anti-hypertensive medication was supposed to be kept stable with medication changes allowed only if deemed clinically necessary.

Among 535 uncontrolled hypertensive patients, 364 patients were blindly allocated to the treatment group and underwent renal denervation across 88 centres in the United States. At 6 months after the procedure, a significant drop in office systolic blood pressure from baseline had occurred in the treatment group; however, this was not statistically significant when compared to the BP fall observed in the sham procedure group (−14.1 ± 23.9 vs −11.7 ± 25.9 mmHg; $p = 0.26$).

In contrast to Symplicity HTN-1 and HTN-2, the reduction of office blood pressure in the treatment group was less pronounced (−14.1 ± 23.9/−6.6 ± 11.9 in HTN-3 vs. −22/−11 mmHg in HTN-1 (28) and −32 ± 23/−12 ± 11 mmHg in HTN-2 (31)). Furthermore, there was a large effect in the sham control group; the drop in office systolic blood pressure was prominent compared to that of HTN-2 (−11.7 ± 25.3 vs. 1 ± 21 mmHg in HTN-2) (31). Although the pretreatment blood pressure was similar, the greater range of standard deviation in the treatment group of HTN-3 indicates a wider variation in response. Interestingly, a pre-specified subgroup analysis revealed that, while no difference in BP changes between RND and sham control were evident in patients with an African-American background, there was a significant difference in non-African Americans, perhaps indicating that racial background may influence the response to the procedure. Of note, patients of African-America descent have been shown to have a less pronounced blood pressure reduction in response to treatment with angiotensin-converting enzyme (ACE) inhibitors and beta-blockers (35).

Concerns have also been raised in regards to the operator experience in this US trial. The procedure of renal denervation in Symplicity HTN-3 was performed by a total of 111 operators throughout the United States. Among them, 31% (34 operators) had done only one procedure, and 85 operators had done less than five procedures (34). Although no significant difference was observed in outcomes between operators who performed less than five procedures and others, this may not eliminate the possible influence of the operators' learning curve on relatively marginal reduction of blood pressure in the treatment group. From this point of view, ineffective renal denervation might be partly attributable to the neutral outcome of this study. However, the absence of tests to assess the degree of renal denervation achieved at all, makes it impossible to investigate this matter further, unlike experimental renal denervation in animal studies.

The results from Symplicity HTN-3 raised some important issues that need to be resolved in future renal denervation studies. The procedure of catheter-based renal denervation is essentially different from traditional experimental denervation in animals, in which total renal denervation is accomplished by visually stripping and by painting phenol or xylocaine around the adventitia of the renal artery. In contrast to animal experiments, a reliable test to confirm that renal denervation is successfully achieved is limited to the renal norepinephrine spillover and muscle sympathetic nerve activity (MSNA) in clinical studies (28).

While the evidence of the utility of renal denervation from experimental animal studies is very strong, it has to be considered together with outcomes of clinical research studies to inform future and better designed clinical trials. In this regard, partial ineffectiveness of current clinical approaches to achieve successful renal denervation is a real possibility.

Irrespective of the results of Symplicity HTN 1–3 the therapeutic concept of renal denervation is likely to be most efficacious in conditions characterized by increased sympathetic drive, such as CKD, end-stage renal disease (ESRD), heart failure, and other cardiac-related disorders. The potential roles of renal denervation in CKD and ERSD from both a clinical and a basic science point of view.

Potential future indications for renal nerve ablation

Insulin resistance Hypertension is more common in diabetes than in the general population and is associated with impaired glucose metabolism and insulin resistance; activation of the SNS may contribute to either condition. Based on these considerations, it is perhaps not surprising that reducing sympathetic activation may beneficially influence glucose homeostasis and insulin resistance. Indeed, a recent report demonstrated potential beneficial effects on glucose metabolism and insulin sensitivity with RDN (36). In this study, 37 resistant hypertensive patients underwent bilateral catheter-based RDN, while 13 untreated patients served as controls. Office blood pressure was reduced by −28/−10 mmHg ($p < 0.001$) and −32/−12 mmHg ($p < 0.001$) at 1 and 3 months in the RDN group. Fasting glucose was reduced from 118 ± 3.4 to 108 ± 3.8 mg/dl ($p = 0.039$) at 3-month follow-up. In addition, insulin levels were decreased from 20.8 ± 3.0 to 9.3 ± 2.5 μIU/ml ($p = 0.006$) and C-peptide levels from 5.3 ± 0.6 to 3.0 ± 0.9 ng/ml ($p = 0.002$). After 3 months, the homeostatic model assessment (HOMA) index decreased from 6.0 ± 0.9 to 2.4 ± 0.8 ($p = 0.001$). Additionally, mean 2-hour glucose levels during oral glucose tolerance test were reduced significantly by 27 mg/dl ($p = 0.012$). In contrast, there were no significant changes in blood pressure or metabolic markers in the control group.

Congestive heart failure Increased sympathetic activity is present in patients with chronic heart failure (CHF) and correlates with functional class. Activation of renal sympathetic efferent nerves causes renin release (37), sodium and water retention (16), reduced renal blood flow (17), and all hallmarks of the renal manifestations of CHF. Effective modulation of renal nerves by RDN might, therefore, be useful to ameliorate the neurohormonal disturbances evident in patients with heart failure. Indeed, experimental studies have demonstrated that surgical RDN could improve both renal and ventricular function (38–41).

In a recent study performed by Brandt et al. (42), in which 46 patients underwent bilateral RDN and 18 untreated patients served as controls, the effects of RDN and cardiac function and structure were assessed. After the procedure, mean interventricular septum thickness reduced significantly from 14.1 ± 1.9 mm to 13.4 ± 2.1 mm and 12.5 ± 1.4 mm ($p = 0.007$), LV mass index decreased from 112.4 ± 33.9 g/m^2 to 103.6 ± 30.5 g/m^2 and 94.9 ± 29.8 g/m^2 ($p < 0.001$) at 1-month and 6-month follow-up, respectively. Whereas, the mitral valve lateral E/E', which indicates reduction of LV filling pressures, decreased from 9.9 ± 4.0 to 7.9 ± 2.2 at 1 month and 7.4 ± 2.7 at 6 months ($p < 0.001$). Furthermore, ejection fraction significantly increased after RDN (63.1 ± 8.1% vs. 70.1 ± 11.5% at 6 months; $p < 0.001$). No significant changes were obtained in control patients. This study for the first time demonstrated that RDN not only reduces blood pressure, but improves heart function and regresses LV hypertrophy, which may be of particular benefit in patients with CHF.

Chronic and end-stage renal failure Hypertension occurs in up to 80% of patients with chronic renal failure and plays a key role in progressive deterioration of renal function and the exceedingly high rate of cardiovascular events in this population (43). Renal nerves are commonly highly activated in this scenario. Accordingly, several experimental studies revealed that sympathetic blockade reduced glomerulosclerosis and progression of renal failure (44, 45).

While patients in the Symplicity HTN-2 trial had a mean eGFR of 77 ml/min/1.73m^2 and patients with chronic kidney disease (CKD) and eGFR<45 ml/min/1.73m^2 were excluded (31), this study is important in the current context since it demonstrated that renal function assessed by serum creatinine, eGFR, and cystatin C concentrations were unchanged at 6 months, suggesting that the procedure itself, and the associated haemodynamic changes, have no adverse effects on the kidneys.

However, whether this approach is safe and effective in patients with an estimated glomerular filtration rate below 45 ml/min/1.73m^2 was unclear. As an appropriate first step to test whether the above mentioned findings from patients with resistant hypertension and normal renal function may also pertain to patients with CKD, a pilot study was initiated and bilateral RDN performed in 15 patients with resistant hypertension and stage 3–4 CKD (mean eGFR 31.2 ± 8.9 ml/min/1.73m^2) (46). Carbon dioxide (CO_2) angiography was used in a subset of patients ($n = 6$) to minimize contrast exposure. Office and ambulatory blood pressure and serum biochemistry were obtained before and at 1-, 3-, 6-, and 12-month follow-up. An average of 5.0 ± 0.7 ablation treatments per artery was delivered without complications in any of the treated patients. Angiographic evaluation directly after renal denervation did not reveal any compromise of treated arteries. Importantly, eGFR remained stable in this patient cohort with five patients being followed up to 12 months. This was irrespective of the use of carbon dioxide angiography. Mean baseline BP was 174 ± 22/91 ± 16 mmHg, despite the use of 5.6 ± 1.3 anti-hypertensive drugs. Office systolic and diastolic blood pressure decreased by −34 ± 13/−14 ± 13, −25 ± 20/−11 ± 10, −32 ± 18/−15 ± 12, −33 ± 20/−19 ± 20 mmHg at 1-, 3-, 6-, and 12-month follow-up, respectively ($p < 0.001$). In contrast to office BP readings, mean 24-hour BP and mean day BP were not significantly reduced after the procedure, possibly related to the limited number of valid ambulatory BP readings available and substantial intra-individual variability. However, radiofrequency ablation treatment had a considerable impact on nocturnal blood pressure control. In addition, significant reduction in the rate of blood pressure rise, blood pressure power surge, and night–day blood pressure ratios were observed. Renal denervation also diminished mean and maximum night-time blood pressure and restored a physiologic dipping pattern in 9 out of 10 patients.

Increased activity of the sympathetic nervous system has also clearly been demonstrated to contribute substantially to elevated blood pressure levels commonly seen in patients with end-stage renal failure (ESRD) on dialysis. Preliminary data on the feasibility of renal denervation and its effects on blood pressure and sympathetic nerve activity in ESRD patients have been reported (47). In this initial safety and proof-of-concept study, RDN was performed in 12 patients with ESRD and uncontrolled blood pressure (BP). Standardized

BP measurements were obtained in all patients on dialysis-free days at baseline and follow-up, and measures of renal noradrenaline spillover and muscle sympathetic nerve activity were available from five patients at baseline and from two patients at 12-month follow-up and beyond. The average office BP was 170.8 ± 16.9/89.2 ± 12.1 mmHg, despite the use of 3.8 ± 1.4 anti-hypertensive drugs in these patients. All five patients in whom muscle sympathetic nerve activity and noradrenaline spillover was assessed at baseline displayed substantially elevated levels, confirming high sympathetic tone in patients with ESRD. Of note, 3 out of 12 patients could not undergo RDN due to atrophic renal arteries, which made it impossible to position the RF treatment catheter appropriately. Compared to baseline, office systolic BP was significantly reduced at 3, 6, and 12 months after RDN (from 166 ± 16.0 to 148 ± 11, 150 ± 14, and138 ± 17 mmHg, respectively), whereas no change was evident in the three non-treated patients. While preliminary in nature, these data indicate that RDN is feasible in patients with ESRD and appears to be associated with a sustained reduction in systolic office BP. In this patient cohort, technical issues may arise owing to atrophic renal arteries, which may pose a problem for application of this technology in some patients with ESRD. Further studies are required to confirm these initial findings and assess the best technical approach to RDN treatment of this patient cohort.

Obstructive sleep apnoea It has been suggested that up to 80% of patients with resistant hypertension suffer from obstructive sleep apnoea (OSA), defined as an apnoea/hypopnoea index (AHI) >5 events per hour (48–50). Current guidelines, therefore, recommend screening for, and treatment of, sleep apnoea in patients with resistant hypertension (51). While several pathophysiological mechanisms have been suggested to contribute to this detrimental relationship, there is general agreement that a major mechanism is an increase in sympathetic activity during the apnoeas (49, 52).

Perhaps not unexpectedly, preliminary data indicate potential favourable effects on sleep apnoea severity in patients with resistant hypertension and concomitant sleep apnoea (51). A recent report by Witkowski and colleagues (53) describes the first experience with renal denervation in patients with resistant hypertension and co-morbid OSA. In this proof-of-concept study, a total of 10 patients with refractory hypertension and sleep apnoea (7 men and 3 women; median age: 49.5 years) underwent renal denervation and completed 3-month and 6-month follow-up evaluations, including polysomnography. Anti-hypertensive regimens were not changed during the 6 months of follow-up. Three and 6 months after the denervation, decreases in office systolic and diastolic BPs were observed (median: −34/−13 mmHg at 6 months; both $p < 0.01$). A decrease in AHI at 6 months after renal denervation was observed in 8 out of 10 patients (median: 16.3 versus 4.5 events per hour; $p = 0.059$).

These preliminary data suggest that catheter-based renal sympathetic denervation may lower OSA severity and confirmed previously described beneficial effects on glucose metabolism, indicating that patients with comorbid resistant hypertension, glucose intolerance, and obstructive sleep apnoea, may specifically benefit from this procedure. While no direct mechanistic insights could be obtained from this study, it is conceivable that renal denervation reduces salt avidity by efferent sympathetic renal nerve disruption and might reduce total body fluid, which is thought to contribute to obstructive episodes through peripharyngeal fluid accumulation that may predispose to upper airway obstruction (54). Furthermore, venous capacitance remains under the control of the sympathetic nervous system and it is likely that renal denervation affects venous capacitance and blood pooling (55), thereby providing a further potential mechanism through which renal denervation could reduce OSA severity in resistant hypertension.

Atrial fibrillation Both animal and human studies suggest that the autonomic nervous system plays an important role in initiation and maintenance of atrial fibrillation (AF). In human studies, Huang et al. (56) suggested that idiopathic paroxysmal AF (PAF) is primarily dependent on vagal withdrawal, while organic PAF is triggered by sympathetic excitation. Some studies observed increased sympathetic tone or a loss of vagal tone before the onset of AF. More recently, Pokushalov et al. (57) reported that RDN reduced AF recurrences when combined with pulmonary vein isolation (PVI). Altogether, 27 hypertensive patients with a history of symptomatic paroxysmal or persistent AF were enrolled, 14 of whom underwent PVI only, and 13 were treated with PVI and RDN. At 12-month follow-up, patients in the PVI + RDN group not only experienced a significant reduction in systolic (181 ± 7 to 156 ± 5; $p < 0.001$) and diastolic blood pressure (97 ± 6 to 87 ± 4; $p < 0.001$), but had a substantially lower rate of recurrence of AF. Nine of the 13 patients (69%) treated with PVI with renal denervation were AF-free versus 4 (29%) of the 14 patients in the PVI-only group ($p = 0.033$). Although optimized blood pressure control might play a considerable role in decreasing the development of recurrence of AF, this study raises the possibility that reducing sympathetic drive with RDN may reduce the rate of AF recurrence in resistant hypertensive patients.

Alternative approaches to achieve renal denervation

The initial promising data on catheter-based RDN and its effects on BP in resistant hypertension have led to the rapid development of several different treatment modalities to achieve renal artery denervation.

Saline-irrigated radiofrequency ablation catheters

The use of catheter-based techniques to achieve functional denervation is not new to the area of interventional cardiology. Saline-irrigated radiofrequency ablation catheters are being used by electrophysiologists for ablation of aberrant cardiac pathways and have been shown to be of value in patients with cardiac arrhythmias for some time. Recently, a report on the use of a saline-irrigated radiofrequency ablation catheter (Celsius Thermocool, Biosense Webster, Diamond Bar, California) for RDN was published. The ablation catheter was manoeuvred within the renal artery to allow energy delivery in a circumferential, longitudinally staggered manner to minimize the chance of renal artery stenosis in 10 patients with resistant hypertension. Energy titration was performed to achieve a

10 to 20% drop in impedance at each location. No more than seven ablation lesions, mean duration 26 ± 6 seconds each, were placed within each renal artery. After 6 months, the systolic/diastolic blood pressure decreased by −21/−11 mmHg, there was no evidence of renal artery stenosis or aneurysm at repeat angiography, and the authors reported a significant decrease in levels of the hormones metanephrine (−12 ± 4; $p = 0.003$), normetanephrine (−18 ± 4; $p = 0.0008$), and aldosterone (−60 ± 33 ng/l; $p = 0.02$) at 3 months follow-up (58).

Radiofrequency ablation catheters

Newer iterations of radiofrequency catheters include:

1 The Vessix V2 RDN system (Vessix Vascular) is a percutaneous radiofrequency balloon catheter. It has received European CE Mark approval for its technology for the treatment of hypertension. A pilot study (REDUCE-HTN clinical study) by Vessix V2 RDN system is ongoing and initial conference abstracts report BP reduction similar in magnitude to those reported in the Symplicity studies.

2 The EnligHTN™ catheter (St. Jude Medical), a basket-like design with four separate electrodes aimed at improving procedural efficiency and decreasing excessive manipulation.

3 Oneshot™ catheter (Maya Medical, Saratoga, California). This catheter is an RF system mounted on a balloon. Gentle inflation of the balloon centres the catheter, which then ablates longer segments of renal artery when activated.

Intra-vascular ultrasound catheters

There are two kinds of intra-vascular catheters for RDN at present:

1 The TIVUS™ catheter (CardioSonic, Tel Aviv, Israel) is a high-intensity, non-focused ultrasonic catheter system. By applying ultrasonic energy, the TIVUS technology enables thermal injury to the adventitia of the renal artery. Swine studies have shown that kidney tissue norepinephrine concentration was reduced by 50% or more at 30- and 90-day follow-up without local tissue damage.

2 The PARADISE™ catheter (ReCor Medical, Inc, Ronkonkoma, NY), is another ultrasound catheter placed inside a low-pressure balloon. Preliminary clinical data for PARADISE were previously reported at EuroPCR 2012 with an average systolic blood pressure reduction of 31 mmHg in seven patients at 60-days follow-up.

Peri-vascular pharmacologic ablation

The Mercator Bullfrog™ catheter (Mercator MedSystems, Inc, San Leandro, CA) is composed of a catheter tipped with a balloon-sheathed microneedle. After advancement of the catheter into the renal artery, the balloon is inflated with saline, securing the system for injection and sliding the microneedle through the vessel wall. Then, guanethidine is delivered through the vessel wall into the adventitia.

Conclusions

Renal denervation has now emerged as a novel treatment option for patients with resistant hypertension, whose BP cannot be controlled by optimal combinations of lifestyle modifications and pharmacotherapy. Both the HTN-1 and HTN-2 studies have shown a favourable safety and long-term efficacy profile (up to 2 years) of RDN achieved by catheter-based radiofrequency ablation, although these findings have been challenged by the results of the sham-controlled Symplicity HTN-3 trial. The potential beneficial effects of RDN appear to be mediated via interference with both efferent and afferent nerves. Based on the mechanisms underpinning several other relevant conditions commonly associated with hypertension, additional benefits beyond improved BP control could potentially be expected in the context of impaired glucose metabolism, heart failure, chronic renal failure, obstructive sleep apnoea, atrial fibrillation, and others. However, at this stage there is not sufficient evidence to support its use in any of these potential indications beyond that of resistant hypertension.

New devices for RDN, including radiofrequency ablation catheters, intra-vascular ultrasound catheters, peri-vascular pharmacologic ablation, and externally applied focused ultrasound are currently being investigated and may demonstrate advantages and disadvantages of various strategies to therapeutically target the renal nerves.

References

1 **Esler M**. The sympathetic nervous system through the ages: from Thomas Willis to resistant hypertension. Exp Physiol 2011;**96**(7):611–22. Epub 2011/05/10.

2 **Ackerknecht EH**. The history of the discovery of the vegatative (autonomic) nervous system. Med Hist 1974;**18**(1):1–8. Epub 1974/01/01.

3 **Adrian ED, Bronk DW, Phillips G**. Discharges in mammalian sympathetic nerves. J Physiol 1932;**74**(2):115–33. Epub 1932/02/08.

4 **Von Euler US**. Sympathin in adrenergic nerve fibres. J Physiol 1946;**105**:26. Epub 1946/09/18.

5 **Cannon WB**. Chemical mediators of autonomic nerve impulses. Science 1933;**78**(2012):43–48. Epub 1933/07/21.

6 **Smithwick RH, Thompson JE**. Splanchnicectomy for essential hypertension; results in 1,266 cases. J Am Med Assoc 1953;**152**(16):1501–504.

7 **DiBona GF, Kopp UC**. Neural control of renal function. Physiol Rev 1997;**77**(1):75–197.

8 **Gao L, Li Y, Schultz HD et al**. Downregulated Kv4.3 expression in the RVLM as a potential mechanism for sympathoexcitation in rats with chronic heart failure. Am J Physiol Heart Circ Physiol 2010;**298**(3):H945–55. Epub 2010/01/02.

9 **Schlaich MP, Lambert E, Kaye DM et al**. Sympathetic augmentation in hypertension: role of nerve firing, norepinephrine reuptake, and Angiotensin neuromodulation. Hypertension 2004;**43**(2):169–75.

10 **Grewal RS, Kaul CL**. Importance of the sympathetic nervous system in the development of renal hypertension in the rat. Br J Pharmacol 1971;**42**(4):497–504.

11 **Masuo K, Rakugi H, Ogihara T, Esler MD, Lambert GW**. Cardiovascular and renal complications of type 2 diabetes in obesity: role of sympathetic nerve activity and insulin resistance. Curr Diab Rev 2010;**6**(2):58–67. Epub 2009/12/26.

12 **Grassi G, Quarti-Trevano F, Seravalle G et al**. Early sympathetic activation in the initial clinical stages of chronic renal failure. Hypertension 2011;**57**(4):846–51. Epub 2011/02/09.

13 **Bertog SC, Sobotka PA, Sievert H**. Renal denervation for hypertension. J Am Coll Cardiol Cardiovasc Interv 2012;**5**(3):249–58. Epub 2012/03/24.

14 **Barajas L, Muller J**. The innervation of the juxtaglomerular apparatus and surrounding tubules: a quantitative analysis by serial section electron microscopy. J Ultrastruct Res 1973;**43**(1):107–32. Epub 1973/04/01.

15 **Kopp UC, Cicha MZ, Smith LA, Mulder J, Hokfelt T**. Renal sympathetic nerve activity modulates afferent renal nerve activity by PGE2-dependent activation of alpha1- and alpha2-adrenoceptors on renal sensory nerve fibers. Am J Physiol 2007;**293**(4):R1561–72.

16 **Bell-Reuss E, Trevino DL, Gottschalk CW**. Effect of renal sympathetic nerve stimulation on proximal water and sodium reabsorption. J Clin Invest 1976;**57**(4):1104–107.

17 **Kirchheim H, Ehmke H, Persson P**. Sympathetic modulation of renal hemodynamics, renin release and sodium excretion. Klinische Wochenschrift 1989;**67**(17):858–64.

18 **Esler M, Straznicky N, Eikelis N, Masuo K, Lambert G, Lambert E**. Mechanisms of sympathetic activation in obesity-related hypertension. Hypertension 2006;**48**(5):787–96.

19 **Grassi G, Cattaneo BM, Seravalle G, Lanfranchi A, Mancia G**. Baroreflex control of sympathetic nerve activity in essential and secondary hypertension. Hypertension 1998;**31**(1):68–72.

20 **Esler M, Jennings G, Biviano B, Lambert G, Hasking G**. Mechanism of elevated plasma noradrenaline in the course of essential hypertension. J Cardiovasc Pharmacol 1986;**8**(Suppl 5):S39–43.

21 **Esler M, Jennings G, Lambert G**. Noradrenaline release and the pathophysiology of primary human hypertension. Am J Hypertens 1989 Mar;**2**(3 Pt 2):140S–146S.

22 **Schlaich MP, Kaye DM, Lambert E, Sommerville M, Socratous F, Esler MD**. Relation between cardiac sympathetic activity and hypertensive left ventricular hypertrophy. Circulation 2003;**108**(5):560–65.

23 **Anderson EA, Sinkey CA, Lawton WJ, Mark AL**. Elevated sympathetic nerve activity in borderline hypertensive humans. Evidence from direct intraneural recordings. Hypertension 1989;**14**(2):177–83.

24 **Kon V**. Neural control of renal circulation. Miner Electrolyte Metab 1989;**15**(1–2):33–43.

25 **Zanchetti AS**. Neural regulation of renin release: experimental evidence and clinical implications in arterial hypertension. Circulation 1977;**56**(5):691–98.

26 **Naraghi R, Geiger H, Crnac J et al**. Posterior fossa neurovascular anomalies in essential hypertension. Lancet 1994;**344**(8935):1466–70. Epub 1994/11/26.

27 **Frank H, Heusser K, Geiger H, Fahlbusch R, Naraghi R, Schobel HP**. Temporary reduction of blood pressure and sympathetic nerve activity in hypertensive patients after microvascular decompression. Stroke 2009;**40**(1):47–51. Epub 2008/10/18.

28 **Krum H, Schlaich M, Whitbourn R et al**. Catheter-based renal sympathetic denervation for resistant hypertension: a multicentre safety and proof-of-principle cohort study. Lancet 2009;**373**(9671):1275–81. Epub 2009/04/01.

29 **Rippy MK, Zarins D, Barman NC, Wu A, Duncan KL, Zarins CK**. Catheter-based renal sympathetic denervation: chronic preclinical evidence for renal artery safety. Clin Res Cardiol 2011;**100**(12):1095–101. Epub 2011/07/29.

30. **Symplicity HTN-1 investigators** Catheter-based renal sympathetic denervation for resistant hypertension: durability of blood pressure reduction out to 24 months. Hypertension 2011;**57**(5):911–17. Epub 2011/03/16.

31 **Esler MD, Krum H, Sobotka PA, Schlaich MP, Schmieder RE, Bohm M**. Renal sympathetic denervation in patients with treatment-resistant hypertension (The Symplicity HTN-2 Trial): a randomised controlled trial. Lancet 2010;**376**(9756):1903–909. Epub 2010/11/26.

32 **Vonend O, Antoch G, Rump LC, Blondin D**. Secondary rise in blood pressure after renal denervation. Lancet 2012;**380**(9843):778. Epub 2012/08/28.

33 **Esler MD, Krum H, Schlaich M, Schmieder RE, Bohm M, Sobotka PA.** Renal sympathetic denervation for treatment of drug-resistant hypertension: one-year results from the Symplicity HTN-2 randomized, controlled trial. Circulation.2012;**126**(25):2976–82. Epub 2012/12/19.

34 **Bhatt DL, Kandzari DE, O'Neill WW et al.** A controlled trial of renal denervation for resistant hypertension. N Engl J Med 2014;**370**(15):1393–401.

35 **Materson BJ, Reda DJ, Cushman WC et al.** Single-Drug Therapy for Hypertension in Men—A Comparison of Six Antihypertensive Agents with Placebo. N Engl J Med 1993;**328**:914–21.

36 **Mahfoud F, Schlaich M, Kindermann I et al.** Effect of renal sympathetic denervation on glucose metabolism in patients with resistant hypertension: a pilot study. Circulation 2011;**123**(18):1940–46. Epub 2011/04/27.

37 **Stella A, Zanchetti A.** Effects of renal denervation on renin release in response to tilting and furosemide. Am J Physiol 1977;**232**(5):H500–507. Epub 1977/05/01.

38 **DiBona GF, Sawin LL.** Role of renal nerves in sodium retention of cirrhosis and congestive heart failure. Am J Physiol 1991;**260**(2 Pt 2):R298–305.

39 **Villarreal D, Freeman RH, Johnson RA, Simmons JC.** Effects of renal denervation on postprandial sodium excretion in experimental heart failure. Am J Physiol 1994;**266**(5 Pt 2):R1599–604.

40 **Nozawa T, Igawa A, Fujii N et al.** Effects of long-term renal sympathetic denervation on heart failure after myocardial infarction in rats. Heart Vessels 2002;**16**(2):51–56.

41 **Clayton SC, Haack KK, Zucker IH.** Renal denervation modulates angiotensin receptor expression in the renal cortex of rabbits with chronic heart failure. Am J Physiol Renal Physiol 2011;**300**(1):F31–39. Epub 2010/10/22.

42 **Brandt MC, Mahfoud F, Reda S et al.** Renal sympathetic denervation reduces left ventricular hypertrophy and improves cardiac function in patients with resistant hypertension. J Am Coll Cardiol 2012;**59**(10):901–909. Epub 2012/03/03.

43 **Converse RL, Jr.**, Jacobsen TN, Toto RD et al. Sympathetic overactivity in patients with chronic renal failure. N Engl J Med 1992;**327**(27):1912–18.

44 **Amann K, Koch A, Hofstetter J et al.** Glomerulosclerosis and progression: effect of subantihypertensive doses of alpha and beta blockers. Kidney Int 2001;**60**(4):1309–23.

45 **Amann K, Rump LC, Simonaviciene A et al.** Effects of low dose sympathetic inhibition on glomerulosclerosis and albuminuria in subtotally nephrectomized rats. J Am Soc Nephrol 2000;**11**(8):1469–78.

46 **Hering D, Mahfoud F, Walton AS et al.** Renal denervation in moderate to severe CKD. J Am Soc Nephrol 2012;**23**(7):1250–57. Epub 2012/05/19.

47 **Schlaich MP, Bart B, Hering D et al.** Feasibility of catheter-based renal nerve ablation and effects on sympathetic nerve activity and blood pressure in patients with end-stage renal disease. Int J Cardiol 2013;**168**(3):2214–20. Epub 2013/03/05.

48 **Logan AG, Perlikowski SM, Mente A et al.** High prevalence of unrecognized sleep apnoea in drug-resistant hypertension. J Hypertens 2001;**19**(12):2271–77. Epub 2001/11/29.

49 **Baguet JP, Barone-Rochette G, Pepin JL.** Hypertension and obstructive sleep apnoea syndrome: current perspectives. J Hum Hypertens 2009;**23**(7):431–43. Epub 2009/01/09.

50 **Ruttanaumpawan P, Nopmaneejumruslers C, Logan AG, Lazarescu A, Qian I, Bradley TD.** Association between refractory hypertension and obstructive sleep apnea. J Hypertens 2009;**27**(7):1439–45. Epub 2009/05/08.

51 **Mancia G, De Backer G, Dominiczak A et al.** 2007 Guidelines for the management of arterial hypertension: The Task Force for the Management of Arterial Hypertension of the European Society of Hypertension (ESH) and of the European Society of Cardiology (ESC). J Hypertens 2007;**25**(6):1105–87.

52 **Narkiewicz K, Somers VK**. Sympathetic nerve activity in obstructive sleep apnoea. Acta Physiol Scand 2003;**177**(3):385–90. Epub 2003/03/01.

53 **Witkowski A, Prejbisz A, Florczak E et al.** Effects of renal sympathetic denervation on blood pressure, sleep apnea course, and glycemic control in patients with resistant hypertension and sleep apnea. Hypertension 2011;**58**(4):559–65. Epub 2011/08/17.

54 **Friedman O, Bradley TD, Chan CT, Parkes R, Logan AG**. Relationship between overnight rostral fluid shift and obstructive sleep apnea in drug-resistant hypertension. Hypertension 2010;**56**(6):1077–82. Epub 2010/11/10.

55 **Pang CC**. Autonomic control of the venous system in health and disease: effects of drugs. Pharmacol Ther 2001;**90**(2–3):179–230. Epub 2001/10/02.

56 **Huang WC, Fang TC, Cheng JT**. Renal denervation prevents and reverses hyperinsulinemia-induced hypertension in rats. Hypertension 1998;**32**(2):249–54. Epub 1998/08/27.

57 **Pokushalov E, Romanov A, Corbucci G et al.** A randomized comparison of pulmonary vein isolation with versus without concomitant renal artery denervation in patients with refractory symptomatic atrial fibrillation and resistant hypertension. J Am Coll Cardiol 2012;**60**(13):1163–70. Epub 2012/09/11.

58 **Ahmed A, Fonarow GC, Zhang Yet al.** Renin-angiotensin inhibition in systolic heart failure and chronic kidney disease. Am J Med 2012;**125**(4):399–410. Epub 2012/02/11.

Chapter 6

Evolution and developments in autonomic control of the heart I: the neurocardiac axis

Mike J. L. DeJongste, Gerbrand J. Groen, and Robert D. Foreman

Key points

1 Developing concepts on the neurocardiac axis.
2 Neural hierarchy in cardiac control.
3 Role of the nervous system in atherosclerosis.
4 The double neurocardiac loop.
5 Pathophysiology of the nervous system in the diseased heart.

Introduction

In the light of the progress that has been made in understanding the interactions among organs, in 'Overview of experimental models of neural hierarchy in *ischaemic* heart disease', we will focus on the evolution and developments in concepts of modulatory exchanges among molecules, cells, and organ systems taking place within the neurocardiac axis.

In 'Overview of experimental models of neural hierarchy in *other* heart diseases', interference in heart–brain interactions will be one of the leitmotivs.

Within the field of neurocardiology, the interest is growing for modulation of, instead of ablating, the delicate nervous system. Since electrical neuromodulation for angina has been accepted as a therapeutic option in cardiology guidelines, investigators have gradually shifted the research focus from clinical studies on efficacy towards using neuromodulation as a tool to provide a better insight into communications between heart and brain.

Historical and evolutionary concepts on the role of the nervous system on cardiac performance

The Greek physician Erasistratus (third century BC) was the first to compare cardiac function with a black smith's bellows. He hypothesized that blood in the arteries was propelled for 'pneuma or spirit' ("breath of life") and in the veins for blood (nourishment) through cardiac contractions, like inflating and deflating a bellows. Galen, who lived in Rome five centuries later, believed that blood was produced in the largest organ of the body, i.e. the liver (1). He believed that blood, after being derived from juices of the gut, flows from liver to veins. His hypothesis was that blood received nutrients from the gut, oxygen from the lungs, and both, 'spirit' and 'warmth', from the heart; from the heart blood flows to organs where it 'disappears'. So, Galen's idea was that the heart was 'resuscitating' blood by adding spirit and warmth to it. Performing autopsies on 30 bodies, Leonardo da Vinci (1452–1519) already obtained elementary knowledge on blood circulation. However, he did not seem to understand the consequences of his findings. To study the circulation, he made drafts and notes, which were finally published late in the nineteenth century. On the threshold of the discovery of the circulation Leonardo da Vinci failed, since he, as a God-fearing person like everyone during that time, believed characteristics of the body could not be expressed in measures and numbers. So, he considered the body as a 'small earth' and the circulation subsequently as 'rivers'. The only exception to this concept was the nervous system, since the earth was not moving and the nervous system was considered to be related to movements. Then, finally, Harvey bridged the gap with exact scientific methods by studying the opened body, using the calculations he made on the 'motor' function of the heart in his '*De motu cordis*' and '*Exercationes de generatione animale*' (1658). In the latter book, he thought that all life came from the egg ('*ovum esse primordium commune, omnibus animalibus*', 1651). By the same token, Nicolaas Hartsoeker published in 1694 '*Essay de dioptrique*' that described the theory of sperm containing a complete little human being, which he therefore referred to as an '*homunculus*'.

In primitive forms of life, usually less than 0.1 mm in size, such as bacteria, no circulation system exists and, therefore, no heart pump is required. In addition to the exchange via diffusion, the only process enabling small organisms to survive, higher forms of life possess the capacity to exchange oxygen and nutrients via the circulation of blood. The main function of the heart in vertebrates is preserving circulation to perfuse organs, enabling all cells of the body to exchange oxygen, nutrients, and warmth against waste. The primitive forms of life also lack a nervous system. In developed forms of life, interaction among organs and tissues to maintain body functions enable the individual to perform personal actions. While primitive lives do not adjust to changes in their environment, higher developed beings become more or less independent of their environment. This emergent process is also the cycle a foetus goes through to reach maturity. In embryonic life a foetus can only survive after 20 weeks (with technical help), when the heart and nervous system are developed to function sufficiently. In this regard, it is of interest that the heart is not able to survive without the intrinsic cardiac nervous system.

Hence, the (autonomic) nervous system is thought to serve as a sort of gatekeeper to maintain the integrity of the cardiomyocyte by enabling the cells, to metabolize oxygen and nutrients from energy sources, more specifically adenosine tri-phosphate (ATP). In the cell, the calcium influx current activates ATP that binds to myosin–troponin bands in which composite bands enable the cell, and subsequently the heart, to contract effectively. Synchronization and adaptation to continuously changing circumstances of subsequent contractions of cardiomyocytes are controlled by the conduction system, which in turn is under control of the hierarchy of the central and peripheral nervous systems. It is surprising that the interaction between the cardiomyocyte and neurones was not defined until the twentieth century. Finally, late in the twentieth century, since the discovery of DNA, the focus changed from haemodynamics and metabolism of cells to genetics. However, since the difference between a human being and a primitive life expressed in the number of genes is not so large as expected, the last decades the research is increasingly focusing on cellular phenotyping and epigenetic regulation (expression and reprogramming).

Pertinent anatomy and physiology (including humoral control) of afferent and efferent autonomic nervous system in cardiac functioning

The Chinese have already recognized the principle of two counteracting forces collaborating in synchronized processes, as a yin yang, as early as the fourteenth century BC. The underlying principle of yin yang is self-evident with regard to the autonomic nervous system in that it helps to define the mutual interactions between the autonomic nervous system and the heart.

Leopoldo Caldani, later followed by his student Luigi Galvani, demonstrated in 1758 that electrical current applied to an isolated muscle from a frog caused contraction of the muscle. Claude Bernard thought that heart rate increased following '*l'influence du grand sympathetic*'. This idea was established in humans by Henle around 1840, when he observed that stimulating vagal nerves of decapitated criminals made the heart stop beating. Once the heart came to a complete stand still, applying current to the sympathetic nerves enabled the heart to start beating again.

Another serendipitous finding was unveiled by Loewi in 1921 who demonstrated that, independent of the nerves, the heart rate slowed when the heart was perfused with acetylcholine.

The autonomic nervous system (ANS) was also referred to as the visceral nervous system when it became apparent that the ANS acts as a control system for visceral organs, such as the heart. The efferent orientated ANS has classically been divided into two limbs: the parasympathetic nervous system and the sympathetic nervous system. A third limb of the ANS makes use of endogenous nitric oxide (NO) as a neurotransmitter and has subsequently been coined the 'non-adrenergic non-cholinergic' part of the ANS. In this regard, humans possess highly specialized cells capable of sensing the oxygen partial pressure in organs, like the enteric nervous system. These cells govern the adjustment of blood supply and so oxygen to organs. In recent years it has been demonstrated that vascular endothelium modulates vascular tone through the release of the pO_2-dependent molecule NO in endothelial cells within the vascular system. So these highly specialized endothelial cells, acting as local oxygen sensors, are closely acting together with NO-dependent neurones to modulate blood flow. The debate is ongoing whether this system, being involved with organs such as the enteric nervous system of the gastrointestinal tract, is part of the ANS or should be considered as an independent system.

The *sympathetic* part of the ANS increases the function of an organ, i.e. cardiac performance, mainly through activation of β-1 adrenergic receptors. Stimulation of β-2 adrenergic receptors results in relaxation of smaller coronary arteries. Constriction of larger coronary arteries is executed through adrenergic stimulation of α-1 receptors, via phospholipase C. The non-smooth muscle α-1 adrenoceptors on the heart are engaged in its inotropic effect. All α–adrenoceptors use G-proteins to employ their effects on Ca^{2+} handling. Like the α-1 adrenoceptors, the α-2 adrenoceptors are involved in smooth muscle contraction; however, these receptors make use of adenylcyclase. In addition, stimulation of the α-2 adrenoceptors induces a negative feedback on norepinephrine release and increases thrombocyte aggregation.

The *parasympathetic* limb of the ANS reduces cardiac performance via muscarine (M_{2-}) receptors (for review see (2)).

Basically, the control and feedback action of the ANS consists of a central nervous part (with the hypothalamus as 'highest' centre) and peripheral components (outside spine and skull). The original division into a sympathetic and parasympathetic part was based upon their motor effects. They differ from the normal motor system in target organs (cardiac muscle and smooth muscle tissue versus skeletal muscle tissue), in their pathway towards the target organ, and in their synapses in between (3).

For the *sympathetic* part of the ANS, the cells of origin are located in the intermediomedial and lateral nucleus of the spinal cord segments C8–L2, for which it is also described as the thoracolumbar part of the ANS. The efferent sympathetic fibres leave the spinal cord via the ventral motor root and enter the sympathetic trunk via (white) rami communicantes. Their fibres have many collaterals that end at sympathetic ganglion cells at various levels: at the level of entrance, after an ascending (synapse in more cranial ganglia) or descending (synapse in more caudal ganglia) course. For the internal organs, including the heart, the postganglionic sympathetic nerve fibres (which lie, however, inside the sympathetic ganglia) supply the organs via visceral branches, called 'splanchnic nerves'. They can originate at every level of the sympathetic trunk, i.e. from cervical, thoracic, lumbar, or sacral ganglia, or from between the ganglia, and reach the target structures either separately or via perivascular routes.

The *parasympathetic* cells of origin are located in the brainstem nuclei (among others in the dorsal nucleus of vagus nerve) and intermediolateral nuclei of the spinal cord segments S2–4. Therefore, this part is also referred to as the bulbosacral part of the ANS. Their preganglionic nerve fibres generally have a small number of collaterals and end upon ganglion cells near or in the wall of the target organ (4).

With regard to heart innervation, sympathetic cardiac nerves are derived from cervical and upper thoracic sympathetic ganglia from both sides, whereas parasympathetic cardiac nerves originate from the left and right vagus nerve, cranial and caudal to the origin of both recurrent laryngeal nerves. They run as separate nerves, along the major vessels towards the heart and end upon the cardiac ganglia and plexuses, which are located in front of the tracheal bifurcation, below and behind the aortic arch, and above the cardiac base and the division of the pulmonary trunk (3). Finally, they all communicate with intrinsic cardiac ganglia (see Chapter 1). The sympathetic adrenergic nerves serve to increase both, heart rate (chronotropy) and contractility (inotropy), augment conduction velocity (dromotropy) and make the relaxation phase faster (lusitropy), whereas the parasympathetic cholinergic nerves have opposite effects on all four effects(5).

The afferent innervation of the heart is as important as the efferent nerve supply. Sensory afferent nerve fibres run along sympathetic and parasympathetic pathways to end in the spinal cord and in the medulla. The afferent nerve fibres that bypass sympathetic pathways have alternative functions and are considered to be responsible for nociceptive conduction during cardiac ischaemia.

Cardiac autonomic nerves

In two large and very detailed reviews, the extrinsic human cardiac innervation is described extensively (6). With regard to the terminology, one should keep in mind that the nerves generally are named according to their origin.

Sympathetic input in the cardiac plexus is by the superior cardiac nerve originating from the superior cervical ganglion and adjacent sympathetic trunk, the middle cardiac nerve originating from the middle cervical ganglion, vertebral ganglion, and adjacent sympathetic trunk, and by the inferior cardiac nerve, which originates from the inferior cervical ganglion (if present) and cervicothoracic or stellate ganglion. The superior cervical ganglion was shown to have connections with primarily C1–C3 spinal nerves, the middle cervical ganglion with the spinal nerves C3 (33%), C4 (90%), C5 (60%), and C6 (15% of cases). The inferior and stellate ganglia primarily were connected to C7–T2 (range C5–T3). The thoracic sympathetic input is by thoracic cardiac nerves that originate from the upper four–five thoracic sympathetic ganglia (5). Lower origins have been described in literature up to T7–9 (3), but were not found by Kawashima in his highly detailed dissections (7).

Parasympathetic input is by the superior and thoracic cardiac branch of the vagus nerve originating proximal and distal to the branching site of the recurrent laryngeal nerve, respectively, and by the inferior cardiac branch of the vagus nerve. All branches were consistently identified (6).

In their trajectory towards the cardiac plexus, both sympathetic and parasympathetic nerves generally run parallel to each other, e.g. the superior cardiac nerve and superior cardiac branch of the vagus nerve run dorsal to the carotid artery toward the aortic arch. The nerves are hard to discern from each other, which may have consequences for cardiovascular surgery that intends to preserve autonomic nerves (6). Furthermore, left–right differences exist (5, 6). The same holds true with regard to the vagal system. Sympathetic control of sinus node and atrioventricular node is done by variable modulation between left and right vagus nerve via three cardiac ganglionated plexuses (4). Also, very recently, it was found in pigs that both left and right stellate ganglia (right more than left) supply the anterior ventricular wall, although electrical stimulation of the left stellate ganglion significantly increased the activation recovery interval (8). The authors concluded that the link between ventricular arrhythmias and sympathetic innervations was further supported. Furthermore, it could clarify why stellate blocks are beneficial in reducing arrhythmias in patients with anterior myocardial scars and ventricular tachyarrythmia storms.

Afferent cardiac nerves

The first description of angina dates back to Heberden (9). In 1772 he accurately reported on the pre-eminent symptoms of angina, commonly experienced as sensations of pressure, heartburn, squeezing, constriction, tightness, or strangling, which typically come to alertness as a vague distress on the chest. Soon after the extensive symptomatic description of cardiac pain, coined as angina pectoris, Heberden received a letter from a 52-year old 'Dr Anonymous' (10), who wrote that his symptoms corresponded exactly with Heberden's account. In addition to the description of the symptoms of his ischaemic heart disease, the English physician seemed to suffer from ventricular arrhythmias. As a consequence of 'the regular shocks at the heart', he wrote that he was expecting to meet with a sudden death.

Angina is intriguing for its wide range of symptom expression, varying from silent myocardial ischaemia to a functional pain syndrome of the heart.

Explanations for this diversity are unknown; however, when angina is 'simply' regarded as a visceral pain state, several rules are compulsory. For example, visceral pain leads to referral in dermatomes that are related to the same spinal cord segments that supply the internal organ, in equal referred pain obeys a segmental rule. Thus, if in a patient angina is felt at the back between the scapulae, this should be regarded as referred pain in dermatomes (±) T4–7. This implies that the ischaemic part of the heart is supplied by the spinal nerves T4–7. Moreover, if angina pain is felt in the jaw, it should be related to dermatome C3, most probably via the cervical sympathetic pathway or via the adjacent superior cardiac vagal pathway, since they have many interconnections. Of course, the nociceptive nerve fibres in that part of the heart need to be stimulated above a certain threshold, but nevertheless this could be regarded as a 'rule of thumb'.

Overview of experimental models of neural hierarchy in ischaemic heart disease

In stable conditions, angina is induced during exercise and abates with rest, or nitroglycerine intake. Due to diffuse innervation of visceral organs, like the heart, ischaemia-provoked sensations are radiated to somatic structures localized on the chest, arms, back, neck, muscles, and sometimes even to the higher abdomen (11). When all three characteristics (in equal localization, radiation, and means of relief) are present, the symptoms are defined as 'typical angina' (12). The diffuse and poorly localized referred symptoms of angina enhance autonomic reflexes, such as sweating, vasomotor symptoms, and muscular rigidity, and are often associated with feelings of unpleasantness. Strong emotional distress may also precede, or is associated with, complaints of pain in the chest. Further, emotional suffering has been associated with increased mortality in patients with coronary artery disease.

Clinical studies suggest that anxiety and depression are prevalent in patients suffering from chest pain with and without underlying cardiac disease (13). Anxiety and/or stress increases circulating levels of corticosteroids, which can act on the glucocorticoid receptors in the amygdala, particularly in the central area (14). The amygdala plays a pivotal role in transforming chronic stressful stimuli into behavioural, visceral, and autonomic responses (15). Experimental studies were conducted to determine if stress induced via the amygdala changes the characteristics of the upper thoracic spinal neurones that process nociceptive afferent information from the heart (16). These studies showed that central sensitization of these neurones occurred in animals that expressed high anxiety resulting from implantation of corticosteroids in the amygdala. In contrast, animals with cholesterol implants expressed low anxiety and the excitability of the spinal neurones did not change. In summary, glucocorticoids manipulate amygdala function by inducing hypersensitivity to nociceptive input from the heart through central sensitization of upper thoracic spinal neuronal activity. Thus, stress and anxiety may play a role in intensifying angina in patients because the neurones of the central nervous system are more sensitive to nociceptive cardiac input.

In some patients angina pectoris is experienced as neck and jaw pain. Clinical reports suggested that this pain was attributed to transmission of nociceptive information in vagal afferent fibres, which were commonly thought to transmit innocuous cardiac sensory information (17, 18). Experimental studies have confirmed this clinical observation (16). Injections of algesic chemicals into the heart activated nociceptive vagal afferent fibres that excited spinothalamic tract cells in the C1–C2 spinal segments; these cells also received somatic input from the neck and jaw regions (16). Thus, these studies confirmed that vagal afferent fibres contribute to the angina that is sometimes expressed in the neck and jaw.

Activation of the spinal afferent nerves with occlusion of the coronary artery or injections of algesic chemicals, such as bradykinin, into the heart, excited spinothalamic tract (STT) cells in the T1–T5 and C5–C6 spinal segments; these cells also received convergent input from the chest and upper arm. However, no visceral input converged onto STT cells in the C7–C8 segments, where the somatic effects are primarily distal and originate from the hand (19). The findings are consistent with the observation from patients that angina commonly occurs in the chest and proximal somatic fields but rarely in the distal aspects of the arm and hand.

Findings over the last 20 years include evidence of convergence of visceral-somatic input to spinothalamic cells and a major role for the vagus nerve in spinal cord processing. Stress-related glucocorticoids may manipulate amygdala function, inducing hypersensitivity to nociceptive input from the heart via central sensitization of upper thoracic spinal neuronal activity.

Cardiac ischaemia depends upon the myocardial oxygen/demand imbalance, in which inadequate myocardial perfusion, hypoxia and metabolic abnormalities, myocardial contractile impairment, and ischaemic ECG changes finally result in symptomatic angina (20). During ischaemic episodes, by anaerobic metabolism, adenosine, bradykinin, and hydrogen ions are released into the circulation, affecting the nociceptive nerve fibres. Capsaicin-sensitive spinal sensory nerves from the heart, which contain transient receptor protein vanilloid-1 (TRPV1) receptors, appear to be important for transmitting nociceptive information from the heart to spinothalamic tract cells (21). Administration of resiniferatoxin (RTX), an ultrapotent capsaicin agonist that targets and desensitizes TRPV1-containing sensory fibres, into the pericardial sac virtually eliminated the nociceptive spinal afferent input to upper thoracic spinal neurones when algesic chemicals excited the cardiac nociceptors.

TRPV1 receptors are non-selective cation channels activated by capsaicin, heat, and hydrogen ions. Especially the activation of TRPV1 ion channels by H^+ ions is considered important, for it leads to an influx of Na^+ and subsequently to a release of substance P and calcitonin gene-related peptide (CGRP), both substances act in nociception and play a role in the pathogenesis of inflammation.

Another ion channel, the acid-sensing ion channels (ASIC) type 3, is also an important mediator of cardiac pain from coronary ischaemia (22). ASICs are proton-gated Na^+-channels, which are present in most, if not all, neurones. The typical ASIC current is transient and is elicited by a rapid drop in the extracellular pH, and especially the ASIC3 type is extremely sensitive to small pH decreases (23). Modest pH shifts (7.4–6.7) during the early onset of myocardial ischaemia can induce sustained activation of ASIC3, whereas lower pH is needed for the activation of TRPV receptors (24). An emerging hypothesis proposes a neurocardiological genetic control during myocardial ischaemia, whereby cardiac nociceptors elicit cardioprotective signals in response to ischaemia (25[editorial]).

In mice it has recently been shown that ASIC3 channels are more sensitive to protons than TRPV1 channels. It was suggested that activation of ASIC3 might prevent ischaemic damage before TRPV1 triggers its nociceptive reflex (26). They further concluded that ASIC3, but not TRPV1, plays a protective role in early ischaemia sensing. Moreover, ASIC3 is preferentially sensitive to lactic acidosis, whereas TRPV1 does not discriminate between lactic acidosis and other forms of acidosis, such as hypercapnea. This hypothesis requires further study, including in humans (vide infra). In summary, experimental studies using animal models have been conducted to elucidate neural mechanisms of angina pectoris, sensitization of cardiac nociceptive stimuli, and neuromodulation of cardiac pain and cardiovascular function (for review see (32)).

The emerging function of the nervous system in the development of atherosclerosis and the putative humoral path from the heart to the brain

The brain governs cardiac functions by means of two controlling efferent pathways: an autonomic nervous pathway and a catecholaminergic humoral pathway. Activation of the efferent pathways induces augmented contractile forces of the heart, increased heart rate, and induced changes in vasomotor status of vessels. Generally, activation of afferent cardiac neural pathways as a consequence of damage resulting from inflammation or myocardial ischaemia, for example, induces symptoms of chest discomfort, labelled as angina pectoris. Furthermore, in addition to an acute coronary syndrome (ACS) or following a coronary artery bypass graft surgery (CABG) many patients experience a period of emotional problems. It is conceivable that both efferent and afferent loops are created to perform neurocardiological interactions between the brain and the heart. Until recently, no reports exist about a humoral afferent pathway from the heart to the brain. For a discussion on how emotional disturbances, following a serious cardiac life event, may be executed by a humoral pathway from the heart to the brain *vide infra*.

Atherosclerotic disease and nervous pathways

In modern times, the rates of change in culture and lifestyle have far exceeded that of biologic evolution, so that the way we live our lives, our life-expectancy, and our disease patterns, are now very different from that of our ancestors. This has become relevant for developed countries, in particular, during the last century and a half. In Western societies, life-expectancy of humans has increased from about 40 years in the mid-nineteenth century to over 80 years at the present time. This improvement in life-expectancy has been made possible through advancements in public health, executed through an interdisciplinary approach, of, among others, physicians, politicians, socio-economic officers, epidemiologists, and industrial participation. The change to a healthier and expected longer-lasting life was mainly the consequence of introducing hygienic facilities (e.g. clean water, bathrooms, sewerage, collecting garbage, etc.), lifestyle changes (e.g. preventive measures with respect to smoking, nutrition, regular exercise, etc.), and better treatment strategies, such as antibiotics. Though cultural changes have improved life-expectancy, significantly, and antibiotics have even reduced mortality further, the complete elimination of infectious plagues does not seem to be realistic, since 'infectious' diseases may have many faces. Maybe as a consequence of the evolutionary capacity of contagious agents to adapt to new ecologic niches, and probably also because evolution has not had time to sort out those individuals with a vulnerability to contemporary diseases, infectious diseases have succeeded in a role in the genesis of chronic degenerative afflictions. So, these newer insights in chronic and often degenerative diseases have caused significant paradigm shifts in our understanding. An example is atherosclerosis, which until recently was considered a 'cultural' disease, whereas our thinking has rapidly changed so that we now consider atherosclerotic diseases to be the result of a chronic (low-grade) inflammation.

The idea whether or not inflammation plays a key role in atherogenesis, i.e. the formation of atheromatous deposits, especially on the innermost layer of arterial wall, led to a controversy in the nineteenth century between Rokitansy ('response to injury' theory followed by inflammation) and Virchow (inflammation as the initiating factor in atherogenesis). This debate seems to be finally settled in favour of the latter. With respect to the initiation of a chronic low-grade inflammatory state, much evidence is provided that many chronic diseases, such as atherosclerosis, 'originate' from an inflammatory status of the gut (27, 28). The inflammatory environment of the gut induces low-grade neuro-inflammatory responses, and among others depends on the nutritive condition of individuals (29). From the available evidence it is further concluded that inflammatory responses of the enteric nervous system of the gut influence brain functions, via a cytokine cascade, specifically via the IL1-activated inflammatory cholinergic nerves. The identified specific pathways (NF kappa-β among others) and involved receptors (Toll-like receptors among others) playing an important role in the gut–brain axis, will not be discussed further in this chapter. In support of the recent literature on the origin of atherosclerosis is the finding that O_2, glucose, and a variety of metabolites are modulating receptors of glomus cells in the gut. When oxygen tension becomes too low, the specialized cells activate the afferent parts of the autonomic reflex system through releasing dopamine and noradrenalin and hence may alter tonic inhibition of the anti-inflammatory–cholinergic pathway (afferent vagus) (30), the so-called gut–brain axis. This afferent humoral pathway is thought to counteract inflammation.

However, during lifetime, the atherosclerotic process proceeds and due to inflammation of larger arterial blood vessels, lipids are deposited as so-called plaques on the arterial wall. The plaques narrow the lumen of the arterial vessels and through hindering blood flow, affect the supply of oxygen and nutrients to organs like the heart, brain, and kidneys. Since, according to recent opinions, atherosclerosis is considered as a generalized inflammatory disease of an individual, it is conceivable that intervening in one affected organ may have an effect on the entire inflammatory state of a person and subsequently influences the function of another organ. Distress in one organ, for instance, following surgery or an infarction, may thus create 'collateral damage'. During myocardial ischaemia, being the underlying cause of cardiac 'pain' in angina pectoris, a cascade of events is triggered that initiates the release of numerous chemical substances into the circulation. All of these chemicals are potential candidates for nociceptor activation and initiation of behavioural and autonomic responses to cardiac pain. Some of the substances released into the circulation may play a role in the humoral interaction between heart and brain. If released chronically, these substances may induce neuropathological modifications, such as anxiety disorders and depression, which frequently are comorbid with ischaemic heart diseases (31). As a consequence of the ischaemic tissue damage in the heart, an immune activation is initiated in which inflammatory response has been found to generate regional blood–brain barrier damage that could be an underlying organic basis for comorbid neuropsychiatric disorders (32). The release of pro-inflammatory cytokines after tissue damage in the heart, therefore, is thought to be the inducer of comorbid neuropsychiatric diseases (33).

Pathophysiology of the nervous system and the heart

Angina and the ischaemic heart: defining the problem of atherosclerotic diseases

In recent years, mortality from cardiovascular diseases has declined significantly, which is credited to the development of a myriad of both therapeutic measures such as medication and revascularization of coronary arteries, and preventive strategies, like tackling risk factors (34). In the entire world, ischaemic heart disease is responsible for 12.8% of all deaths, followed by stroke and other cerebro-vascular diseases, causing 10.8% of all deaths (35). The decline in mortality in the industrial world during the last 60 years, from 450 to 120 per 100,000 inhabitants, is irrespective of population growth (36). As a consequence, more and more people survive the (sequelae of their) heart diseases and so the presence of atherosclerotic disease (i.e. the morbidity) has become a disease burden with huge economic consequences for Western societies. Furthermore, quality of life has become an even more vital issue for the survivors of atherosclerotic diseases. Therefore, characteristics of quality of life have to be taken into account as an end-point in future studies concerning both surgery of the ANS and neuromodulation techniques, such as spinal cord stimulation (see Chapter 9) (37).

Angina and atherosclerotic disease

According to the haemodynamic conception, myocardial ischaemia occurs when the demand of oxygen and nutrients of the myocardial tissue exceeds the required oxygen supply (38). This mismatch may either result from an increased demand (pathologically high heart rates or extremely thickened myocardium), but is most often due to a decreased blood supply through atherosclerotic plaque formation. In the presence of narrowed coronary arteries, the discrepancy between myocardial oxygen consumption and demand is most frequently induced during exercise. The subsequent metabolic changes in the myocyte stimulate the release of a variety of chemicals that activate, among others, specific receptors in the heart. The activated cardiac receptors excite diffuse fibre endings in the myocardium that convey alerting signals via afferent fibres to spino-thalamic tracts that ascend to the cortex, where angina pectoris ultimately becomes cognizant. In addition, the release of chemicals from ischaemic myocytes affects the function of endothelial cells, and so causes vasomotor responses.

Chronic refractory angina

In general, myocardial ischaemia and its symptomatic presentation as angina is adequately treated with (a combination of) pharmacotherapy and revascularization procedures. The latter treatments are executed by percutaneous coronary intervention (PCI) and coronary artery bypass surgery (CABS). However, increasing numbers of patients have become resistant to these conventional therapies. Hence, maximum doses of anti-ischaemic drugs do not adequately reduce complaints of angina. In addition, these patients are not suitable for revascularization procedures, any longer (39). Patients suffering from chronic refractory angina are defined as therapeutically resistant to conventional strategies, when these treatments become depleted (40). The majority of these patients are between 60 and

70 years old, predominantly of the male gender, have received at least one revascularization procedure, have a long history of cardiovascular disease, have experienced at least one myocardial infarction, and have a left ventricular ejection fraction of greater than 40% (41). In addition, complaints of angina have to exist for at least 3 months and myocardial ischaemia has to be documented. Since the exercise capacity of patients suffering from chronic refractory angina is severely restricted, they experience difficulties in performing daily activities. These severe physical limitations and frequently present comorbidities commonly result in symptoms of anxiety or depression (42). Unfortunately, the impact of chronic refractory angina on patients' quality of life and social life is devastating and habitually underestimated (43). Patients suffering from refractory angina are considered to have an altered perception of angina as a result of sensitization of receptors in the myocardium (16, 44, 45). Animal models for angina support the latter (32). When chronic myocardial ischaemia stimulates the mechanical and chemical receptors of the myocardium too frequently, the threshold of these receptors decreases—so-called sensitization (46). It is debatable whether the sensitized nerves exaggerate the symptoms of angina and so dramatically inflate the meaning of a 'warning' signal for a cardiac event, particularly in the absence of an acute coronary syndrome (vide infra).

The exact prevalence and incidence of refractory angina is unknown today; however, it has been estimated that between 100,000 and 900,000 patients are suffering from this condition and another 50,000 new cases could be diagnosed each year in the USA (47, 48). The numbers are still increasing, as mortality from cardiovascular diseases is still declining. So, given the increasing number of patients and the implications of chronic refractory angina, it is for these patients' benefits to offer new therapies focusing on the reduction of both angina and ischaemic burden.

Acute coronary syndromes

The term acute coronary syndrome (ACS) encompasses a group of unstable cardiac conditions, during which a coronary artery is obstructed and the myocardium becomes severely jeopardized. Contrarily to stable angina, the symptoms occurring at rest are not relieved by the use of nitroglycerine, and are commonly accompanied by vaso-vegetative and emotional sensations. The latter symptom may be accompanied with a feeling of dying. Standard therapies to prevent irreversible tissue damage following acute coronary occlusion are aimed at restriction of the duration and extent of myocardial ischaemia.

Both, pharmacotherapy and coronary interventions, mainly percutaneous executed, have demonstrated to significantly improve the outcomes of patients with ACS with regard to morbidity and mortality. Though the nervous system is of paramount importance in controlling cardiac function in the presence of an ACS and more specifically the intrinsic cardiac nervous system, scarce literature is available on modulation of the nervous system during an ACS (49).

Overview of experimental models of neural hierarchy in other heart diseases

Arrhythmias

In Greek mythology, after fighting a war with the Persians, a soldier died immediately after running 42.2 km from Marathon to Athens to tell the administration that the war was won. After training, to date, tens of thousands of persons run marathons, without dying. A properly trained body with a balanced ANS enables us to perform these endeavours and prevent arrhythmias. The ANS is a prominent factor in the induction of both atrial and ventricular arrhythmias. The power of the ANS is known since ancient history. Already in the Bible, Ananias, a member of the early Christian church, died suddenly after being accused of falsehood, which tragedy was followed by the sudden death of his wife Sapphire after hearing the news that her husband had died, unexpectedly (Acts of Apostles: 5).

Irrespective of an underlying (structural) heart disease, sudden death in adults most often results from lethal arrhythmia (50). Therefore, research is directed toward the prevention of serious arrhythmias through modulation of the cardiac nervous system. Modulation of autonomic arrhythmic activity during pathophysiological cardiac conditions, so-called 'autonomic modulation', executed through either autonomic nerve stimulation or autonomic denervation, is suggested to be even effective in the treatment of pharmacotherapeutically refractory arrhythmias.

Heart failure

Circulation of oxygen rich blood is initiated by recurrent contractions of the left ventricle. The cardiac output is the product of stroke volume and heart rate and contraction force. Deterioration of output, AS determined through THESE components, may cause heart failure. Stroke volume and heart rate depend on the state of the autonomic nervous system, which also affects the left ventricle ideally builds up blood pressures to about 120 mmHg. This pressure is sufficient to overcome the distance from left ventricle to brain, against gravity. Then blood pressure gradually drops to a mean of 80 mmHg, which is optimal as filling pressure for oxygen and carbon dioxide exchange in the capillaries. From the capillaries, the oxygen-poor blood returns to the right ventricle through active skeletal muscle contractions and the relatively low pressure in the right heart. The right ventricle pumps the oxygen-poor blood to the lungs for gas exchange at a pressure of about 20–30 mmHg. So, when pressures, volumes, or contraction force change significantly, heart failure comes into sight.

Heart failure is defined as a clinical syndrome characterized by the inability of the heart to supply sufficient blood to the body for subsequently dealing with the metabolic demands of the organs. The symptoms of heart failure depend upon the affected side of the heart. The most important symptoms of heart failure result from either pooling of blood (backward failure) or a reduction in output of the hampered ventricle (forward failure). An impaired function of the left ventricle gives rise to exaggerated feelings of fatigue and shortness of breath, especially during exercise when motor neurones are activated (51).

Malfunction of the right ventricle may cause swelling (oedema) of the lowest parts of the body (frequently feet and legs). In addition to right and left ventricular failure, when the heart has a reduced contractility and so fails to pump sufficient blood into the circulation, the condition is coined as systolic heart failure. In contrast, when the heart fails to return enough blood (resulting from an impaired relaxation of the heart muscle or from abnormal ventricular filling), the cardiac state is termed diastolic failure or heart failure with preserved ejection fraction (HFPEF).

In contrast to heart failure with reduced ejection fraction (HFREF), the role of ANS in HFPEF is not well established (52). According to the American Heart Association, about 5.1 million Americans suffer from all of the above-mentioned types of heart failure; about half of them are females (53). Heart failure in women is frequently the result of long-term high blood pressure, yielding to heart failure with a preserved output, and in men heart failure is most often the outcome of coronary artery disease. As a consequence of improved survival of coronary artery disease, more patients will develop heart failure. Albeit that much progress has been made to develop therapeutic strategies for heart failure related to improvements in lifestyle, medication, and devices, patients with this medical condition face a bad prognosis with a poor quality of life. Furthermore, for some severely restricted patients with decreased cardiac functioning and a subsequent increased risk on developing arrhythmias, current treatment options have become exhausted.

References

1 **Boylan M**. Galen: on blood, the pulse, and the arteries. J Hist Biol 2007;**40**;207–30.

2 **Olshansky B, Sabbah HN, Hauptman PJ et al**. Parasympathetic nervous system and heart failure. Circulation 2008;**118**:863–71.

3 **Langley JN**. The autonomic nervous system. Brain 1903;**26**;1–26.

4 **Mitchell GAG**. Anatomy of the autonomic nervous system. Livingstone Ltd: Edinburgh, London; 1953:1–20, 237–56.

5 **Hildreth V, Anderson RH, Henderson DJ**. Autonomic innervation of the developing heart: origins and function. Clin Anat 2009;**22**:36–46.

6 **Kawashima T**. The autonomic nervous system of the human heart with special reference to its origin, course, and peripheral distribution. Anat Embryol (Berl) 2005;**209**:425–38.

7 **Kawashima T**. Anatomy of the cardiac nervous system with clinical and comparative morphological implications. Anat Sci Int 2011;**86**:30–49.

8 **Vaseghi M, Zhou W, Shi J et al**. Sympathetic innervation of the anterior left ventricular wall by the right and left stellate ganglia. Heart Rhythm 2012. Epub. http://dx.doi.org/10.1016/j.hrthm.2012.03.052.

9 **Heberden W**. Some account of the breast. Med Trans 1772;**2**:58–67.

10 **Kligfield P**. The frustrated benevolence of 'Dr. Anonymous'. Am J Cardiol 1981;**47**:185–87.

11 **Garrison DW, Chandler MJ, Foreman RD**. Viscerosomatic convergence onto feline spinal neurons from esophagus, heart and somatic fields: effects of inflammation. Pain 1992;**49**:373–82.

12 **Diamond GA and Forrester JS**. Probability of coronary artery disease. Circulation 1982;**65**:641–42.

13 **Sheps DS, Creed F, Clouse RE**. Chest pain in patients with cardiac and noncardiac disease. Psychosom Med 2004; **66**:861–67.

14 **Shepard JD, Barron KW, Myers DA.** Corticosterone delivery to the amygdala increases corticotropin-releasing factor mRNA in the central amygdaloid nucleus and anxiety-like behavior. Brain Res 2000;**861**:288–95.

15 **Rozen JB, Schulkin J.** From normal fear to pathological anxiety. Psychol Rev 1998;**105**:325–50.

16 **Foreman RD, Qin C.** Neuromodulation of cardiac pain and cerebral vasculature: neural mechanisms. Cleve Clin J Med 2009;**76**(Suppl. 2):S75–79.

17 **Lindgren I, Olivecrona H.** Surgical treatment of angina pectoris. J Neurosurg 1947; **4**:19–39.

18 **White JC, Bland EF.** The surgical relief of severe angina pectoris: methods employed and end results in 83 patients. Medicine 1948;**27**:1–42.

19 **Foreman RD.** Mechanisms of cardiac pain. Annu Rev Physiol, 1999;**61**:143–67.

20 **Rosen, SD.** From heart to brain: the genesis and processing of cardiac pain. Can J Cardiol 2012;**28**:S7–19.

21 **Qin C, Farber JP, Miller KE et al.** Responses of thoracic spinal neurons to activation and desensitization of cardiac TRPV1-containing afferents in rats. Am J Physiol Regul Integr Comp Physiol 2006;**291**:R1700–707.

22 **Sutherland SP, Benson CJ, Adelman JP et al.** Acid-sensing ion channel 3 matches the acid-gated current in cardiac ischemia-sensing neurons. Proc Natl Acad Sci 2001;**98**:711–16.

23 **Gründer S, Chen X.** Structure, function, and pharmacology of acid-sensing ion channels (ASICs): focus on ASIC1a. Int J Physiol Pathophysiol Pharmacol 2010;**2**;73–94.

24 **Yagi J, Wenk HN, Naves LA et al.** Sustained currents through ASIC3 ion channels at the modest pH changes that occur during myocardial ischemia. Circ Res 2006;**99**:501–09.

25 **Bolli R, Abdel-Latif A.** No pain, no gain: The useful function of angina. Circulation 2005;**112**:3541–43.

26 **Chenq CT, Chen IL, Chenq MH et al.** Acid-sensing ion Channel 3, but not capsaicin receptor TRPV1, plays a protective role in isoproterenol-induced myocardial ischemia in mice. Circulation J 2011;**75**:174–78.

27 **Mayer EA.** Gut feelings: the emerging biology of gut-brain communication. Nat Rev Neurosci 2011;**12**:453–66.

28 **McLean PG, Bergonzelli GE, Collins SM et al.** Targeting the microbiota-gut-brain axis to modulate behavior: Which bacterial strain will translate best to humans? Proc Natl Acad Sci U S A. 2012;**109**(4):E174; author reply E176. doi: 10.1073/pnas.1118626109. Epub 2012 Jan 13.

29 **Kinross JM, Darzi AW, Nicholson JK.** Gut microbiome-host reactin in health and disease. Genome Med 2011;**3**:14.

30 **Tracey KJ.** Reflex control of immunity. Nature Reviews 2009, **9**:418–28.

31 **Tully PJ, Penninx BW.** Depression and anxiety among coronary heart disease patients: can affect dimensions and theory inform diagnostic disorder-based screening? J Clin Psychol. 2012 Apr;**68**(4):448–61. doi: 10.1002/jclp.21828. Epub 2012 Feb 3

32 **DeJongste MJ, Terhorst GJ, Foreman RD.** Basic research models for the study of underlying mechanisms of electrical neuromodulation and ischemic heart-brain interactions. Cleve Clin J Med 2009 Apr;**76**(Suppl. 2): S41–46 (Review).

33 **Liu H, Luiten PG, Eisel UL et al.** Depression after myocardial infarction: TNF-α-induced alterations of the blood-brain barrier and its putative therapeutic implications. Neurosci Biobehav Rev 2013 May;**37**(4):561–72. doi:10.1016/j.neubiorev.2013.02.004. Epub 2013 Feb 13 (Review).

34 **Hoyert D.** 75 years of mortality in the United States, 1935–2010. NCHS Data B 2012;**88**:1–8.

35 World Health Organization link: http://www.who.int/mediacentre/factsheets/fs310/en/index.html.

36 **Nabel EG, Braunwald E.** A tale of coronary artery disease and myocardial infarction. N Engl J Med 2012;**366**:54–63.

37 **Anderson VC, Carlson C, Shatin D.** Outcomes of spinal cord stimulation: patient validation. Neuromodulation 2001;**4**:11–17.

38 **Bing RJ.** Coronary circulation and cardiac metabolism. In: Fishman AP and Richards DW (eds) Circulation of the Blood: Men and Ideas. New York: Oxford University Press, 1964:199–264.

39 **Mannheimer C, Camici P, Chester MR et al.** The problem of chronic refractory angina. Eur Heart J 2002;**23**:355–70.

40 **Jessurun GAJ, Meeder JG, DeJongste MJL.** Defining the problem of intractable angina. Pain Reviews 1997;**4**:89–99.

41 **Ten Vaarwerk IAM. Jessurun GAJ, DeJongste MJL et al.** On behalf of the working group neurocardiology. Baseline characteristics of patients with refractory AP treated with SCS. Heart 1999;**82**:82–89.

42 **Josephus Jitta DJ, DeJongste MJL, Kliphuis CM, et al.** Multimorbidity, the predominant predictor of quality-of-life, following successful spinal cord stimulation for angina pectoris. Neuromodulation 2011;**14**:13–18.

43 **Vulnink NCC, Overgaauw DM, Jessurun GAJ et al.** The effects of spinal cord stimulation on quality of life in patients with therapeutically refractory angina pectoris. Neuromodulaton 1999;**2**(1):29–36.

44 **Svorkdal N.** Treatment of inoperable coronary disease and refractory angina: spinal stimulators, epidurals, gene therapy, transmyocardial laser, and counterpulsation. Semin Cardiothorac Vasc Anesth 2004;43–58.

45 **Ji RR, Kohno T, Moore KA, Woolf CJ.** Central sensitization and LTP: do pain and memory share similar mechanisms? Trends Neurosci 2003;**26**:696–705.

46 **Sylvén C.** Neurophysiological aspects of angina pectoris. Z Kardiol 1997;**86** Suppl 1:95–105.

47 **Manchanda A, Aggarwal A, Aggarwal N, Soran O.** Management of refractory angina pectoris. Cardiology J 2011;**18**: 343–51.

48 **Henry TD, Satran D, Jolicoeur EM.** Nat Rev Cardiol 2014 Feb;**11**(2):78–95. doi:10.1038/nrcardio.2013. 200. Review. Erratum in: Nat Rev Cardiol. 2014 Feb;11(2):i. Treatment of refractory angina in patients not suitable for revascularization.

49 **de Vries J, DeJongste MJ, Zijlstra F, Staal M.** Long-term effects of electrical neurostimulation in patients with unstable angina: refractory to conventional therapies. Neuromodulation. 2007 Oct;**10**(4):345–8. doi: 10.1111/j.1525-1403.2007.00121.x.

50 **Hookana E, Junttila MJ, Puurunen VP et al.** Causes of nonischemic sudden cardiac death in the current era. Heart Rhythm 2011;**8**:1570–75.

51 **Ranieri F1, Di Lazzaro V.** The role of motor neuron drive in muscle fatigue. Neuromuscul Disord 2012;(Suppl. 3):S157–61. doi: 10.1016/j.nmd.2012.10.006.

52 **Patel H, Ozdemir BA, Patel M et al.** Impairment of autonomic reactivity is a feature of heart failure whether or not the left ventricular ejection fraction is normal. Int J Cardiol 2011 Aug 18;**151**(1):34–39. doi: 10.1016/j.ijcard.2010.04.054. Epub 2010 May 18.

53 **Go AS, Mozaffarian D, Roger VL et al.** Heart disease and stroke statistics—2013 update: a report from the American Heart Association. Circulation 2013;**127**:e6–e245.

Chapter 7

Evolution and developments in autonomic control of the heart II: therapeutical interventions

Mike J. L. DeJongste, Michiel Kuijpers, Gerbrand J. Groen, and Robert D. Foreman

Key points

1. Refractory therapeutical cardiovascular diseases.
2. Recent developments in neuro-ablative surgery.
3. Recent developments in electrical neuromodulation therapies.
4. (Potential) cardiac indications for neuromodulation.
5. Mechanism of action of electrical neuromodulation.

Introduction

In the wake of the dilemma of improved survival in coronary artery disease and the subsequent increase in morbidity (see Chapter 6), a variety of adjuvant therapies have been developed for patients suffering from chronic (refractory) angina. Newer therapies can be divided into four groups: pharmacological (e.g. Ranalozine®, a drug that is thought to prevent calcium overload by affecting the late sodium-dependent current in the presence of myocardial ischaemia and Ivabradine®, a selective inhibitor of the sinus node—the inhibition is executed via specific I_f channels); invasive non-pharmacological procedures, such as local injection into the heart with stem cells, or with growth factors to induce angiogenesis; non-pharmacological non-invasive (e.g. transcutaneous neurostimulation and external enhanced counter-pulsation); and non-pharmacological invasive (laser therapy and spinal cord stimulation, (SCS) or nerve ablative strategies (1, 2).

Given the differences in outcome measures, such as efficacy, safety, cost-effectiveness, the lack of direct comparative studies, and the different safety profiles, electrical neuromodulation is considered in the algorithm for refractory angina as one of the first additional therapies to be chosen (2). Of the additional therapies, electrical neuromodulation has further been shown to be one of the most effective and safest (3).

In this chapter, the focus is on ablative and electrical neuromodulation for the treament of a variety of cardiac diseases. Electrical neuromodulation can be performed through stimulation (or blocking/ablation) of the stellate ganglion, transcutaneous electrical nerve stimulation (TENS), SCS, sub-cutaneous electrical nerve stimulation (SENS, also coined peripheral nerve [field] stimulation and subQ stimulation), and vagal nerve stimulation (VNS). To date, an increase in research effort in the field of cardiology is directed onto the autonomic nervous system and its role in myocardial ischaemia, arrhythmias, and heart failure. Modulation of these three components will be further discussed in this chapter.

Brief historical perspective of neuromodulation for cardiac diseases, executed by ablative therapies and modulation of neurones

Surgery of the autonomic system

The cardiovascular system is directed to adjust sufficient blood supply to meet the metabolic requirements of organs through changes in heart rate, blood pressure, and contractile force. The neural hierarchy in cardiac control enables the function of organs, among others the heart, to meet conditions requiring adjustment in metabolism to maintain organ function. To prevent the nervous system from affecting the function of visceral organs like the heart, the involved signals can be modified by dissection of the nerve itself. This rather crude, irreversible method of interrupting the nervous system was originally accomplished by performing a true sympathectomy, thus surgical removal of a section of the sympathetic chain using open surgical techniques. This type of surgery has been performed since the very end of the nineteenth century, when Alexander operated on the upper sympathetic system to treat various conditions, including epilepsy, glaucoma, causalgia, hyperhidrosis, and also angina pectoris, two decades later (4). Different approaches to disrupt nerve function have been developed since the 1920s, resulting in the 'minimally invasive' video-assisted thoracoscopic surgery (VATS) sympathectomy or endoscopic thoracic sympathectomy (ETS) in 1990 (5). This VATS procedure has been recently developed as the method of choice for sympathectomy.

There is on-going debate about the preferred method of sympathicolysis with respect to the side-effects of the method, the appropriate level of dissection, and how selective the nerve should be dissected. The conventional sympathectomy is more and more replaced by a sympathicotomy, that is dividing, however, not excising, the sympathetic chain at certain levels, and hence sparing the ganglia (Fig. 7.1). While presumed equally effective, the sympathicotomy is thought to produce fewer side-effects on cardio-respiratory function (6). Classically, ETS is performed using three thoracic entry-ports for camera and surgical instruments. Recently, experience has been obtained with truly minimal invasive surgical techniques, requiring just one single 7 mm trans-axillary surgical access-port (7).

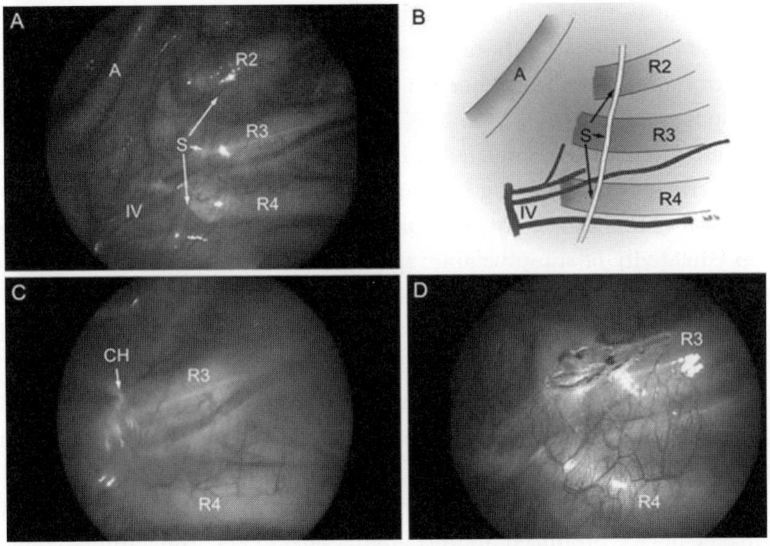

Fig. 7.1 Intra-operative view of a single-port VATS sympathicotomy. The lung is collapsed, offering full view of the operative field. (A, B) The sympathetic chain can be seen through the parietal pleura, running along the neck of the second, third and fourth rib. (C) Cauterization of the chain by diathermy on a high costal level (third rib). (D) Close-up of situation after sympathicolysis. Through the opened parietal pleura, the divided sympathetic chain is visible, the transection is extended 2 cm laterally over the rib to transect possible accessory nerve fibres, and an active search for Kuntz's nerve is performed. Such a nerve is transected when present.

However, even the most selective sympathetic denervation procedure remains by nature an irreversible and destructive treatment modality, and almost uniformly requires general anaesthesia. Moreover, since the procedure is executed by a thoracic, vascular, or neurosurgeon, this denervation method necessitates both referral and interdisciplinary teamwork. Complications with respect to the surgical procedure are scarce, but include, among others, pneumothorax and Horner's syndrome. In addition, re-innervation may occur.

Modulation of the autonomic system

As an alternative to ablation, much evidence is provided with respect to stimulation of nerves for a variety of indications. Electrical stimulation of dorsal columns of the spinal cord, spinal cord stimulation (SCS), has been used to treat patients with angina pectoris that cannot be treated with conventional therapies. This will be discussed in much greater detail in subsequent sections. The concept of SCS is based on the model of the 'Gate Control Theory', as postulated by Melzack and Wall in their landmark study, in 1965 (8). They proposed that large myelinated Aβ-fibres affect nociceptive information processed in unmyelinated (C-fibres) and relatively slow-conducting Aδ-fibres, via inter-neurones. So, stimulation of the myelinated afferent fibres decreases the amount of information coming from the nociceptive afferent nerves to reduce the nociceptive sensation, via the closing of a neuronal 'gate' in the dorsal horn of the spinal cord. The proposed model provides a scientific base for stimulation of myelinated fibres to induce electro-analgesia through electrical neuromodulation. Introduced in 1967, electrical neurostimulation was found to effectively suppress pain (9).

Animal studies have been conducted to better understand the possible neural mechanisms that underlie SCS for treating patients with refractory angina pectoris (10). Spinal cord stimulation of the T1–T2 dorsal columns in an anaesthetized animal model significantly reduced activity of spinothalamic tract neurones in response to activation of the cardiac nociceptors with an algesic chemical bradykinin (see Chapter 6). The limiting factor of this study was using animals with normal hearts; study of hearts with previous infarction or ischaemic hearts would be more relevant, clinically. Nevertheless, this study shows that nociceptive cardiac information transmitted in the spinothalamic tract is significantly decreased during SCS, because SCS activated inhibitory mechanisms in the spinal grey matter.

In 1967, Braunwald et al. reported that stellate ganglion stimulation by means of a modified pacemaker device produced an anti-angina effect (11). The authors coincidentally observed a normalization of the ST–T segment shift in response to electrical stimulation in a patient experiencing a myocardial infarction (12). However, in spite of beneficial anti-anginal effects, stimulation of the stellate ganglion as therapy for angina was gradually abandoned, since in the seventies coronary artery bypass surgery came into vogue. Following the initial encouraging results of stellate ganglion stimulation as novel treatment for angina, a decade later some patients developed angina that could not be relieved any longer by bypass surgery. As a consequence, newer neuromodulation techniques have been developed. In 1982, TENS was reported for the first time as an effective method to reduce both intensity and frequency of angina attacks and to increase exercise capacity (13, 14). Even though TENS is an effective, safe, and rather cheap therapy, the disadvantage of this external device, is that gel pads come off easily on hairy chests and during perspiration, and that it frequently induced skin irritation (15, 16). Due to these disadvantages, the use of the transcutaneous method of electrical stimulation increasingly shifted to a fully implanted spinal cord stimulating systems. SCS initially was also referred to as dorsal column stimulation (DCS) or epidural spinal cord electrical stimulation (ESES).

Furthermore, retrospective studies have shown that SCS appears to have a more sustained effect than TENS (17). Outcomes of studies on the anti-angina effect of SCS were first published in 1987 (18). In their observational study, the authors reported a reduction of both frequency and intensity of angina attacks and decreased the need for short-acting nitrates in patients with angina and SCS. Since then many studies have been published (vide infra) advocating the beneficial effects of SCS in patients with refractory angina. Albeit that SCS is accepted in both European and American guidelines, many potential candidates are not being treated with SCS, since cardiologists have not greatly accepted neuromodulation methods. This lack of enthusiasm appears to be related to, among others, cardiologists who do not perform the implants themselves, but have to refer patients to an implanter, most often an anaesthesiologist or a neurosurgeon. In addition, cardiologists often deny the problem of refractory angina. Moreover, after an estimate of 10,000 SCS implants for angina, worldwide, the underlying mechanisms of electrical neuromodulation are only clarified in part. Finally, follow-up has to be carefully executed by a dedicated technician or physician. These arguments may be an explanation for the lack of SCS implants with respect to the referral of potential candidates. To overcome part of the under-use of SCS for angina, we and others, performed studies to assess the feasibility of sub-cutaneous electrical nerve stimulation (SENS), also referred to as (sub-cutaneous) peripheral nerve stimulation, peripheral field stimulation, sub-cutaneous target stimulation, or sub-cutaneous electrical nerve stimulation (19). In a pilot study we have demonstrated that SENS may be a feasible alternative to TENS and SCS (20). Our preliminary results on the efficacy of SENS in the treatment of refractory angina have recently been substantiated by another small study (21). So, in addition to the relatively simple surgery that can easily be carried out by trained physicians, like cardiologists, SENS theoretically carries lower complication risks when compared to SCS. Further, SENS is thought to employ the convenience of SCS, and is able to sustain at least a similar efficacy as SCS (22). However, before SENS can be applied as a routine treatment, the preliminary studies have to be repeated in a large, randomized controlled setting.

Rationale for target selection and approach of modulation of the nervous system in the management of cardiac diseases

To assess measures like efficacy, safety, and costs of the different methods, double-blind, randomized, controlled trials (RCTs) are required. RCTs for comparison of the different electrical neuromodulation modalities or to compare the different adjunct methods in the treatment of angina are difficult to perform because the patient is aware of the paresthesias and the physician may observe the artefacts on the ECG. However, it is feasible to randomize patients to a treatment group, receiving active neurostimulation via the implanted device, and a control group, also receiving the implanted device but no neurostimulation for a given period of time.

In clinical studies, after an arbitrary period of 6–26 weeks, the device in the control group is switched to the active mode. From this moment, the study is no longer randomized and the entire group can be followed-up. Regarding the study design, a real placebo study can theoretically be executed when the stimulation does not provoke artefacts on the ECG. Sub-threshold neurostimulation has been shown to have comparable effects as neurostimulation-induced paresthesias. However, recently studies addressing sub-threshold neurostimulation resulted in conflicting outcomes, with respect to efficacy (23, 24). Subsequently, blinding of both the subject and the investigator remains a problem in studies on neuromodulation and angina.

In general, the function of the heart can be examined through several investigative approaches, depending on the cardiac disease. In brief, in addition to history and physical examination for angina assessment of outcomes measures are executed by means of cost/benefit assessments, perceived quality of life (studied by means of diaries and questionnaires), and functional tests. To study the efficacy of electrical neuromodulation for cardiac diseases, all of the following additional tools have been used: exercise stress testing, ambulatory ECG monitoring, right atrial pacing, echocardiography, nuclide tracing studies on myocardial perfusion, and coronary angiography (including flow studies). To evaluate the pumping function of the heart, exercise stress tests, echocardiography, cine-angiography, and magnetic resonance imaging are performed. Finally, with reference to previous tests, assessment of arrhythmias is done through ambulatory ECG registrations (Holter monitoring), stress exercise testing, and electrophysiological studies.

Accepted and emerging cardiac indications for electrical neuromodulation

Angina and electrical neuromodulation and patient selection

Adequate selection of patients results in 80% overall success rate of SCS after 4 years. In agreement with the care algorithm, treatment of chronic refractory angina starts with non-invasive electrical neuromodulation, performed by using TENS (2, 25). If TENS is successful but adverse events occur, such as the frequently observed skin irritation through an ortho-ergic contact dermatitis (15, 16), treatment with SCS or SENS is instigated. In the past, research on the anti-angina effect of the different modalities of electrical neuromodulation has been carried out. To date, TENS, SCS, or SENS all have been proven to be successful within the armamentarium for the treatment of angina. The predominant inclusion criterion is that the patient must be capable to execute (switching the device 'on' and 'off' and comprehend) the therapy (see also screening tools).

Heart failure and electrical neuromodulation

When the heart fails to meet the metabolic demands of the body, usually as a result of ischaemic heart disease, the hampered systolic left ventricular function and over-stressed neuro-hormonal activation reflect a poor prognosis. Therefore, treatment strategies to reduce symptoms and improve the prognosis of patients with heart failure have been developed during the last decades. Among others, present standard therapies for heart failure include lifestyle changes (fluid and salt intake restrictions), pharmacotherapeutics (β-blockers, diuretics, and renin–angiotensin system modifiers), and devices. The implantable cardioverter defibrillators (ICD) and cardiac resynchronization therapy (CRT) have been shown to reduce mortality. However, not every patient suffering from heart failure is suitable for these devices. Nevertheless, there is a considerable need for new therapies, because mortality from heart failure remains high. The encouraging effects of electrical neuromodulation in the treatment of patients suffering from angina pectoris may also be applicable to patients suffering from other cardiac diseases, such as heart failure, since the autonomic nervous system also has a dominant role in heart failure. (26)

Arrhythmias and electrical neuromodulation

Patients with congenital or acquired structural changes of the heart may encounter serious arrhythmias. Initiated by a trigger (usually an extra-systole) and in the presence of a modifying factor (frequently the autonomic nervous system) the structural altered myocardial substrate becomes the matrix for (fatal) arrhythmias. Acquired symptomatic arrhythmias, most often of ventricular origin, usually result from inhomogeneous activation of the heart as a consequence of an inherited or ischaemically induced, unstable electrical activation of the heart. Since the autonomic nervous system is involved in the genesis of arrhythmias, preventive treatment of these serious arrhythmias can be performed by pharmacotherapeutics, such as anti-arrhythmic agents or β-blocking agents. Because most anti-arrhythmic agents have been shown to increase mortality, they have been largely abandoned (27). In contrast, to date β-blocking is still frequently used to constructively affect the sympathetic limb of the autonomic nervous system.

Technical details of neurostimulation procedures

To apply transcutaneous electrical nerve stimulation (TENS) requires placing small pads with gel on the skin of the chest covering the area where the patient is experiencing angina. The pads are wired to a small box containing a chip, software, and batteries having a size of about 6 × 4 cm. The delivered current induces a tingling sensation. The modality is considered to be simple and safe. In addition, the method is reversible and provides a long-term effect of about 60% after 4 years in a group of well-selected patients. Training to get used to the method and improve condition by means of a rehabilitation programme is recommended (2, 25).

The implantable nerve stimulating device delivers electrical current (amps or volts) to surrounding structures, such as nerves. Under light sedation, the neurostimulation device is connected to one or more leads containing 4–16 electrodes. For the treatment of angina with SCS, the electrodes of the lead are usually placed between C7 and T2. The device is most often implanted in the abdomen at the left lateral side just above the belt position. The surgical procedure of an SCS device implantation is comparable to the implantation of a cardiac pacemaker. Surgery is most often performed by a trained neurosurgeon or anaesthesiologist, making use of fluoroscopic control during the procedure. A multidisciplinary collaboration between cardiologist, pain specialist, implanter, and technician is essential during selection of the patients, assistance during the surgical procedure, and follow-up.

Patients have to be competent to switch the neurostimulation device to an 'on' or 'off' position. So, they have to be capable of using the patient programmer or magnet. Activation of the device induces paresthesias over the site where the electrodes are positioned. Habitually, the paresthesias correspond with the area where angina is experienced, even though controversy exists as to whether covering the entire region of angina is really necessary (23, 24). SCS also has found to have long-term benefical effects on cost-effectiviness.

SCS as an accepted therapy for refractory angina requires correct placement of leads and electrodes into the epidural space for covering the area where angina is felt. Furthermore, some patients are not eligible for SCS due to anomalies of the spinal cord anatomy or, for instance, because of the threat of a myocardial infarction or cerebral vascular accident when anticoagulants are withheld, peri-operatively.

The SENS method is another approach to relieve refractory angina. With this method leads containing 4–8 electrodes are placed sub-cutaneously along the sternum, at the site where the patient feels angina. Leads are connected to a neurostimulation device implanted in the upper abdominal wall or at the left-upper thoracic site. In general, sub-cutaneous lead implantation is easier and theoretically has less serious complications, compared to SCS. In addition, an (interventional) cardiologist can safely perform the sub-cutaneous lead and neurostimulator implantation.

Outcomes of spinal cord stimulation on cardiac diseases

As a consequence of improved survival, an increasing number of patients with cardiac diseases have become refractory to standard therapies. In this review of the literature we discuss electrical neuromodulation for treatment of chronic heart diseases, such as chronic refractory angina and heart failure. Extensive reviews on underlying mechanisms of neuromodulation have been published elsewhere (10, 28, 29).

Chronic angina refractory to standard therapies

Screening tools for patients

Habitually, patients with refractory angina also suffer from comorbidities, which may influence the results of SCS (30). Furthermore, the personality of these patients may affect the efficacy of electrical neuromodulation therapies (31). Before applying neuromodulation, screening of these parameters may further improve the outcomes.

Efficacy

In, observational studies, registries and randomized studies on SCS, improvement in quality of life was found (23, 24, 30) even if patients were treated with neuromodulation for unstable refractory angina (32). Making use of diaries and questionnaires, quality of life measures are usually expressed as a reduction in complaints of angina in conjunction with a decrease in nitroglycerine intake and an increase exercise tolerance. In addition to clinical studies, experimental studies have provided suggestions for the underlying mechanisms for the decrease in myocardial ischaemia (33) during electrical neuromodulation. Finally, neuromodulation has no adverse effect on mortality (34, 35). With respect to the latter, electrical neuromodulation does not block complaints of angina, but defers the sensitized threshold for angina (36). As a consequence, evidence is provided on the failure of SCS to block complaints of angina during an acute myocardial infarction (37). Several studies have demonstrated that the encouraging outcomes of SCS on angina are maintained long-term (30, 32, 34, 38). Thus, SCS has been accepted in the

American Heart Association/American College of Cardiology guidelines on angina, for a decade (39).

A recent review on observational studies provides evidence for the consistent beneficial effects of SCS (40) in the 'real world', used as adjunct treatment, for patients with refractory angina (2, 41). In addition, two meta-analyses of seven randomized studies on SCS, applied in patients suffering from refractory angina, have substantiated the outcomes of observational studies (42, 43).

Safety

A favourable aspect of electrical neuromodulation is that the effects of all of these modalities are reversible, since stimulation can be withheld at any time and, when required, the implanted device can be removed. The combination of an implantable neuromodulation device with cardiac pacemakers, or implantable cardio-defibrillators (ICD), appears to be safe, when preventive measures are taken into account, such as bipolar stimulation and executing a testing procedure encompassing the creation of conditions of potential interference (44, 45). However, there is a potential danger of inhibiting a potential appropriate ICD shock, specifically when TENS is used (46). Further, the implanted neuromodulation device may trigger the ICD to deliver an inappropriate shock. Potential interferences are not only related to output and sensing, but also depend on the position of the body. Therefore, since not all circumstances can be simulated to address medico-legal and safety concerns, combining devices is still debatable (47).

Regarding the latter, it remains imperative not to use a method that abolishes complaints of angina during acute coronary events. However, according to the available literature patients do experience symptoms of angina in the presence of active electrical neuromodulation during an acute myocardial infarction (37, 48–51). Moreover, during active stimulation in the presence of an acute myocardial infarction, myocardial ischaemia was reduced (vide infra) (12, 52). Experimental evidence is provided by a study showing that propagation of impulses from heart to brain is not suppressed (36). Finally, electrical neuromodulation has not been shown to affect morbidity and mortality adversely (50, 53).

Mechanisms of action

Both, clinical and basic studies have reported on the underlying mechanisms of electrical neuromodulation to employ its anti-ischaemic effects (23, 54–58). Moreover, electrical neuromodulation has been shown to affect the catecholamine metabolism (59), improve lactate metabolism (33), and affect local myocardial turnover of β-endorphin and calcitonin-gene-related peptide (60). In contrast, naloxone was unable to antagonize the anti-ischaemic effects of SCS (61).

In summary, anti-anginal effects and anti-ischaemic properties of electrical neuromodulation in ischaemic cardiac conditions have been demonstrated to be the result of modulation of the processing of cardiac nociceptive stimuli within the neural hierarchy of cardiac control (62, 63) and the enhancement of ischaemic tolerance, resulting from improvement in collateral perfusion and myocardial preconditioning (56, 57).

Acute coronary syndromes

In many clinical studies, the authors reported that electrical neuromodulation employs anti-ischaemic effects and so favourably affects the consequences of myocardial ischaemia, (reviews 1, 3, 29, 58) even in the presence of a myocardial infarction (12, 52). We therefore have studied patients experiencing an acute myocardial infarction. With active TENS, a significant decrease in ST–T elevation was observed, when compared to a control group without TENS, after the primary percutaneous coronary intervention was performed in 38 patients with a ST–T elevation myocardial infarction (STEMI) (52). To assess the underlying mechanism of the protective effect of electrical neuromodulation on myocardial ischaemia, we examined the effect of 5 minutes of TENS on collateral perfusion during coronary occlusion performed through percutaneous coronary intervention (PCI) in 60 randomized patients with chronic stable angina (64). The latter study showed that application of TENS, only 5 minutes before PCI, significantly improved both, collateral perfusion and myocardial ischemia (i.e. ST-T elevation).

It is yet unknown whether this reduction in change of ST–T segment following an acute myocardial infarction has an impact on the prognosis. Furthermore, in 21 out of 26 patients with unstable refractory angina, during long-term follow-up (6.6 ± 4.1 years) excellent results were reported with respect to angina complaints and hospital admissions (32). In addition, in a randomized, controlled study, the outcomes of the retrospective study were confirmed (65). The clinical observations corroborate with experimental findings of a rabbit study by Southerland et al. (57). The researchers demonstrate that pre-emptive SCS reduces the risk zone of a myocardial infarction. Moreover, the authors showed a cardioprotective effect of SCS, mediated by modulation of α-sympathetic cardiac neurones and an increased phosphorylation of cardiac protein kinase C. The latter is an important mediator in ischemic preconditioning (66).

In conclusion, it is very well conceivable that the deleterious consequences of myocardial ischaemia, specifically in the presence of a myocardial infarction, are limited through active pre-emptive electrical neuromodulation, resulting in normalization of the exaggerated activity of the intrinsic cardiac nervous system and improvement in ischaemic tolerance of the cardiac myocyte.

Heart failure

For an increasing number of patients with heart failure, current treatment options are unsatisfactory. These patients are disabled due to a severe decrease in exercise capacity in conjunction with an increased risk to develop (fatal) arrhythmias. Until very recently, only one clinical study was published on SCS and heart failure (67). The authors reported a reduction in the deterioration in left ventricular function during adenosine provocation with SCS. It is debatable whether this observation should be judged as the result of an altered modulation of adenosine handling or to a direct improvement in ejection fraction, following active SCS.

Notwithstanding the lack of evidence on alterations of indices of ventricular function in studies with electrical neuromodulation assessed in patients with refractory angina, experimental studies making use of heart failure models have shown that SCS employs favourable effects on ventricular functioning and reduces the risk for ventricular arrhythmias. The common denominator in SCS for treating cardiac diseases is the autonomic nervous system. Therefore, it is feasible that modulation of the autonomic nervous system may provide beneficial changes in the outcomes of patients with heart failure. At present, related to the slow progress made in the development of newer pharmacological agents to treat heart failure, the interest in neuromodulation for treating heart failure is growing. In this regard, results of a pre-clinical randomized SCS study in a canine model of heart failure are relevant (68). The left ventricular ejection fraction (LVEF) improved from a mean of 18 to 45% after 5 weeks of active neurostimulation in the SCS group but not in the control or medication group. In a second study, making use of the same heart failure model, the improvement in LVEF was sustained for 10 weeks.

In an experimental study, Zamotrinsky et al. observed beneficial effects of vagal nerve stimulation in patients with coronary artery disease (69). The authors found that vagal nerve stimulation induces dilatation of cardiac micro-circulatory vessels and subsequently improved left ventricular contractility in patients with severe coronary artery disease. In 2008, Schwartz et al. were the first to report an improvement in left ventricular performance and dyspnoea in a feasibility study of eight patients with systolic heart failure after 6 months of stimulation of the right vagal nerve (70).To date, application of electrical neuromodulation in patients with heart failure is the subject of several on-going clinical studies to assess the effect of nervous modulation on systolic heart failure (among others: NECTAR-HF (71); SCS-Heart (72); DEFEAT-HF [SCS] (73); INOVATE [vagal nerve stimulation] (74); TensIC (75)). In contrast to both, basic studies (68) and observational studies (67, 72) the results of randomized studies are disappointing (71, 73). However, combination of SCS and ICD was found to be safe (76).

It seems, however, too early to draw definite conclusions whether or not electrical neuromodulation is successful as adjunct therapy for patients with heart failure since sample size and end points of the studies differ.

Arrhythmias

Recent work by Issa *et al.* found that in an experimental model autonomic stimulation prevents ventricular arrhythmias (77). Others observed an additional improvement of the left ventricular function (68). In a recent review on autonomic modulation of the heart, Stavrakis *et al* reported that stimulation of intrinsic cardiac neurones affects all kind of arrhythmias (78). In this regard it is conceivable that electrical neuromodulation may also prevent serious arrhythmias. In a recent experimental study, pigs were randomized to SCS or sham control, following a 45-minute occlusion of a coronary artery (79). The incidence of ventricular arrhythmias was significantly reduced in the group with SCS when compared to controls. Their findings corroborate another study on canine post-ischaemia-induced heart failure. In the group with active SCS, the overall incidence of ischaemic-induced ventricular arrhythmias was reduced from 59 to 23% (77).

In summary, there is paucity of information about the clinical efficacy of electrical neuromodulation on ventricular arrhythmias (80). This may be related to bias in the study population, since patients suffering from end-stage coronary artery disease are considered as survivors of their disease. These patients with refractory angina most often maintain their left ventricular function and do not experience serious arrhythmias.

Regarding the autonomic nervous system, electrical neuromodulation is thought to mediate its advantageous achievements through an effect on (α-) sympathetic or on the parasympathetic nervous system. Earlier publications advocated a sympathicolytic effect of SCS (81). This hypothesis was soon challenged by clinical studies that did not show a change in heart rate variability (HRV), a measure of autonomic function (82–84). However, the latter findings are in contrast with a recent study using only 30 minutes of SCS to significantly influence the sympathetic–parasympathetic balance, resulting in a reduction of the sympathetic modulation (85). Of note, the latter investigators have used another HRV measure and different neurostimulation parameters. In a clinical study, researchers failed to demonstrate a change in cardiac norepinephrine spill-over during SCS (86). Finally, two studies with positron emission tomography were unable to demonstrate changes in cardiac sympathetic function cardiac innervation following SCS (87, 88).

In contrast to studies addressing the sympathetic limb of the autonomic nervous system, in an experimental study performed in 47 dogs, SCS was found to enhance parasympathetic activity via vagal nerve stimulation (89). Their findings corroborate the encouraging effects of electrical neurostimulation on ventricular arrhythmias. In a recent review, Brack et al. discussed the promising findings of vagal nerve stimulation on both improvement of cardiac performance and increased threshold for ventricular fibrillation (90).

Irrespective of the parasympathetic or sympathetic modulation, the common mechanistic denominator is the intrinsic cardiac nervous system (63, 91, 92). Recently, it was found that electrical neurostimulation of the right inferior ganglionated plexus, which selectively innervates the atrioventricular node, reduces the ventricular rate during atrial fibrillation (93). In this respect, a recent study is of interest. Disproportionate stimulation of mediastinal nerves on the superior vena cava activated the intrinsic cardiac neurones, resulting in 78% of the cases in atrial arrhythmias, leading to atrial fibrillation. When pre-emptive SCS was applied, stabilization of the intrinsic cardiac local circuit neurones was found with a subsequently reduction in atrial arrhythmias (94).

The future: further improvements in integrative approaches on interfaces between heart and nervous system

The potential power of the autonomic nervous system on cardiac performance remains underestimated and so therapies aiming to modulate the autonomic nervous system are under-utilized. It is, therefore, to be expected that in the near future cardiac indications are extended to heart failure and maybe even to therapeutically refractory tachyarrhythmias.

Furthermore, the more delicate modulation of the autonomic nervous system, when compared to ablative therapies, provides more insights into (pathophysiological) interactions between brain and heart. Therefore, neuromodulation can also be used to study basic and clinical questions related to neurocardiology.

Basic questions, among others, refer to the part of the nervous system involved in neural hierarchy of cardiac control and it is feasible that in the future electrical neuromodulation will enable neurones to deliver precisely the desired concentration of neuro-active chemicals to the heart.

Clinical issues are related to questions such as how to improve cardiac outcomes of patients suffering from end-stage coronary artery disease and heart failure.

Moreover, preventive neuromodulation may improve the quality of life of patients fearing the shock induced by the implantable cardioverter defibrillator. So, we are suggesting that integration of devices, for instance, combining a spinal cord stimulator with an implantable cardioverter defibrillator, have a promising future.

Conclusions

The on-going research in the field of neurocardiology has considerably upgraded our knowledge about the cardiac–brain axis. The consequence is that we are capable of treating our patients better. In particular, in patients with chronic refractory angina, in whom conventional therapies fail to improve their debilitating symptoms, electrical neuromodulation, independent of the applied modality, has been demonstrated in many randomized control trials to be highly effective and safe. Furthermore, several studies have observed that electrical neuromodulation has improved left ventricular ejection fraction and reduced the occurrence of arrhythmias.

Since many studies with SCS showed improvements in indices of quality of life, symptoms of depression, and anxiety disorders, it is important to screen for comorbidities. SENS seems to be a promising method of electrical neuromodulation in the treatment of refractory angina; however, further clinical and basic studies on this subject are required.

References

1 **Henry TD, Satran D, Jolicoeur EM**. Treatment of refractory angina in patients not suitable for revascularization. Nature Reviews Cardiology 2014 Feb;**11**(2):78–95. DOI:10.1038/nrcardio.2013.200. Review. Erratum in: Nat Rev Cardiol. 2014 Feb;11(2):i.

2 **Mannheimer C, Camici P, Chester MR et al**. The problem of chronic refractory angina. Report from the ESC Joint Study Group on the Treatment of Refractory Angina. European Heart Journal 2002;**23**:355–70.

3 **DeJongste MJ, Tio RA, Foreman RD Chronic therapeutically refractory angina pectoris**. Heart 2004; **90**:225–30.

4 **Hashmonai M, Kopelman D**. History of sympathetic surgery. Clinical Autonomic Research 2003 Dec;**13**(Suppl. 1):I6–9.

5 **Göthberg G, Hyltander A, Claes G**. Endoscopic thoracic sympathectomy. A surgical method employed in severe hand sweating. Lakartidningen 1990;**87**:3318–19.

6 **Fiorelli A, D'Aponte A, Canonico R et al**. T2-T3 sympathectomy versus sympathicotomy for essential palmar hyperhidrosis: comparison of effects on cardio-respiratory function. Eur J Cardiothorac Surg 2012;**42**:454–61.

7 **Kuijpers M, Klinkenberg TJ, Bouma W et al.** Single-port one-stage bilateral thoracoscopic sympathicotomy for severe hyperhidrosis: prospective analysis of a standardized approach. J Cardiothorac Surg 2013;**8**:216.

8 **Melzack R, Wall PD.** Pain mechanisms: a new theory. Science 1965;**150**:971–79.

9 **Shealy CN, Taslitz N, Mortimer JT et al.** Electrical inhibition of pain: experimental evaluation. Anesth Analg 1967;**46**:299–305.

10 **Chandler MJ, Brennan TJ, Garrison DW et al.** A mechanism of cardiac pain suppression by spinal cord stimulation: implications for patients with angina pectoris. Eur Heart J 1993:96–105.

11 **Braunwald E, Epstein SE, Glick G et al.** Relief of angina pectoris by electrical stimulation of the carotid-sinus nerves. New Engl J Med 1967;**277**:1278–83.

12 **Braunwald E.** Personal reflections on efforts to reduce ischemic myocardial damage. Cardiovasc Res 2002;**56**:332–38.

13 **Mannheimer C, Carlsson CA, Ericson K, Vedin A, Wilhelmsson C.** Transcutaneous electrical nerve stimulation in severe angina pectoris. Eur Heart J 1982;**3**:297–302.

14 **Mannheimer C, Carlsson CA, Emanuelsson H et al.** The effects of trans- cutaneous electrical nerve stimulation in patients with severe angina pectoris. Circulation 1985;**71**:308–16.

15 **Strobos MA, Coenraads PJ, De Jongste MJ et al.** Dermatitis caused by radio-frequency electromagnetic radiation. Contact Dermatitis 2001;**44**:309.

16 **Llamas M, Santiago D, Navarro R et al.** Unusual allergic contact dermatitis produced by a transcutaneous electrical nerve stimulator. Contact Dermatitis 2010;**62**:189–90.

17 **Deer TR, Mekhail N, Provenzano D et al.** The appropriate use of neurostimulation of the spinal cord and peripheral nervous system for the treatment of chronic pain and ischemic diseases: the Neuromodulation Appropriateness Consensus. Committee.Neuromodulation. 2014 Aug;**17**(6): 515–50; discussion 550. doi: 10.1111/ner.12208. PMID: 25112889.

18 **Murphy DF, Giles KE.** Dorsal column stimulation for pain relief from intractable angina pectoris. Pain 1987;**28**:365–68.

19 **Levy R.** Differentiating the leaves from the branches in the tree of neuromodulation: The state of peripheral nerve field stimulation. Neuromodulation 2011;**14**:201–05.

20 **Buiten MS, DeJongste MJL, Beese U.** Subcutaneous electrical nerve stimulation: a feasible and new method for treatment of patients with refractory angina. Neuromodulation 2011;**14**:258–64.

21 **Goroszeniuk T, Kothari S.** Subcutaneous target stimulation or peripheral subcutaneous field stimulation: that is the question. Neuromodulation 2011;**14**:185–85.

22 **Goroszeniuk T.** Neuromodulation 2011:**14**:486 (letter to the editor).

23 **Eddicks S, Maier-Hauff K, Schenk M et al.** Thoracic spinal cord stimulation improves functional status and relieves symptoms in patients with refractory angina pectoris: the first placebo-controlled randomised study. Heart 2007;**93**:585–90. Epub 2007 Jan 19.

24 **Lanza GA, Grimaldi R, Greco S et al.** Spinal cord stimulation for the treatment of refractory angina pectoris: a multicenter randomized single-blind study (the SCS-ITA trial). Pain 2011;**152**:45–52.

25 WWW.Angina.Org. Care pathway.

26 **Chatterjee NA, Singh JP.** Novel Interventional Therapies to Modulate the Autonomic Tone in Heart Failure. JAAC Heart Fail, 2015;**10**:786–802. Doi: 10.1016/j.jchf.2015.05.008. Epub 2015 Sep 9. Review])

27 The Cardiac Arrhythmia Suppression Trial (CAST) Investigators. Preliminary report: effect of encainide and flecainide on mortality in a randomized trial of arrhythmia suppression after myocardial infarction. N Engl J Med 1989;**321**:406–12.

28 **Wu M, Linderoth B, Foreman RD.** Putative mechanisms behind effects of spinal cord stimulation on vascular diseases: a review of experimental studies. Auton Neurosci 2008 Feb 29;**138**(1–2):9–23. Review.

29 **DeJongste MJL and Foreman RD**. Spinal cord stimulation for refractory angina. In: Krames ES, Packham PH, Rezai AR (eds) Neuromodulation, vol **2**. Elsevier: Amsterdam; 2009:ch.69.

30 **Andréll P, Yu W, Gersbach P et al**. Long-term effects of spinal cord stimulation on angina symptoms and quality of life in patients with refractory angina pectoris—results from the European Angina Registry Link Study (EARL). Heart 2010;**96**:1132–36.

31 **De Vries J, DeJongste MJ, Versteegen G et al**. Personality: predictor of neurostimulation outcomes in patients with chest pain. Neuromodulation, 2006;**9**:123–7.

32 **de Vries J, DeJongste MJ, Zijlstra F et al**. Long-term effects of electrical neurostimulation in patients with unstable angina: Refractory to conventional therapies Neuromodulation, 2007;**10**:345–348.

33 **Mannheimer C, Eliasson T, Andersson B et al**. Effects of spinal cord stimulation in angina pectoris induced by pacing and possible mechanisms of action. Br Med J 1993;**307**: 477–80.

34 **Di Pede F, Lanza GA, Zuin G et al**. Immediate and long-term clinical outcome after spinal cord stimulation for refractory stable angina pectoris. Investigators of the Prospective Italian Registry of SCS for angina pecoris. Am J Cardiol 2003;**91**:951–55.

35 **Börjesson M, Andréll P, Mannheimer C**. Spinal cord stimulation for long-term treatment of severe angina pectoris: what does the evidence say? (Review). Future Cardiol 2011;**7**:825–33.

36 **Hautvast RW, ter Horst GJ, DeJong B et al**. Relative changes in regional cerebral blood flow during spinal cord stimulation in patients with refractory angina pectoris. Eur J of Neuroscience 1997; **9**:1178–83.

37 **Andersen C, Hole P, Oxhøj H**. Does pain relief with spinal cord stimulation for angina conceal myocardial infarction? Br Heart J. 1994 May;**71**(5):419–21.

38 **Bagger JP, Jensen BS, Johannsen G**. Long-term outcome of spinal electrical stimulation in patients with refractory chest pain. Clin Cardiol 1998;**21**:286–88.

39 **Gibbons RJ, Abrams J, Chatterjee K**. ACC/AHA 2002 guideline update for the management of patients with chronic stable angina—summary article: a report of the American College of Cardiology/American Heart Association Task Force on Practice Guidelines (Committee on the management of patients with chronic stable angina). Circulation 2003;**107**:149–58.

40 **Lanza GA, Barone L, Di Monaco A**. Effect of Spinal Cord Stimulation in patients with refractory angina: evidence from observational studies. Neuromodulation 2012 Feb 24. DOI: 10.1111/j.1525-403.2012.00430.x. [Epub ahead of print.] DOI 10.2217/fca.11.58 (doi:10.2217/fca.11.58)

41 **Jessurun GA, Meeder JG, DeJongste MJ**. Defining the problem of intractable angina. Implications for therapeutical approaches in the relief of ischemic cardiac pain. Pain Rev 1997;**4**:89–99

42 **Taylor RS, De Vries J, Buchser E et al**. Spinal cord stimulation in the treatment of refractory angina: systematic review and meta-analysis of randomised controlled trials. BMC Cardiovasc Disord 2009;**25**:9–13.

43 **Börjesson M, Andrell P, Lundberg D et al**. Spinal cord stimulation in severe angina pectoris—a systematic review based on the Swedish Council on Technology assessment in health care report on long-standing pain. Pain 2008;**140**:501–508.

44 **Enggaard TP, Andersen C, Scherer C**. Spinal cord stimulation for refractory angina in patients implanted with cardioverter defibrillators: five case reports. Europace 2010;**121**:336–37.

45 **Iyer R, Gnanadurai TV, Forsey P**. Management of cardiac pacemaker in a patient with spinal cord stimulator implant. Pain 1998;**74**:333–35.

46 **Holmgren C, Carlsson T, Mannheimer C et al**. Risk of interference from transcutaneous electrical nerve stimulation on the sensing function of implantable defibrillators. Pacing Clin Electrophysiol 2008;**31**:151–58.

47 **De Vries J, Staal MJ, DeJongste MJL**. Is there a future for combinations of implantable devices in human bionics? Neuromodulation 2002;**5**:131–32.

48 **Jessurun GAJ, TenVaarwerk IAM, DeJongste MJL et al**. Sequalae of spinal cord stimulation for refractory angina pectoris. Reliability and safety profile of long-term clinical application. Cor Artery Dis 1997;**8**:33–37.

49 **Gonzalez-Darder JM, Gonzalez-Martinez, V; Canela-Moya, P**. Cervical spinal cord stimulation in the treatment of severe angina pectoris. Neurosurgery Q 1998;**8**(1):16–23

50 **Murray S, Carson KG, Ewings PD et al**. Spinal cord stimulation significantly decreases the need for acute hospital admission for chest pain in patients with refractory angina pectoris. HEART 1999;**82**(1):89–92

51 **Zipes DP, Svorkdal N, Berman D et al**. Spinal Cord Stimulation Therapy for Patients With Refractory Angina Who Are Not Candidates for Revascularization. Neuromodulation, 2012;**15**(6):550–559. DOI: 10.1111/j.1525-1403.2012.00452.x

52 **De Vries J, Svilaas T, DeJongste MJ et al**. Impact of electrical neurostimulation on persistent ST elevation after successful reperfusion by primary percutaneous coronary intervention. J Electrocardiol 2007;**40**(6):522–26.

53 **Ten Vaarwerk IA, Jessurun GA, DeJongste MJ et al**. Clinical outcome of patients treated with spinal cord stimulation for therapeutically refractory angina pectoris. HEART 1999;**82**(1):82–88.

54 **Hautvast RW, DeJongste MJ, Staal MJ et al**. Spinal cord stimulation in chronic intractable angina pectoris: a randomized, controlled efficacy study. Am Heart J 1998;**136**:114–20.

55 **Eliasson T, Mannheimer C, Waagstein F et al**. Myocardial turnover of endogenous opioids and calcitonin-gene-related peptide in the human heart and the effects of spinal cord stimulation on pacing-induced angina pectoris. Cardiology 1998;**89**:170–77.

56 **Hautvast RW, Blanksma PK, DeJongste MJ et al**. Effect of spinal cord stimulation on myocardial blood flow assessed by positron emission tomography in patients with refractory angina pectoris. Am J Cardiol 1996;**1**;77:462–67.

57 **Southerland EM, Milhorn DM, Foreman RD et al**. Preemptive, but not reactive, spinal cord stimulation mitigates transient ischemia-induced myocardial infarction via cardiac adrenergic neurons. Am J Physiol Heart Circ Physiol 2007;**292**:H311–17.

58 **DeJongste MJL**. Chapter 7: Neuromodulation and the heart with special emphasis on myocardial ischemia. In: Carrillo-Ruiz JD (ed.) Topics in Neuromodulation Treatment. InTech, Rijeka; Croatia;2012:143–66

59 **Emanuelsson H, Mannheimer C, Waagstein F et al**. Catecholamine metabolism during pacing-induced angina pectoris and the effect of transcutaneous electrical nerve stimulation. Am Heart J 1987;**114**:1360–66.

60 **Eliasson T, Mannheimer C, Waagstein F et al**. Myocardial turnover of endogenous opioids and calcitonin-gene-related peptide in the human heart and the effects of spinal cord stimulation on pacing-induced angina pectoris. Cardiology 1998;**89**:170–77.

61 **Mannheimer C, Emanuelsson H, Waagstein F**. The effect of transcutaneous electrical nerve stimulation (TENS) on catecholamine metabolism during pacing-induced angina pectoris and the influence of naloxone. Pain 1990;**41**:27–34.

62 **Albutaihi IA, Hautvast RW, DeJongste MJ et al**. Cardiac nociception in rats: neuronal pathways and the influence of dermal neurostimulation on conveyance to the central nervous system. J Mol Neurosci 2003;**20**:43–52.

63 **Foreman RD, DeJongste MJL and Linderoth B**. Intergrative control of cardiac function by cervical and thoracic spinal neurons. In: Armour JA, Ardell JL (eds) Basic and Clinical Neurocardiology. Oxford University Press: New York, USA; 2004:ch.5.

64 **De Vries J, Anthonio RL, DeJongste MJ et al.** The effect of electrical neurostimulation on collateral perfusion during acute coronary occlusion. BMC Cardiovasc Disord,2007; **7**:18–36.

65 **Börjesson M, Eriksson P, Dellborg M et al.** Transcutaneous electrical nerve stimulation in unstable angina pectoris. Coron Artery Dis 1997;**8**:543–50.

66 **Yang Z1, Sun W, Hu K.** Molecular mechanism underlying adenosine receptor-mediated mitochondrial targeting of protein kinase C. Biochim Biophys Acta. 2012 Apr;**1823**(4):950–8. doi: 10.1016/j.bbamcr.2011.12.012. Epub 2011 Dec 31.

67 **Kujacic V, Eliasson T, Mannheimer C et al.** Assessment of the influence of spinal cord stimulation on left ventricular function in patients with severe angina pectoris: an echocardiographic study. Eur Heart J 1993;**14**:1238–44.

68 **Lopshire JC, Zhou X, Dusa C et al.** Spinal cord stimulation improves ventricular function and reduces ventricular arrhythmias in a canine postinfarction heart model. Circulation, 2009:**120**:286–94.

69 **Zamotrinsky AV, Kondratiev B, de Jong JW.** Vagal neurostimulation in patients with coronary artery disease. Auton Neurosci 2001 Apr 12;**88**(1–2):12109–16.

70 **Schwartz PJ, De Ferrari GM, Sanzo A et al.** Long term vagal stimulation in patients with advanced heart failure: first experience in man. Eur J Heart Fail 2008;**10**:884–91.

71 **Zannad F, De Ferrari GM, Tuinenburg AE et al.** Chronic vagal stimulation for the treatment of low ejection fraction heart failure: results of the neural cardiac therapy for heart failure (NECTAR-HF) randomized controlled trial. Eur Heart J 2014 Aug 31. pii: ehu345. Epub ahead of print.

72 **Tse HF, Turner S, Sanders P et al.** Thoracic Spinal Cord Stimulation for HEArt Failure as a Restorative Treatment (SCS HEART Study): First-in-man Experience. Heart Rhythm 2014 Dec 11. **pii**: S1547–5271(14)01422-2. DOI: 10.1016/j.hrthm.2014.12.014. Epub ahead of print.

73 **Wang S, Zhou X, Wang Z.** et al. DEFEAT-HF Trial: The potential causes for the negative result . INT J OF CARDIOL, 2015:**191**:271–72.

74 **Hauptman PJ, Schwartz PJ, Gold MR et al.** Rationale and study design of the INcrease Of Vagal TonE in Heart Failure study: INOVATE-HF Am Heart J 2012;**163(6)**:954–62.

75 **WWW**.ClinicIaTrials.Gov. (search key words: nerve and heart failure)

76 **Torre-Amione G1, Alo K, Estep JD et al.** Spinal cord stimulation is safe and feasible in patients with advanced heart failure: early clinical experience. Eur J Heart Fail 2014 Jul;**16**(7):788–95. DOI: 10.1002/ejhf.107. Epub 2014 Jun 24.

77 **Issa ZF, Zhou X, Ujhelyi MR et al.** Thoracic spinal cord stimulation reduces the risk of ischemic ventricular arrhythmias in a postinfarction heart failure canine model. Circulation 2005;**111**: 3217–20.

78 **Stavrakis S, Scherlag BJ, Po SS.** Autonomic Modulation: An Emerging Paradigm for the Treatment of Cardiovascular Diseases. Circulation Arrhythm Electrophysiol 2012;**5**:2 247–48.

79 **Odenstedt J, Linderoth B, Bergfeldt L et al.** Spinal cord stimulation effects on myocardial ischemia, infarct size, ventricular arrhythmia, and noninvasive electrophysiology in a porcine ischemia-reperfusion model. Heart Rhythm 2011;**8**:892–98.

80 **Ziad FI, Zipes DP.** Antiarrhythmic effects of targeted cardiac neuromodulation: Is it time for clinical application? Heart Rhythm 2005;**2**:1363–64.

81 **Meglio M, Cioni B, Rossi GF et al.** Spinal cord stimulation affects the central mechanisms of regulation of heart rate. Appl Neurophysiol 1986;**49**:139–46.

82 **De Jongste MJ, Haaksma J, Hautvast RW et al.** Effects of spinal cord stimulation on myocardial ischaemia during daily life in patients with severe coronary artery disease. A prospective ambulatory electrocardiographic study. Br Heart J 1994;**71**:413–18.

83 **Hautvast RW, Brouwer J, DeJongste MJ et al.** Effect of spinal cord stimulation on heart rate variability and myocardial ischemia in patients with chronic intractable angina pectoris—a prospective ambulatory electrocardiographic study. Clin Cardiol 1998;**21**:33–38.

84 **Di Pede F, Zuin G, Giada F et al.** Long-term effects of spinal cord stimulation on myocardial ischemia and heart rate variability: results of a 48-hour ambulatory electrocardiographic monitoring. Ital Heart J 2001;**2**:690–95.

85 **Anselmino M, Ravera L, De Luca A et al.** Spinal cord stimulation and 30-minute heart rate variability in refractory angina patients. Pacing Clin Electrophysiol 2009;**32**:37–42.

86 **Norrsell H, Eliasson T, Mannheimer C, et al.** Effects of pacing-induced myocardial stress and spinal cord stimulation on whole body and cardiac norepinephrine spillover. Eur Heart J 1997;**18**:1890–96.

87 **Fricke E, Eckert S, Dongas A et al.** Myocardial sympathetic innervation in patients with symptomatic coronary artery disease: follow-up after 1 year with neurostimulation. J Nucl Med 2008;**49**(9):1458–64.

88 **Spinelli A, Lanza GA, Calcagni ML et al.** Effect of spinal cord stimulation on cardiac adrenergic nerve function in patients with cardiac syndrome X. J Nucl Cardiol 2008;**15**:804–10.

89 **Olgin JE, Takahashi T, Wilson E et al.** Effects of thoracic spinal cord stimulation on cardiac autonomic regulation of the sinus and AV nodes J Cardiovasc Electrophysiol 2002;**13**:475–81.

90 **Brack KE, Winter J, Ng GA.** Mechanisms underlying the autonomic modulation of ventricular fibrillation initiation-tentative prophylactic properties of vagus nerve stimulation on malignant arrhythmias in heart failure. Heart Fail Rev. 2013 Jul;**18**(4):389–408. doi: 10.1007/s10741-012-9314-2. Review.

91 **Foreman RD, Linderoth B, Ardell JL et al.** Modulation of intrinsic cardiac neurons by spinal cord stimulation: implications for its therapeutic use in angina pectoris. Cardiovasc Res 2000 Aug;**47**(2): 367–75.

92 **Armour JA, Linderoth B, Arora RC et al.** Long-term modulation of the intrinsic cardiac nervous system by spinal cord neurons in normal and ischaemic hearts. Auton Neurosci 2002 Jan10;**95**(1–2):71–79.

93 **Mischke K, Zarse M, Schmid M et al.** Chronic augmentation of the parasympathetic tone to the for ventricular rate control during atrial fibrillation. J Cardiovasc Electrophysiol 2010 Feb;**21**(2):193–99. Epub 2009 Oct 5.

94 **Gibbons DD, Southerland EM, Hoover DB et al.** Neuromodulation targets intrinsic cardiac neurons to attenuate neuronally mediated atrial arrhythmias. Am J Physiol Regul Integr Comp Physiol 2012;**302**:R357–64.

Chapter 8

Periarterial sympathectomy in the treatment of upper extremity peripheral vascular disease

Christian E. Sampson

Key points

1 Upper extremity sympathectomy first reported in 1949.
2 Current principles advocate periadventitial stripping as a key to long-term success.
3 Digital ischaemia pathophysiology is the interplay of several factors: vasospasm, endothelial intimal proliferation, and mechanical compression secondary to arterial fibroplasias.
4 Patient selection and technique of periarterial sympathectomy involves use of standard microsurgical principles.
5 Outcome largely dependent on patient selection.

Introduction

This chapter will discuss the management of upper extremity ischaemia due to vasospastic and vaso-occlusive disorders in the upper extremity by periarterial sympathectomy. Periarterial sympathectomy for the management of ischaemia of the upper extremity, as manifest in the majority of cases by ischaemia in the hand and digits, has been performed for more than 50 years. This chapter will review the history of periarterial sympathectomy, how the procedure has evolved, and the current pathophysiologic understanding of its mechanism of action. Patient selection methods, operative technique, and outcome studies will also be presented.

History of periarterial sympathectomy

Sympathectomy of the upper extremity was first performed by Barcroft and Walker (1) who demonstrated a six-fold increase in blood flow in normal hands. Long-term results, however, were disappointing as reported by Flatt (2). Sympathetic nerve fibres travel along peripheral nerves in the extremity and one reason why proximal sympathectomy in some cases did not have long-lasting results was given by Pick (3). He showed that the brachial plexus does not receive its rami communicantes exclusively from the cervico-sympathetic trunk, but that there are accessory nerve pathways. Other nerves bypass the sympathetic trunk including the sino-vertebral nerve, carotid plexus, nerve of Kuntz, and the intermediary sympathetic ganglia in the spinal nerve roots. These alternate sympathetic pathways may account for residual sympathetic nerve activity in the upper extremity after proximal, cervico-thoracic sympathectomy.

In the distal part of the upper extremity, Pick demonstrated that the radial artery is innervated by a small branch from the superficial branch of the radial nerve and by eight additional twigs from the lateral cutaneous nerve of the forearm. He also showed that the distal third of the ulnar artery receives three branches from the ulnar nerve and a branch from the medial cutaneous nerve of the forearm, which is typically on the volar aspect of the ulnar artery and can be seen at the wrist level. The deep palmar arch receives two branches from the deep branch of the ulnar nerve and one from the median nerve. The superficial palmar arch receives approximately 12 branches from the common digital nerves. The digital arteries receive 3 to 12 small branches from the proper digital nerves.

Mitchell (4) demonstrated that sympathetic nerve fibres branch within the adventitia. Morgan et al. (5) studied the sympathetic nerves in the hand and digits using dark field microscopy of sections of arteries and nerves immersed in glyoxylic acid to excite fluorescence of catecholamine-containing nervous tissue. Their results proved that sympathetic nerves travel with the peripheral nerves and send frequent branches to the adjacent arteries. Furthermore, they showed that the sympathetic axons are located within the epineurium of the peripheral nerves, and that the branches to adjacent arteries penetrate only the adventitia of the vessel, not reaching the media. Also, sympathetic innervation was greater in the median nerve distribution as compared to the ulnar nerve distribution.

Flatt used the anatomic information provided by Pick, Mitchell, and Morgan to formulate the principles of distal digital periarterial sympathectomy, which he reported in 1980. The principle reasoning he employed was that the more distal the sympathectomy is performed, the more effective it will be in improving perfusion. His procedure was to strip 3 to 4 mm of adventitia from the proper digital arteries, distal to the junction of the distal perforating artery with the common digital artery. He included eight patients with digital vascular insufficiency due to frostbite, crush injury, scleroderma, and Raynaud's disease. Follow-up was from 1 to 17 years and digital ulcers did show evidence of healing, there was reduction of pain (less in the crush injury group), and digital temperature increased 1–3 degrees.

Current principles of periarterial sympathectomy

The use of periarterial sympathectomy is considered a salvage procedure in most cases of vasospastic and occlusive disorders. Medical treatment is the usual first choice for pain, and digital ulcerations in the extremity due to peripheral arterial disorders. Calcium channel blockade therapy is the primary medical treatment. Nifedipine, both short-acting and long-acting forms, is often used first. Other medications include alpha-1 blockers (prazosin and terazosin), tricyclic antidepressants (elavil), selective serontonin re-uptake inhibitors (prozac, zoloft), iloprost (prostacyclin analogue), prostaglandin E1, and more recently sildenafil (Viagra) and tadalafil (Cialis). Interestingly, onabotulinumtoxin A (Botox) has been used successfully to alleviate symptoms (6, 7). But some patients remain refractory to medical management, and medical therapy may not have consistent, long-term benefit, as well as having unacceptable side-effects, including orthostatic hypotension and dizziness. Other non-surgical treatments are available, including biofeedback, acupuncture, and behavioural modification. In the subset of patients who do not improve with conservative medical management, and in those with impending tissue loss, periarterial sympathectomy (PAS) is a surgical option to consider. PAS has also been employed in the management of acute ischaemia following trauma with positive results (8).

Wilgis (9, 10) extended Flatt's concept of circumferential adventitial stripping to also include identification and division of the sympathetic branches arising distally from the digital nerves. He reported results from 18 digits in 10 patients with chronic ischaemia. Pre-operatively, all patients showed an increase in digital perfusion after a digital block. Post-operatively, all but one patient had improved digital circulation as measured with pulse volume recordings and radioisotope study. Pain was relieved and ulcerations healed within 2 weeks. Egloff et al. (11) reported their results in 13 patients with Raynaud's disease with a 3- to 13-month follow-up. All patients had improvement in their symptoms with only one complication of digital pulp hypoesthesia.

Reisman (12) published results of 51 periarterial sympathectomies in 42 patients, which included those patients in Wilgis et al.'s study. Average follow-up was 26 months and 49 digits (96%) had complete relief of symptoms and ulcers healed in 3 weeks, and there were no recurrent symptoms in the follow-up period. Blood flow showed a marked increase, as measured by pulse volume recordings and radionuclide scans. The temperature of the operated digits showed increases of up to 6°C within 1 to 2 weeks. The only complications were delayed wound healing in patients on steroids and/or in patients with scleroderma. One conclusion was that PAS should only be performed in those patients who show an increase in pulse volume recording after digital nerve block. This, however, is not currently advocated as studies by Ruch (13) have shown that improvement can occur after PAS without an increase in digital temperature. This suggests that total blood flow may not be improved after PAS, but that there is enough improvement in nutritional blood flow to produce positive results. El-Gammal et al. (14) reported their experience with PAS in 3 patients (11 digits) suffering from chronic ischaemia secondary to Raynaud's disease, CREST syndrome, or traumatic ulnar artery thrombosis. They performed a more extensive, multi-level, PAS by including 2 cm of the common digital arteries, the bifurcation, and 1 cm of the proper digital arteries, as well as 2 cm of adventitia from the ulnar and radial arteries at the wrist and from the dorsal branch of the radial artery. By employing this approach they hoped to provide a more complete sympathetic denervation of the digits. They showed pain relief in all patients, complete in two patients, and partial in the patient with ulnar artery thrombosis. All ulcers healed by 3 months, including several that were infected. They also recommended routine use of the operating microscope in order to perform a more thorough sympathectomy and to avoid complications such as inadvertent arteriotomy.

Koman et al. (15) further extended the concept of distal multi-level periarterial sympathectomy by stripping the superficial palmar arch in addition to the common and proper digital arteries, and the radial and ulnar arteries at the wrist. In 2002 he reported 46-month follow-up results (13). Of 22 patients, 18 reported a decrease in pain, subjective

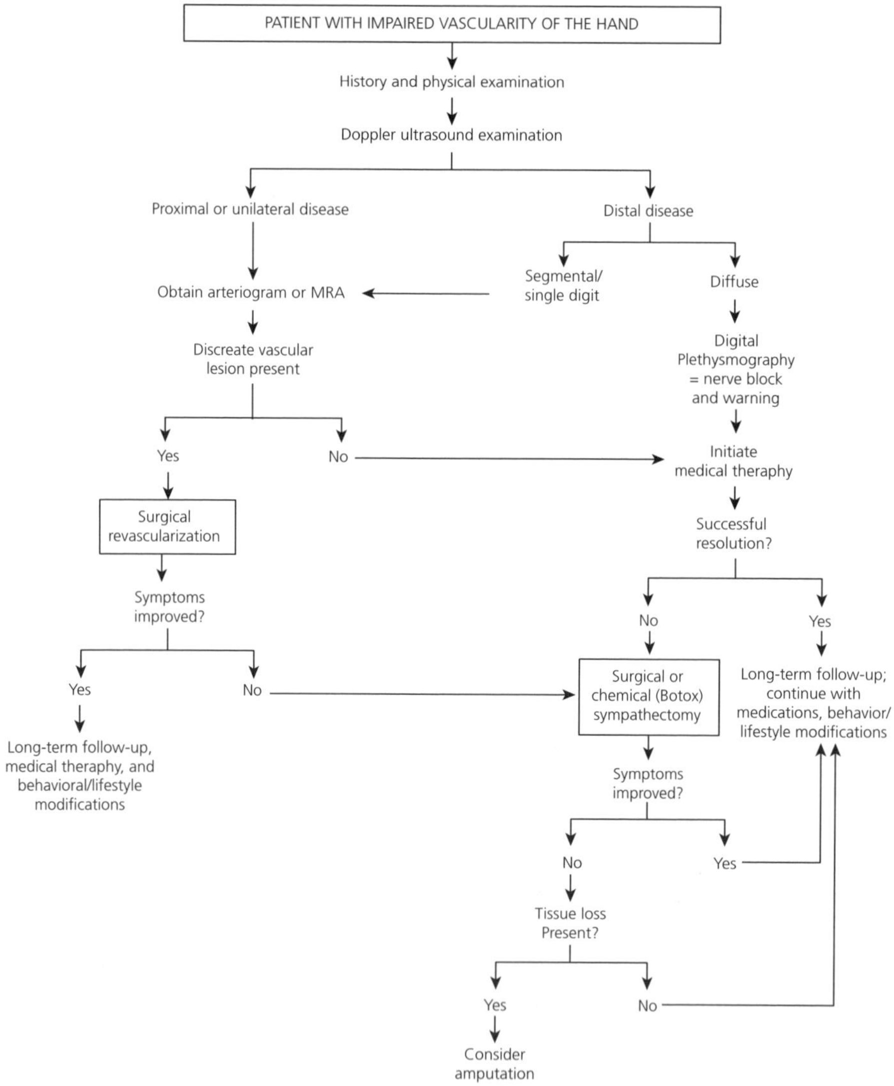

Fig. 8.1 Impaired vascularity treatment algorithm.

improvement in ulcer healing, and reduction in ulcer occurrence; 6 patients reported no new ulcerations; distal fingertip amputations were performed in 3 patients (14%).

The data available regarding periarterial sympathectomy leaves many questions unanswered. While algorithms are available for the management of digital ischaemia (Fig. 8.1), no algorithm will encompass all clinical scenarios, and the treatment plan must be individualized. Specifics regarding the anatomic level of the sympathectomy, extent of periadventitial stripping, and peri-operative management have not been studied in a randomized, prospective fashion. Thus, these management issues are left up to the experience and personal preference of the surgeon. However, the current standard PAS procedure is to include the radial and ulnar arteries at the wrist, superficial palmar arch, and common and proper digital vessels. In cases of isolated, single-digit ischaemia, common and proper digital artery PAS may be considered.

Pathophysiology

Digital ischaemia is due to the interaction of three factors that can reduce blood flow, namely: vasospasm, abnormal endothelium secondary to intimal proliferation, and mechanical compression secondary to arterial fibroplasias (8). In vasospastic conditions, it is the result of changes in the vascular structure and/or inappropriate vascular control mechanisms (16). Adequate tissue perfusion requires:

1 Blood flow to nutritional capillary beds adequate to meet metabolic demand.
2 Adequate oxygen-carrying capacity.
3 Adequate diffusion of oxygen through intra-vascular spaces to functioning cellular structures.

In the majority of patients, the oxygen- and nutrient-carrying capacity of the peripheral vascular system is adequate to meet metabolic demand. In the absence of an occlusive process or cell death, ischaemic symptoms are due to the inadequate delivery of nutrients and oxygen. Vasospasm decreases total blood flow and/or shunts blood through non-nutritional thermoregulatory pathways. In the case of vascular injury, local and systemic factors can produce inappropriate vasospasm that decreases large-vessel collateral flow and shunts existing flow in small vessels into non-nutritional channels. Koman has devised a classification based upon physiologic staging that allows vasospastic conditions to be categorized (17). Group I patients are those with idiopathic Raynaud's disease characterized by normal vascular architecture, no identifiable underlying aetiology, and the presence of vasospasm. Group II patients are those with Raynaud's phenomenon secondary to collagen vascular disease and can be divided into those with normal circulation (A), and those with compromised circulation (B). Group III patients are those with vasopasm secondary to vascular injury and may be divided into those with normal collateral flow (A) and those with abnormal collateral flow (B). Group IV patients are those without pre-existing or acquired structural vascular abnormality, and have vasospasm secondary to an isolated or combined injury of nerves, soft tissue, or bone. PAS is typically performed in patients comprising groups I and II, and less commonly in group III and IV patients.

Tissue ischaemia secondary to vasospastic conditions is due to inadequate nutritional perfusion, including inadequate delivery of oxygen and metabolites to cellular structures, which leads to the development of an anaerobic and acidotic tissue environment, and ultimately cell death. Pollock et al. (18), showed that PAS did not improve overall total blood flow in patients with vaso-occlusive disease but that it could improve nutritional and thermoregulatory flow in the microcirculation by dilating the distal cutaneous microcirculatory vessels. Others have also shown that cutaneous circulation is improved following distal sympathectomy (10, 11, 14). Pollock et al. (18), using the central auricular artery in a rabbit ear model, measured blood flow via laser Doppler perfusion imaging. Their results showed the artery became dilated immediately after sympathectomy, and was followed 30 minutes later by dilation of arterioles, arteriovenous anastomoses, and venules. The laser Doppler perfusion imaging values and ear temperature increased while core body temperature remained stable. They concluded that acute PAS reduces vascular tone and increases total microcirculatory perfusion, both cutaneous and thermoregulatory, by both venular and arteriolar dilation.

Patient selection and technique

Candidates for PAS are those patients with ischaemic symptoms due to vaso-spastic or vaso-occlusive disorders refractory to conservative medical therapy. They may have chronic, non-healing ulcers, and pain (Figs 8.2 and 8.3).

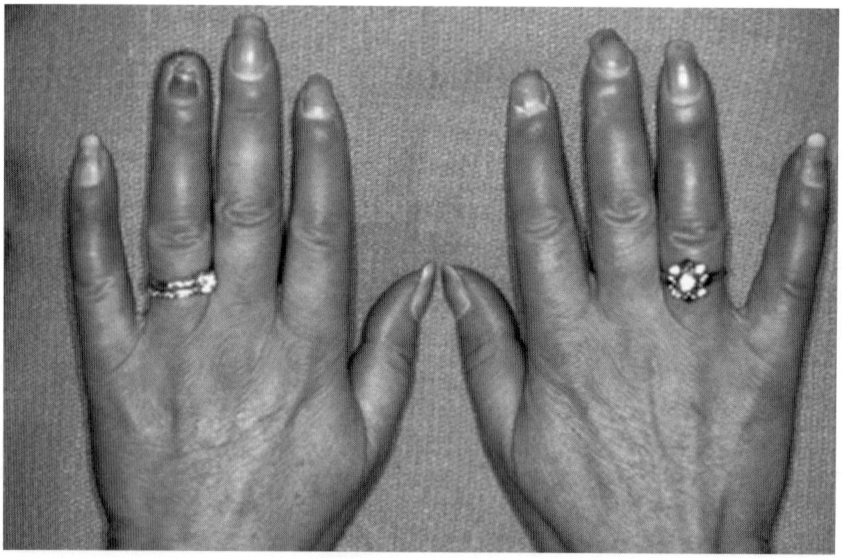

Fig. 8.2 Clinical appearance of acute Raynaud's vasospasm.

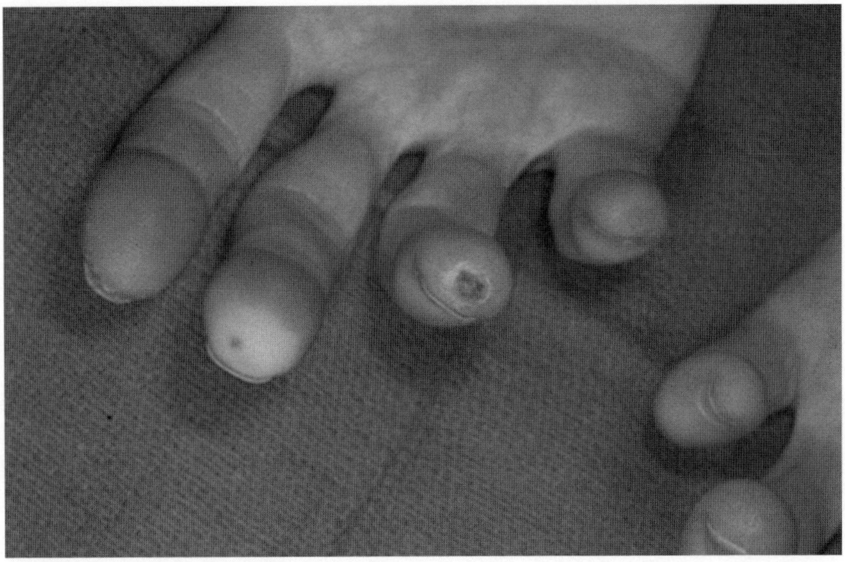

Fig. 8.3 Raynaud's digital ulcerations.

There may be impending tissue loss or gangrene necessitating amputation, in addition to PAS. The underlying disease process may be Raynaud's disease or Raynaud's phenomenon secondary to a number of processes, typically including frostbite, trauma, scleroderma, discoid lupus, systemic lupus erythematosus, mixed connective tissue disorders, and undifferentiated rheumatic diseases. Cigarette smoking has a detrimental effect on digital perfusion (19–24) and patients should stop smoking before surgery and be given appropriate counselling in the post-operative period. PAS can be used in patients who are still smoking but I do not recommend performing vascular reconstructive procedures in active smokers. Arteriography with magnification views should be routinely obtained, except in patients with renal insufficiency or intra-venous contrast allergy (Fig. 8.4).

Any lesion deemed amenable to reconstruction should be so treated. In many cases, digital run-off is difficult to assess due to poor flow. Magnetic resonance angiography, with the proper surface coils and software analysis, can provide detailed images of hand and digit arterial anatomy, but the resolution is still not as good as conventional arteriography. Pre-operative testing modalities include isolated cold stress testing ICST (16), laser Doppler fluxmetry (LDF), and pulse volume recording with and without digital blockade. LDF is an extremely sensitive, non-invasive method of examining cutaneous peripheral microcirculation through the use of a monochromatic low-energy laser beam. Of these, pulse volume recordings are the easiest to perform and the most readily available. Some patients will have a history of extreme cold sensitivity and ICST should be used with caution in this subset of patients, as the experience can be unpleasant. In

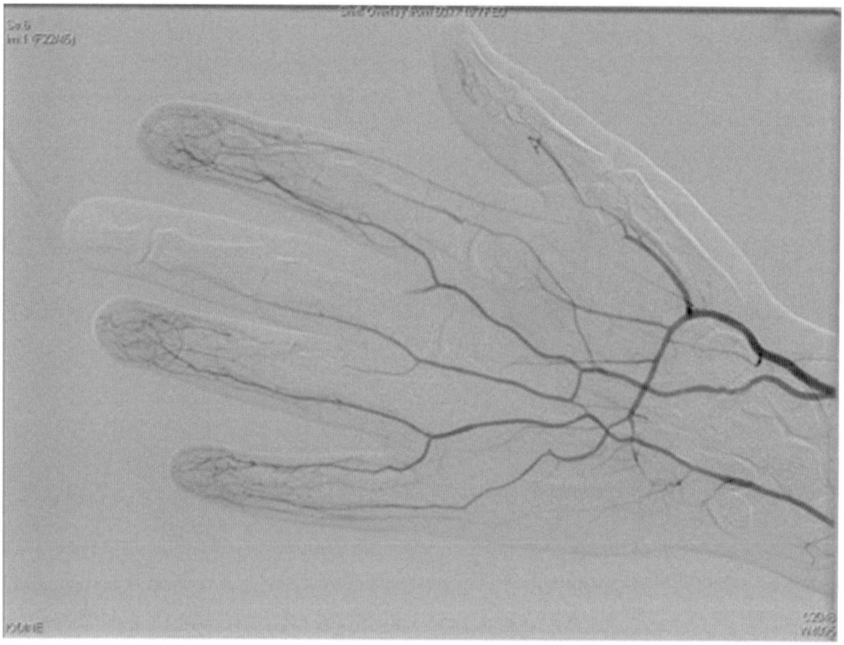

Fig. 8.4 Digital subtraction ateriogram in patient with middle-finger digital ischaemia showing radial and ulnar digital artery cut-off.

cases where multiple digits are involved, PAS should be performed at the palmar and wrist level.

The surgical technique has been well described by Jones et al. (25) and Koman et al. (15), and requires three incisions. A transverse palmar incision is used to gain access to the superficial palmar arch and common digital vessels, and longitudinal incisions are made over the ulnar and radial arteries at the wrist, respectively (Fig. 8.5).

The procedure is typically performed utilizing a regional anaesthetic, which has the benefit of providing sympathetic blockade. The operating room should be warmed prior to receiving the patient, and kept warm during the procedure. A tourniquet is used and an operating microscope is used to perform the actual circumferential peri-adventitial dissection. Skin flaps should be handled very carefully and undermining should be performed only to the extent needed for adequate exposure, in order to minimize skin flap ischaemia and subsequent wound-healing complications. Meticulous haemostasis, using a bipolar cautery, is needed. When cauterizing small branches on the arch, common and proper digital arteries, the cautery should be set to a very low setting to avoid thermal injury to the main vessel. Because intra-operative findings do not always correlate with the pre-operative arteriogram, the surgeon should always be prepared to perform a direct revascularization or bypass with a reversed vein graft, if

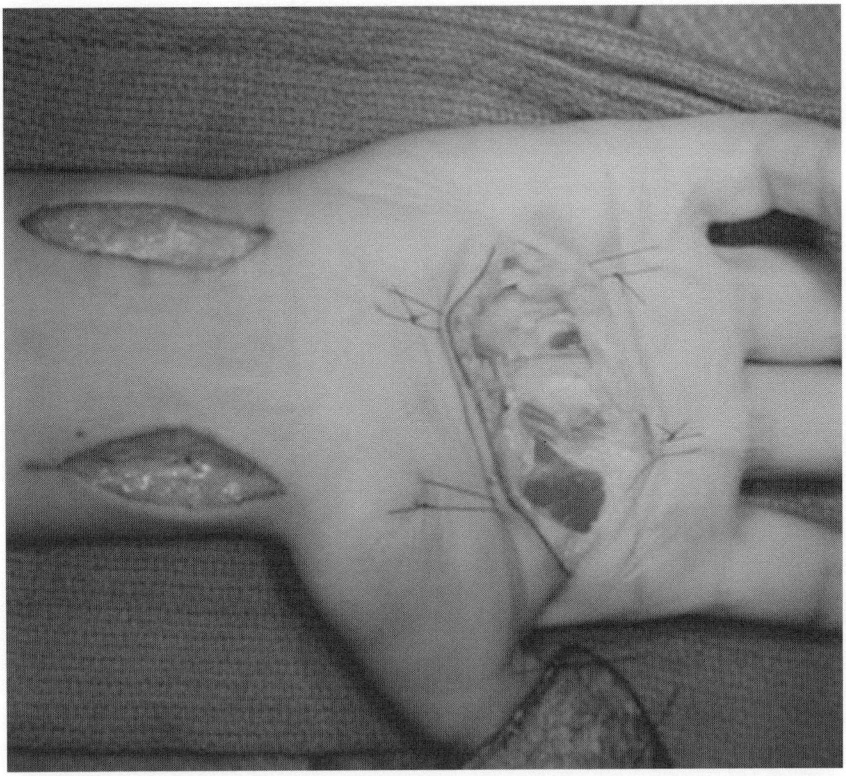

Fig. 8.5 Intra-operative view depicting surgical approach for palmar and wrist sympathectomy.

necessary. This would include resection of thrombosed arterial segments with end-to-end repair, where possible. PAS can be likened more to an adventectomy than removal of nervous tissue from the adventitia. As such, the amount of tissue removed from the vessel can be quite substantial. The surgeon should always be prepared to repair an inadvertent arteriotomy, if needed. A minimum length of 1 cm should be stripped from the radial and ulnar arteries, superficial palmar arch, and common digital arteries (Fig. 8.6).

I prefer 2 to 3 cm of stripping, when possible, in order to reduce the possibility of recurrent symptoms due to regeneration of the sympathetic nerves. A drain is routinely used. Post-operative anticoagulation is usually needed only if a vascular reconstructive procedure was performed. Aspirin therapy can be used post-operatively, and in my practice, if a vascular reconstructive procedure is performed, I routinely place the patient on aspirin (325 mg daily) for 6 to 12 weeks post-operatively. A bulky dressing is applied and a splint is used for 1 to 2 weeks to protect the skin incisions. Sutures are removed at 10 to 14 days.

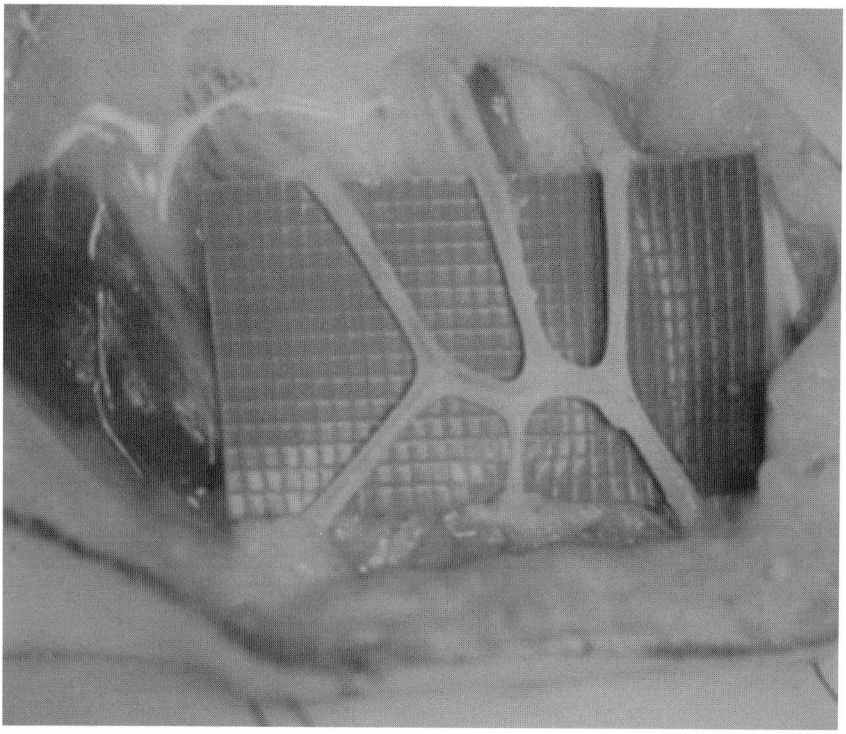

Fig. 8.6 Close-up of completed sympathectomy of palmar vessels.

Outcome

Peripheral arterial sympathectomy must be regarded as a palliative procedure. The course of the underlying disease process is not being fundamentally altered. Nevertheless, the procedure does offer relief of symptoms, ulcer healing, and improved quality of life in the short term. It is, however, not without complications. Reisman (12) reported delayed wound healing in scleroderma patients. O'Brien et al. (26) found recurrence of superficial digital ulcerations in 4 out of 13 patients with scleroderma or Raynaud's phenomenon. Ruch et al. (13), after a mean follow-up period of 46 months, reported 75% of patients had additional ulcerations and/or gangrene. In this study there was subjective improvement, as patients experienced fewer new ulcers and had less pain. In a retrospective study performed by Kalliakmanis et al. (27), it was found that PAS led to ulcer healing in all 16 digits operated on, with a mean time to healing of 5 weeks. There were no recurrent ulcerations at a mean follow-up of 24–80 months. Mean pain score (0 = no pain, 1 = mild pain, 2 = moderate pain, 3 = severe pain) fell from 3.6 before surgery to 2.9 after surgery. The overall improvement following surgery was scored from 0 to 3 (0 = no improvement, 1 = slight improvement, 2 = moderate improvement, 3 = great improvement); the mean score was 1.90. Kotsis and Chung (28) performed a meta-analysis of digital sympathectomy reported in the English language literature between 1966 and 2002. They reported 14% of all patients required amputation and 18% of patients had recurrent ulceration. In patients with scleroderma, there was a 37% complication rate. They stressed that differences in surgical technique, the multiple causes of digital ischaemia, and variations in outcome measurement, made direct comparisons difficult. Their conclusion was that until a randomized, prospective study with standardized pre- and post-operative metric analysis is performed, the true effectiveness of PAS will not be known. Hartzell et al. (29) compared long-term results of periarterial sympathectomy in patients with digital vasospasm secondary to either an autoimmune disease or generalized atherosclerotic disease. The average follow-up period was 96 months. They reported that PAS led to complete digital ulcer healing or reduced number of ulcers in 15 of 20 patients in the autoimmune group, whereas only one out of eight patients had complete digital ulcer healing or reduced number of ulcers in the atherosclerotic group. The conclusion was that PAS is beneficial in autoimmune disorders, whereas it is of little or no benefit in patients with atherosclerotic disease. When counselling patients, it can be said that the data supports the conclusion that there is often improvement in symptoms with reduction in pain, ulcer healing, and improved quality of life. Some patients may not respond at all, but this probability is low in properly selected patients. Recurrent symptoms are the result of multiple factors. Regeneration of the divided sympathetic nerves is possible. Other factors are progression of disease and trauma, which is often mild and occurs in performing activities of daily living. Applying strict criteria guidelines to patient selection is controversial (17). Increased digital temperature and blood flow after digital blockade is indicative of inappropriate sympathetic tone that can be treated by PAS. However, patients with vaso-occlusive disease with adequate collateral flow will not have the same response to blockade. Nevertheless, Ruch (13) has shown that these patients will often benefit more from PAS, which maximizes nutrient blood flow by decreasing inappropriate arteriovenous shunting.

Conclusions

Periarterial sympathectomy is a microsurgical technique that has been shown to be of benefit in patients with digital ischaemia secondary to a variety of vasospastic and vaso-occlusive disorders. The typical patient is one with Raynaud's disease, or Raynaud's phenomenon secondary to autoimmune connective tissue diseases, but it has also been shown to be of benefit in the setting of acute trauma. An important understanding is that, in pre-operative evaluation, patients do not need to have improved total blood flow, as measured by techniques such as either pulse volume recording or digital temperature after digital blockade with a local anaesthetic in order to be considered a candidate for PAS. Although PAS can improve total digital blood flow, improved digital nutritional blood flow in these patients, not measured by pulse volume recording or digital temperature, is often sufficient to allow healing of ulcers, and reduce or eliminate pain.

References

1 **Barcroft, H. Walker, A. J.** Return of The Tone in Blood Vessels of The Upper Limb After Sympathectomy. *Lancet* 1949;**1**:1035–9.

2 **Flatt, A. E.** Digital artery sympathectomy. *Journal of Hand Surgery*, 1980;**5**(6):550–56.

3 **Pick, J.** *The Autonomic Nervous System*. Philadelphia: J.B. Lippincott 1970.

4 **Mitchell, G.** *Anatomy of the Autonomic Nervous System*. Edinburgh: E. S. Livingstone 1953.

5 **Morgan, R. F. Reisman, N. R. Wilgis, E. F.** Anatomic localization of sympathetic nerves in the hand. *Journal of Hand Surgery* 1967;**8**(3):283–8.

6 **Czop, C. Koman, A. L. Rauck, R. Smith, T. L.** The Pharmacologic Approach To The Painful Hand. *Hand Clinics* 1996;**12**:633–42.

7 **Gear, J. L. Lim, P. K. Pritzker, M. R. Van Beek, A. L.** Management of Vasospastic Disorders with Botulinum Toxin A. *Plastic and Reconstructive Surgery* 2007;**119**:217.

8 **Henry, M. L. Levaro, F. Masson, M.** Periarterial Sympathectomy Salvage of the Acutely Ischemic Hand. *Journal of Reconstructive Microsurgery*, 2003;**19**(1):7–10.

9 **Wilgis, E. F.** Evaluation and Treatment of Chronic Digital Ischemia. *Ann Surg* 1981;**193**:693–8.

10 **Wilgis, E. F.** Digital sympathectomy for Vascular Insufficiency. *Hand Clinics* 1985;**1**:361–7.

11 **Egloff, D. V. Mifsud R. P. Verdan, Cl.** Superselective Digital Sympathectomy In Raynaud's Phenomenon. *The Hand* 1982;**15**(1):110–14.

12 **Reisman, N. R.** Surgical management of Raynaud's phenomenon. *Texas Medicine* 1984;**80**:44–9.

13 **Holden, M. Koman, A. L. Ruch, D. S. Smith, B. P. Smith, T. L.** Periarterial Sympathectomy in Scleroderma Patients: Intermediate-term Follow-up. *Journal of Hand Surgery* 2002;**27A**:258–64.

14 **Blair, Wr. El-Gammal, T. A.** Digital periarterial sympathectomy for ischaemic digital pain and ulcers. *Journal of Hand Surgery* 1991;**16B**:382–5.

15 **Koman, L. S. Pollock, D. Pollock, E. F. Russell, G. B. Smith, B. P. Smith, T. L.** The Microcirculatory Effects of Peripheral Sympathectomy. *Jourbal of Hand Surgery* 1995;**20A**:868–72.

16 **Koman, L. A. Smith, B. P. Smith, T. L.** Stress Testing in the Evaluation of Upper Extremity Perfusion. *Hand Clinics*, 1993;**1**:59–83.

17 **Koman, L. A. Li, Z. Ruch, D. S. Smith, B. P. Smith, T. L.** Vascular Disorders. In S. W. Wolfe, *Green's Operative Hand Surgery, 6th Edition* (p. 66). Philadelphia: Elsevier Churchill Livingsone 2011.

18 **Koman, A. L Krome, J. Li, Z. Pollock, D. C.** Rosencrance, E. Acute Effects of Periarterial Sympathectomy on the Cutaneous Microcirculation. *Journal of Orthopaedic Research* 1997;**15**:408–13.

19 **Bornmyr, S. Svensson. H.** Thermography and laser-Doppler flowmetry for monitoring changes in finger blood flow upon cigarette smoking. *Lin Physiol* 1991;**11**:135–41.

20 **Fulcher, S. M. Holden, M. Koman, A. L. Smith, B. P. Smith, T. L.** The Effect of Transdermal Nicotine on Digital Perfusion in Reformed Habitual Smokers. *Journal of Hand Surgery*, 1998;**23A**:792–9.

21 **Krupski, W. C.** The Peripheral Vascular Consequences of Smoking. *Ann Vasc Surg* 1991;**5**:291–304.

22 **Blair, W. F. Brown, T. D. Gable, R. H. Morecraft, R. B.** Acute Effects of Smoking on Digital Artery Blood Flow in Humans. *Journal Hand Surgery* 1994;**19A**:1–7.

23 **Heggers, J. P. Reus, W. F. Robson, M. C. Zachary, L.** Acute effects of tobacco smoking on blood flow in the cutaneous micro-circulation. *Br J Plast Surg* 1984;**37**:213–5.

24 **van Adrichem, L. N. Hovius, S. E. R. van der Meulen, J. C. van Strik, R.** The acute effect of cigarrete smoking on the micricirculation of a replanted digit. *J Hand Surg* 1992;**17A**:230–34.

25 **Jones, N. F.** Acute and chronic ischemia of the hand: Pathophysiology, treatment, and prognosis. *J Hand Surg*, 1991;**16A**:1074–83.

26 **Kumar, P. A. V. Mellow, C. G. O'Brien, B. McC. Oliver, T. V.** Radical Microarteriolysis in The Treatment of Vasospastic Disorders of The Hand, Especially Scleroderma. *J Hand Surg* 1992;**17B**:447–52.

27 **Gerostathopoulos, N. Ignantiadis, J. Kalliakmanis, A. P. Petratos, D.** Digital Periarterial Sympathectomy for Severe Ischemia of Raynaud's Syndrome. *Vascular Disease management*, 2007;**4**(1):27–30.

28 **Chung, K. C. Kotsis, S. V.** A Systematic Review of the Outcomes of Digital Sympathectomy For the Treatment of Chronic Digital Ischemia. *J Rheumatol* 2003;**30**(8):1788–92.

29 **Hartzell, T. L. Makhni, E. Sampson, C. E.** Long-term Results of Periatrterial Sympathectomy. *J Hand Surg*, 2009;**34A**:1454–60.

Chapter 9

Spinal cord stimulation for complex regional pain syndrome I: mechanisms

Tim McCormick and Stana Bojanic

Key points

1. Spinal cord stimulation (SCS) mechanism of action appears to be predominantly via GABAergic inhibitory inter-neurones at a spinal segmental level.
2. SCS acts by restoring 'normal' pain processing in awakened or sensitized nociceptive pathways.
3. Complex regional pain syndrome (CRPS) is a chronic neuropathic pain state with complex pathophysiology demonstrating peripheral and central mechanisms that may vary over time and between patients.
4. Few treatments for CRPS have proven effective and currently therapy is focused around 'four pillars of treatment'
   - (a) Patient information and education to support and self-management.
   - (b) Physical and vocational rehabilitation.
   - (c) Psychological intervention.
   - (d) Pain relief (medications and procedures).
5. SCS has established itself as an effective, cost-efficient therapy for CRPS.

Historical perspective

Analgesia from electrical stimulation is not a new concept. In fact analgesia from electricity, albeit a form of piscine electrotherapy, was known about before electricity itself. The therapeutic effects of the Nile catfish (*Malopterurus electicus*) decorated Egyptian tomb reliefs (2750 BC), whilst the philosopher Aristotle (384–382 BC) and Scribonius Largus, physician to the Roman Emperor Claudius (47 AD), praised the torpedo ray's (*Torpedo marmorata*) ability to numb and relieve gout pain, respectively (1, 2).

The development of the first electrostatic generator in 1650, and subsequently the Leyden Jar, extended the possible applications of electrotherapy as physicians then had a way of generating, storing, and discharging electricity at will (1).

The popularity of electrotherapy was at its height in the nineteenth century when it was used for many ailments, even in cases of rather dubious benefit. This lack of clinical rigor led to increased scepticism and electrotherapy was even compared to a form of 'medical quackery'. The Flexner report on medical education in 1910 extinguished the electrotherapy spark by stating that it was scientifically insupportable and electrotherapy was subsequently legally excluded from clinical practice (3).

The spark was reignited following further research on the electrical stimulation of the nervous system (4), and the theory of central inhibition of pain transmission by non-painful stimuli. This work culminated in Melzack and Wall's Gate Control Theory (GCT) of Pain in 1965 (5).

Prior to the GCT there were two mutually exclusive pain theories:

1 Specificity theory, which stated that pain was a specific modality and specific pain receptors relayed their signal through dedicated pain pathways to the thalamus.
2 Pattern theory, which stated that intense stimulation of non-specific receptors produced a nerve impulse pattern that coded for pain.

Neither theory was able to provide a satisfactory theory for pain transmission. The GCT hypothesized that the Substantia Gelatinosa (SG) within the dorsal horn (DH) functioned as a gate that modulated afferent nerve impulse patterns before onward transmission (see Fig. 9.1). This gate could be opened by an excess of nociceptive small-fibre activity and closed by an excess of non-nociceptive large-fibre activity or from descending fibres from higher centres. The theory stated that pain transmission was subject to modulation. This reduced the therapeutic emphasis from destruction of neural pathways to pain control by modulation and the birth of neuromodulation (6).

The first attempts at neuromodulation started with the stimulation of peripheral nerves and yielded positive results with reports of partial or complete analgesia during stimulation (7, 8). It was then a natural step to develop more invasive procedures and attempt to

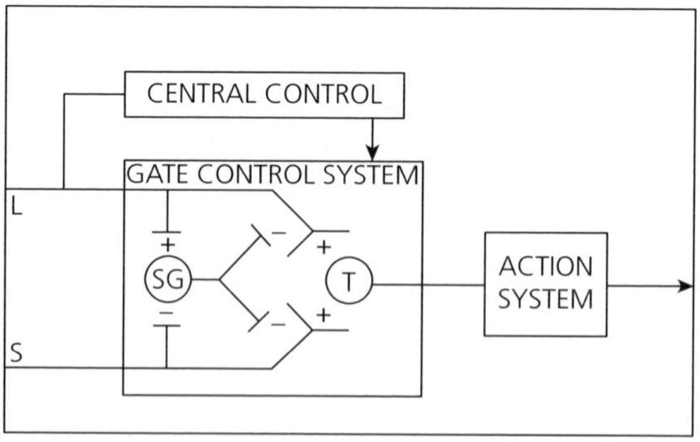

Fig. 9.1 Gate Control Theory.
Reproduced from Science, 150 (3699), Ronald Melzack and Patrick Wall, Pain mechanisms: a new theory, p. 971–979, Copyright (1965), with permission from AAAS.

stimulate the dorsal columns directly. This was first reported as a novel analgesic technique by Shealy in 1967 (9). The early implants involved intra-dural electrodes, with an electrode being placed directly on the dorsal columns. This represented a major surgical undertaking and procedures were fraught with complications and hardware failure. Complications were reduced with a switch to epidurally placed electrodes, but indiscriminate use and poor results led the technique to fall into disrepute (10).

In the last decade there has been a growing consensus that SCS could be a reasonably effective treatment for chronic neuropathic pain where other therapies have failed. This reflects less indiscriminate use, improved electrodes and hardware design, and psychological screening. These factors have resulted in an increase in success, a reduction in complications, and a rise in efficacy (11).

Anatomy, physiology, and disease pathophysiology

The nociceptive pathway

It would be difficult to fully appreciate the mechanism of action of SCS without an understanding of the anatomy and physiology of the somatosensory system and the spinal cord. An in-depth review of this is beyond the scope of this chapter, but the nociceptive pathway (pain being an emotional experience, nociception being the physiological activation of neural or 'pain' pathways) will briefly be reviewed.

A (potentially) harmful stimulus or injury in the form of a type of energy (mechanical, heat, chemical, etc.) occurs in the periphery. This causes release of chemicals and is the first step in the nociceptive pathway (transduction). The chemicals form an 'inflammatory soup', which has a myriad of effects. The predominant causes are alterations in blood flow, tissue permeability, and direct activation or increased excitability of nociceptors (rubor, calor, tumor, and dolor) (see Fig. 9.2).

The activation of nociceptors, provided it is of sufficient magnitude, results in the second stage in the pain pathway (transmission). This is where energy that has been transduced from its initial form to electrical activity, is transmitted through the periphery along the primary afferent or sensory neurone towards the dorsal horn. At the dorsal horn, the primary afferent neurone then synapses with second-order neurones.

Activation of this pain pathway can result from tissue damage causing the 'inflammatory soup' or from damage to the primary afferent nerve itself (neuropathic pain), where the characteristic signs of inflammation or injury may be absent.

The primary afferent fibres are classified according to their conduction velocities and the cutaneous stimuli to which they respond. The intensity of the stimulus is relayed by the frequency of impulses. The primary afferent fibres responsible for nociception are the A delta and C fibres, and their receptors respond to extreme temperatures, and mechanical and chemical stimuli. A delta fibres can be further be subdivided into fast/slow adaptors and low/high threshold varieties (13) (see Table 9.1).

The nociceptive primary afferents predominantly synapse in the dorsal horn in a highly organized way. The dorsal horn is organized into laminae (laminae of Rexed). The C fibres

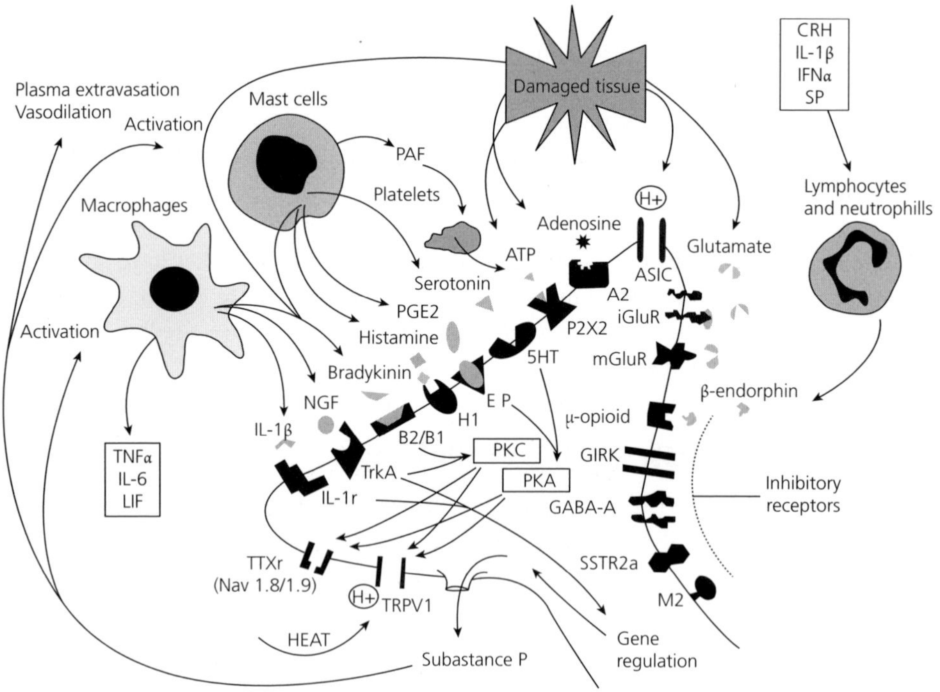

Fig. 9.2 Schematic diagram of the neurochemistry of somatosensory processing at peripheral sensory nerve endings.

Table 9.1 Primary afferents reviews

Afferent Fibres	A beta	A delta	C
Diameter	Large, 6–20 μm	Small, 1–5 μm	Small, 0.2–0.5 μm
Myelin	+ +	+	–
Conductance	80–120 m/s	35–75 m/s	0.5–2 m/s
Activation stimuli	Non-noxious	Non-noxious/noxious	Polymodal noxious
Dorsal Horn termination	Lamina III	Lamina I, IV	70%—peptidergic, Trk A +, lamina I/II 30%—non-peptidergic, IB4 +, lamina II/III

A beta = Large myelinated Light touch, pressure, hair movement III, IV, V.

A delta = Thinly myelinated Pain sharp intense tingling first pain I, II, IV, V.

C = Small un-myelinated Pain predominant (>75%) prolonged

burning second pain I, II

terminate in the outer laminae, I and II, whilst A delta synapse in I, III, IV, and V (see Fig. 9.3).

The majority of primary afferent neurones synapse to inter-neurones or second-order neurones, which allows significant modulation to occur before their ultimate projections. There are two predominant second-order neurones—wide dynamic range (WDR) neurones and nociceptive-specific (NS) neurones. The WDR are concentrated in the deeper laminae (III–IV) and receive input from A beta, A delta, and C fibres, i.e. both noxious and non-noxious stimuli, but their response is graded so noxious stimuli evoke a greater response. NS neurones only respond to noxious stimuli and are found in the superficial laminae (I, II) (12).

Development of neuroimaging techniques has increased our understanding of how pain is represented centrally. Pain was initially thought to be relayed to the somatosensory cortex via the thalamus, but it is now known that nociceptive inputs have a more complex path. The axons of both WDR and NS cross the mid-line near the level of the cell body and ascend in the contralateral spinothalamic tract to the thalamus. There are also direct connections to the medulla (spinoreticular and spinomesencephalic tract) and hypothalamus (spinohypothalamic tract). Nociceptive inputs activate a number of cortical structures—anteriorly cingulate cortex, insula, frontal cortices, and somatosensory cortex S1 and S2. These regions are referred to as the pain matrix (13).

The nociceptive signal may be altered along its pathway, a process known as modulation. The inflammatory soup not only serves as an initiating event, it can also produce

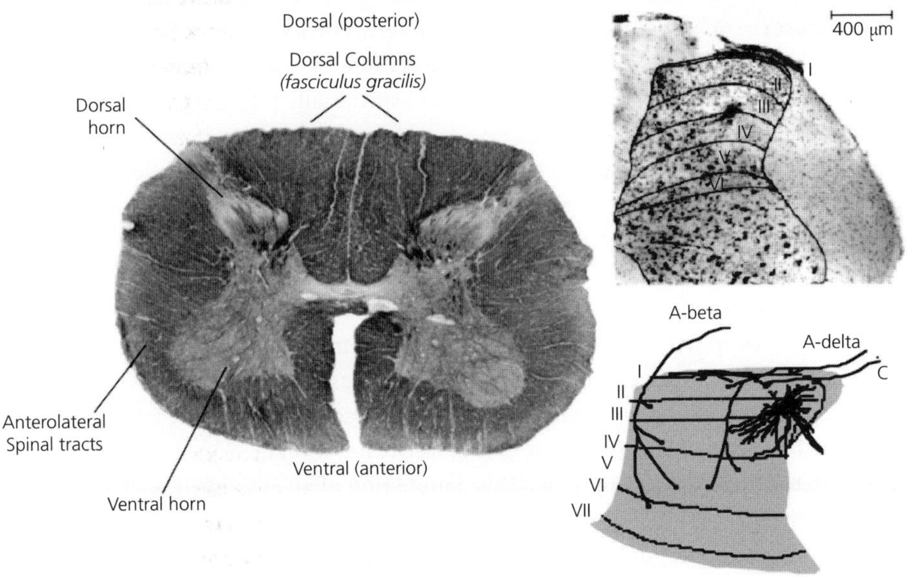

Fig. 9.3 Rexed laminae.

Reproduced from Honorio T. Benzon, Essentials of Pain Medicine, Third Edition, Copyright (2011), with permission from Elsevier.

more enduring changes in the peripheral sensory neurone. These changes include phosphorylation of transducer molecules and ion channels, thereby making the neurone more excitable and capable of spontaneous discharge. The magnitude of its response is then increased. This is known as peripheral sensitization.

A second major site of modulation is in the dorsal horn. The dorsal horn receives inputs from the periphery but there are also descending tracts from the brainstem that can modulate the nociceptive signal. The inputs from higher centres are generally thought of as inhibitory but can have an anti- or pro-nociceptive influence, i.e. result in an augmented or reduced signal. The response from the peripheral input is also dynamic, i.e. a nociceptive input can induce plastic changes within the DH resulting in dysfunctional inhibition and a prolonged state of hyperexcitability, thereby amplifying the pain signal (hyperalgesia) and creating a state where neurones are capable of spontaneous discharge (spontaneous pain) (14). Non-nociceptive low-threshold A beta fibres can also be recruited from a non-nociceptive role to become inputs that feed into the nociceptive pathway (allodynia). This plasticity in the DH can also result in an increase in the nociceptive neuronal receptive field causing the area where pain is felt to increase (12).

How does SCS work?

The mechanism of SCS is complex and current theories are, at times, contradictory. This is perhaps understandable as the pain it appears to suppress is also only partly understood. Despite this, it does appear that SCS is intricately linked with spinal segmental mechanisms at the dorsal horn.

The analgesic potential of neuromodulation was borne out of the GCT (5), so naturally the mechanism of SCS was initially thought of in terms of activation of the large-diameter fibres and the subsequent stimulation of inhibitory inter-neurones. Indeed, since the proposed site of action was the dorsal column, SCS was initially referred to as dorsal column stimulation.

Early clinical reports questioned the GCT theory as a mechanism as, contrary to the proposed mechanism, SCS appeared to have little effect on acute, chronic, or experimental nociceptive pain. Thresholds were significantly increased though in sites displaying hyperalgesia and allodynia. These findings were supported by Quantitative Sensory Testing and if a brief consideration is given to what SCS has been successfully used for (CRPS, neuropathic pain), it supports the theory that SCS has had more success treating neuropathic pain rather than nociceptive or inflammatory pain (15, 16).

The mechanisms of allodynia and cutaneous hypersensitivity are areas of ongoing research but the effects of SCS may be related to the restoration of a 'normal' equilibrium to this disordered pain-processing state. This dampening of an awakened nociceptive pathway can be seen experimentally as SCS can reduce spontaneous discharge of WDR and decreases augmented responses seen in neuropathic pain models (17).

It is generally accepted that with most systems, paraesthesia, indicating stimulation of the dorsal column, is necessary for pain relief, and lesion studies have shown that a large proportion of the analgesic effect is mediated via the dorsal column (14). However, this may not be the only site of action. Antidromic action potentials have been recorded over major peripheral nerves during SCS, with a reduction in primary afferent conduction velocity (7, 18), and a reduction in electrical activity from neuromas has also been noted. These mechanisms suggest that SCS can block afferent activity and may have a peripheral action. There are also experimental studies that suggest SCS may act through modulation of supraspinal mechanisms (19).

Local neurochemistry

The clinical finding that analgesia persists after cessation of stimulation (post-stimulation analgesia) implies a modulation of neural activity and transmitter substances. Application of an electrical current onto the spinal cord causes a wealth of transmitter release and subsequent interactions (20–22)—which are pivotal for the attenuation of pain, is not known. What is known, is that the mechanism does not involve the opioid system, as SCS effects are not affected by naloxone.

Gamma-aminobutyric acid (GABA)

Utilizing micro-dialysis techniques, SCS has been found to increase the inhibitory neurotransmitter gamma-aminobutyric acid (GABA) in the dorsal horn, whilst the release of the excitatory neurotransmitters, glutamate and aspartate, were decreased (20, 21, 23). It is also known that after peripheral nerve injury, GABA inhibitory control mechanisms are attenuated, whilst the release of the excitatory neurotransmitters are enhanced (22). GABA appears to be of special interest as the increase in levels were only seen in rats that responded to SCS (20) and its importance is also supported by the GABA agonist baclofen. Intrathecal baclofen markedly enhanced the effects of SCS (23) and converted non-responding rats into responders. Further support for GABA comes from experiments where allodynia, responsive to SCS, could be counteracted by intrathecal injection of a GABA receptor antagonist or, more specifically, a GABA B receptor antagonist. Elevated levels of GABA persisted after cessation of stimulation, which matches the clinical picture (21), and a reduction in WDR neuronal hyperexcitability was closely related to the raised GABA levels, suggesting that SCS can 'normalize' abnormal central nociceptive processing by increasing or restoring GABA levels.

Serotonin

Another neurotransmitter of interest is serotonin, which is known to be intricately linked to descending inhibitory pain pathways. SCS has been found to induce serotonin release and, similar to GABA, this increase was only seen in animals responsive to SCS. Nerve injury is known to cause changes in the expression and function of serotonin neurones and its receptor subtypes and SCS may reverse this dysfunction. Intrathecal serotonin enhances SCS affects, whilst GABA B antagonists partially blocked the effects, suggesting serotonin effects were mediated via the GABAergic pathways.

Acetylcholine (ACh) and noradrenaline

SCS has also been found to induce release of ACh and noradrenaline and again this was only seen in responsive animals; this analgesia could be reversed by intrathecal muscarinic antagonists. Intrathecal clonidine, an alpha adrenoceptor agonist, is thought to exert its anti-nociceptive effects by increasing dorsal horn ACh (24). Muscarinic and alpha 1 adrenoceptors are located on GABAergic inter-neurones, so the proposed action is again via GABAergic inter-neurones (14, 22). Other substances known to be involved included substance P, which is released by SCS (25), and adenosine, which can abolish neuropathic pain acutely (26).

Summary of SCS mechanism

In summary, SCS appears to have its predominant effects on sensitized nociceptive pathways. Its analgesic effect is predominantly achieved at a segmental spinal level by reducing the effects of central sensitization, namely the exaggerated responses and spontaneous activity in the dorsal horns by second-order neurones. This is thought to be due to a dysfunction in GABAergic systems and SCS may act by restoring the normal levels of the inhibitory GABA.

Disease pathology of CRPS

Complex regional pain syndrome, or the entity known as CRPS, has been known by various names. It was first reported, by Weir Mitchell, as causalgia in American Civil War veterans with peripheral nerve damage and a continuous burning pain. Wier Mitchell is also credited with documenting phantom limb pain in the subsequently erroneously amputated limbs. Sudeck observed bone demineralization and muscle wasting after infections in limbs in 1900—hence Sudeck's dystrophy—and in 1947, Evans postulated sympathetic nervous system involvement and reflex sympathetic dystrophy was conceived.

Historically, diagnosis of CRPS was often made from clinical experience or by a variety of non-standardized systems, which resulted in inconsistent diagnosis and treatment (27).

In 1994, an International Association of the Study of Pain (IASP) Consensus Group met in Florida to address this discrepancy. This group created the new name and diagnostic criteria for complex regional pain syndrome (Table 9.2) (28).

Table 9.2 CRPS criteria, as outlined by the IASP

The presence of an initiating noxious event, or a cause of immobilization†
Continuing pain, allodynia, or hyperalgesia in which the pain is disproportionate to any known inciting event
Evidence at some time of oedema, changes in skin blood flow, or abnormal sudomotor activity in the region of pain (can be a sign or symptom)
This diagnosis is excluded by the existence of other conditions that would otherwise account for the degree of pain and dysfunction

Reproduced from Merskey H, Bogduk N, Classifications of chronic pain, Second Edition, Copyright (1994), with permission from IASP Press.

†Not required for diagnosis; 5–10% of patients will not have this. Must have criteria 2, 3, and 4 for diagnosis.

Table 9.3 Table of Budapest Criteria

Continuing pain, which is disproportionate to any inciting event
Must report at least one symptom in three of the four following categories:
Sensory
Vasomotor
Sudometor/Oedema
Motor/Tropic
Must display at least one sign at time of evaluation in two or more of the following categories:
Sensory
Vasomotor
Sudometor/Oedema
Motor/Tropic
There is no other diagnosis that better explains the signs and symptoms

Although these criteria were thought to be sensitive, they lacked the required sensitivity and the diagnostic criteria were further refined into the Budapest Criteria in 2007 (Table 9.3).

Aetiology and epidemiology

CRPS describes an array of painful conditions with continuing disproportionate pain usually occurring, but not necessarily, after an initiating event or trauma (29). It has a slight female preponderance and generally affects patients from 36 to 42 years (range 9–85) and there are approximately 50,000 new cases per year in the USA (30). In the majority of cases, the onset of symptoms is after 1 month and 15% of sufferers will have unrelenting pain and impairment 2 years after onset (31, 32). The hallmarks of CRPS are abnormal sensory, motor, sudomotor, vasomotor, or trophic findings in addition to the characteristic neuropathic pain symptoms (spontaneous pain, hyperalgesia, and allodynia). Type I and II CRPS only differ by the presence (type II) or absence (type I) of an identifiable nerve injury, but it is now generally accepted that some form of nerve trauma, albeit trivial, is the trigger in both (33). Previously, CRPS was considered to be a sympathetically mediated pain condition but it is now apparent that there are multiple pathophysiological mechanisms occurring both at the periphery and centrally that are not yet fully understood. Previous implication of the sympathetic nervous system followed the beneficial response of sympathetic blockade but it cannot be guaranteed that all patients will respond to such blocks, and now CRPS is generally thought of as either sympathetically maintained pain (SMP) or sympathetically independent pain (SIP). It should be noted that patients of both SMP and SIP can benefit from SCS.

Pathophysiology

Although CRPS type I was thought not to be associated with a nerve injury, in skin biopsies from affected limbs, significantly lower densities of epidermal neurites were found, compared with the unaffected limb. These changes were predominantly in primary nociceptive fibres and were not seen in non-CRPS pain (33). Decreased density of A delta and C fibres have also been reported in CRPS I in another study (34). These findings demonstrate that in CRPS I, even with the absence of any apparent nerve injury, there was still significant neuronal loss.

Peripheral sensitization

Tissue trauma elicits a local response with the release of pronociceptive substances that trigger a nociceptive impulse. The resulting inflammatory soup can also increase the background frequency of nociceptive signals, increase that magnitude of response to nociceptive inputs, and reduce the threshold for thermal and mechanical stimuli, i.e. peripheral sensitization. These explain some of the hallmarks of CRPS, namely spontaneous pain, hyperalgesia, and allodynia (35, 36).

Central sensitization

A constant barrage of nociceptive input to the spinal cord results in an amplification of the signal at the dorsal horn—central sensitization. Release of neuropeptides (substance P, glutamate, etc.) act on N-methyl-D-aspartic acid receptors and result in exaggerated response to non-noxious stimuli (allodynia) and noxious stimuli (hyperalgesia). This can be objectively measured by increased excitability or windup. In windup, a short, repeated stimulus results in increased excitability in the spinal cord. Significantly greater windup is seen on affected limbs with CRPS compared to the unaffected limb; it is not known if this is a consequence or cause of CRPS.

Sympathetic nervous system

Altered sympathetic function, although no longer thought to be the sole mechanism, still has a role to play. Nerve trauma in animal studies results in adrenergic receptors being expressed on nociceptive fibres, thereby creating a mechanism of sympathetically maintained pain and sympatho-afferent coupling, where SNS activation increases CRPS pain intensity (30); but the traditional notion that features of chronic CRPS were due to SNS excess are erroneous.

Genetic factors

Familial CRPS indirectly supports a genetic contribution but currently, there is no consistent compelling evidence for specific genetic factors. The potential importance of genetic factors is suggested by some of the mechanisms believed to contribute to CRPS having a genetic link.

Brain plasticity

Several neuroimaging studies suggest a reorganization of somatosensory maps in CRPS, specifically a reduction in the size of the representation of the CRPS affected limb.

Interestingly, this can return to normal size after successful treatment. These central changes have meaningful effects, the degree of somatotrophic reorganization correlates with the pain intensity and degree of hyperalgesia and impaired two-point discrimination (37–41).

Inflammatory factors

Several small trials indicated benefit of steroids in patients with acute CRPS, suggesting an inflammatory mechanism. This is thought to arise from classic inflammatory mechanism and neurogenic inflammation (42, 43). Neurogenic inflammation occurs from the release of pro-inflammatory neuropeptides directly from the nerve fibres. These neuropeptides can cause the warm red oedematous extremity of acute CRPS. One neuropeptide, TNF-alpha, appears to be key in this process, and administration of a TNF-alpha antibody (infliximab) may reduce symptoms in some patients (44).

Psychological factors

It is clear that purely psychogenic factors were never necessary or capable of producing the signs of CRPS but, in theory, psychogenic factors could exacerbate symptoms. Depression, anxiety, and anger can all increase catecholamine levels (45, 46) and alter immune function (47–49), and thereby theoretically perpetuate signs and symptoms of CRPS, although there is no data to support this hypothesis.

Treatment overview

Many treatments for CRPS have been tried but few have proven effective. This may have been due, in part, to a continuing lack of detailed understanding on the pathophysiological mechanisms in play. Current treatment is based around 'four pillars of treatment' and a prompt diagnosis (50). A rapid diagnosis of CRPS is important, as response to treatment appears to be adversely affected by delay (51). Despite this, it is not uncommon for patients to experience a significant delay. The 'four pillars of treatment' are:

1 Patient information and education to support and self-management.

2 Physical and vocational rehabilitation.

3 Psychological intervention.

4 Pain relief (medications and procedures) (50).

In the context of a chronic disease, where full recovery can be difficult to achieve, information is of paramount importance. Physicians can help by educating, setting goals, and agreeing treatment plans with patients. Patients should be offered physical therapies as early as possible, and occupational therapy for assessment of functional needs and to access regional support services. CRPS is not associated with a history of psychological issues prior to the pain (52–54) but these may be present, or develop, and should be addressed, where appropriate. Pain relief can be pharmacological, simple analgesia and anti-neuropathic medication (though no drugs currently hold a UK license for CRPS), or interventional. Interventional techniques included intravenous regional sympathetic blocks (IVRSB), once widely practiced, but now not routinely used as four randomized controlled trials failed to demonstrate any benefit (50). Other procedures, such as nerve plexus blocks and catheters, are used in some centres but the supportive evidence is anecdotal. SCS should be considered in patients who have not responded to appropriate integrated management.

SCS and CRPS

A series of observational studies found that pain was significantly reduced in CRPS with SCS (55–58). A subsequent prospective RCT of CRPS I, randomized patients to receive spinal cord stimulation (SCS) and physical therapy (PT) or PT alone. It found a greater reduction in pain and an improvement in global perceived health in SCS and PT treatment group compared to PT treatment alone at 6 months. Although no functional improvement was observed, the authors comment that the patients were severely disabled at baseline and with such severe disability, with advanced contractures and muscle atrophy, functional improvement was unlikely (59). The favourable pain results were maintained at 24-month follow-up (60). A cost-analysis based on the above RCT found that, despite the initial outlay for the implant (SCS and RT costs in year 1 were double that of PT alone), the average costs declined significantly in the SCS and PT group but remained high in the PT alone group; the two lines crossing each other after three years (61). So, in summary, SCS currently represents good value in terms of quality-adjusted-life-years (QALYs) (62, 63).

SCS and sympathetic nervous system

SCS is known to have an effect on the sympathetic nervous system, as manifested in its anti-anginal, anti-ischaemic effects. The vasodilatory effects of SCS may be due to an inhibition of vascular tone, and antidromic activation of primary afferents may also play a role, although the mechanism is not yet fully understood (64–65).

Some pain conditions (notably CRPS) can be subdivided into sympathetically maintained pain (SMP) and sympathetically independent pain (SIP) (66). In cases of CRPS, SCS has been shown to be an effective treatment in SIP and SMP.

What the future holds

As our understanding of the mechanism of SCS and underlying disease processes increases, so do therapeutic options. New strategies can be developed to enhance the analgesic effects of SCS and greater understanding of the effects of SCS; for example, effects on the vascular system may broaden SCS indications.

It is known that by utilizing adjunct pharmacology, not only can the analgesic effects of SCS can be augmented, but previous non-responders can be switched to responders. Baclofen has been shown to enhance SCS effects, as has adenosine, serotonin, gabapentin, pregabalin, and clonidine.

The frequency of stimulation affects neurotransmitter release and the most effective parameters from SCS have not been systematically investigated. SCS analgesia may involve different mechanisms at different frequencies, thus it may be possible to alter effects by utilizing different frequencies.

Other sites of neuromodulation also warrant future consideration. An area of interest is the Dorsal Root Ganglion (DRG), stimulation of which has the advantage of being an assessable structure with the potential to target more specific areas, i.e. a single dermatome.

Conclusions

SCS has been in the physician's armamentarium for more than 40 years and has been used to treat a variety of pain syndromes in that time. It is a treatment modality that is more effective at treating neuropathic pain, rather than nociceptive pain. Modulation of the autonomic nervous system has been demonstrated but does not appear to be a prerequisite for analgesia; indeed, SCS has been proven effective for SMP and SIP CRPS.

Effects of SCS are mediated by a complex set of interactions at multiple levels, although a restoration of the neurotransmitter GABA, in the dorsal horn, appears pivotal.

The pathophysiological mechanisms of CRPS are multi-factorial in nature. They may include inflammation, altered sympathetic function, reduced representation in the somatosensory cortex, genetic factors, psychophysiologic interactions, and peripheral and central sensitization. The degree to which individual mechanisms contribute to CRPS may differ from patient to patient and even within one patient over time.

A better understanding of the pathophysiological processes at work in CRPS and the mechanisms of SCS is key to progress. This will enable risk factors to be identified and the signs and symptoms of CRPS to be linked to underlying processes. Improved diagnosis and treatment protocols could then be developed with interventions, such as SCS, applied appropriately and promptly to reduce the duration or even development of symptoms in the first place.

References

1 **Kane K, Taub A**. A history of local electrical analgesia. Pain 1975;**2**:125–38.
2 **Gildenberg PL**. History of electrical neuromodulation for chronic pain. Pain Med 2006;**7**(S1):S7–13.
3 **Krabbenbos IP, van Dongen EPA, Nijhuis HJA, Liam AL**. Mechanisms of spinal cord stimulation in neuropathic pain. In: Carrillo-Ruiz JD (ed) Topics in Neuromodulation Treatment. InTech; 2012:89–110.
4 **Light R, Chaffee EL**. Electrical excitation of the nervous system—introducing a new principle: remote control. Preliminary report. Science 1934;**79**(2048):299–300.
5 **Melzack R, Wall P**. Pain mechanisms: a new theory. Science 1965;**150**(3699):971–79.
6 **Dickerson A**. Gate Control Theory of pain stands the test of time. Br J Anaesth 2002;**88** (6):755–57.
7 **Wall PD, Sweet WH**. Temporary abolition of pain in man. Science 1967;**155**:108–109.
8 **Wall P**. The discovery of transcutaneous electrical nerve stimulation. Physiotherapy 1985;**71**:348–50.
9 **Shealy C, Mortimer J, Resnick J**. Electrical inhibition of pain by stimulation of the dorsal columns. Journal of Int Anesth Res Soc 1967;**46**:489–91.
10 **Mailis-Gagnon A, Furlan A, SAndoval J, Taylor R**. Spinal cord stimulation for chronic pain. Cochrane Datab Syst Rev 2004, Issue 3. Art No. CD003783.

11 **Cameron T**. Safety and efficacy of spinal cord stimulation for the treatment of chronic pain: a 20-year literature review. J Neurosurg 2004;**100**:254–67.

12 **Ralevic V, Burnstock G**. Receptors for purines and pyrimidines. Pharmacol Rev 1998; **50**:413–92.

13 **Brooks J, Tracey I**. From nociception to pain perception: imaging the spinal and supraspinal pathways. J Anat 2005;**207**:19–33. Review.

14 **Guan Y**. Spinal cord stimulation: neurophysical and neurochemical mechanisms of action. Curr Pain Headache Rep 2012;**16**:217–25.

15 **Nashold B, Somjen G**. Paraesthesia and EEG potentials evoked by stimulation of the dorsal funiculi in man. Exp Neurol 1972;**36**:273–87.

16 **Lindbolm U, Meyerson B**. Influence on touch, vibration and cutaneous pain of dorsal column stimulation in man. Pain 1975;**1**:257–70.

17 **Yakhnista V**. Effects of spinal cord stimulation on dorsal horn neuronal activity in a rat model of mononeuropathy. Pain 1999;**79**:223–33.

18 **Wall PD**. The past and future of local nerve and brain stimulation. Presented at: International Congress of the International Neuromodulation Society; Rome; 1992.

19 **Roberts M, Rees H**. Physiological basis of spinal cord stimulation. Pain Rev 1994;**1**:184–98.

20 **Stiler C**. Release of gamma-aminobutyric acid in the dorsal horn and suppression of tactile allodynia by spinal cord stimulation in mononeuropathic rats. Neurosurgery 1996;**39**:367–74.

21 **Cui J**. Spinal cord stimulation attenuates augmented dorsal horn release of excitatory amino acids in mononeuropathy via the GABAergic mechanism. Pain 1997;**73**:87–95.

22 **Schechtmann G**. Cholinergic mechanisms involved in the pain relieving effect of spinal cord stimulation in a model of neuropathy. Pain 2008;**139**:136–45.

23 **Cui J**. Effects of spinal cord stimulation on touch evoked allodynia involve GABAergic mechanisms. An experimental study in the mononeuropathic rat. Pain 1996;**66**:287–95.

24 **Xu Z**. Role of muscarinic and nicotinic receptors in clonidine induced nitric oxide release in rat model of neuropathic pain. Brain Res 2000;**861**:390–98.

25 **Linderoth B**. Dorsal column stimulation induces release of serotonin and substance P in the cat dorsal horn. Neurosurgery 1992;**28**:187–95.

26 **Cui J**. Adenosine receptor activation suppresses tactile hypersensitivity and potentiates effects of spinal cord stimulation in mononeuropathic rats. Neurosci Lett 1997;**223**:173–76.

27 **Harden R, Bruehl S, Stanton-Hicks M**. Proposed new diagnostic criteria for complex regional pain syndrome. Pain Medicine 2007;**8**(4):326–31.

28 **Merskey H, Bogduk N**. Classification of Chronic Pain: Descriptions of Chronic Pain Syndromes and Definitions of Pain Terms. Second edition. Seattle: IASP Press; 2002.

29 **Fukui S, Shigemori S, Nosaka S**. Beneficial effects of electroconvulsive therapy on clinical features and thalamic blood flows in a CRPS type 1 patient. Br J Anaesth 2002;**16**(3):248–50.

30 **Bruehl S, Chung O**. How common is complex regional pain syndrome Type-I? Pain 2007;**129** (1–2).

31 **Mirone G, Natale M, Rotondo M**. Peripheral median nerve stimulation for the treatment of iatrogenic complex regional pain syndrome (CRPS) type II after carpal tunnel surgery. J Clin Neuroscience 2009;**16** (6):825–27.

32 **Placzek JD, Boyer MI, Gelberman RH, Sopp B, Goldfarb CA**. Nerve decompression for complex regional pain syndrome type II following upper extremity surgery. J Hand Surg Am 2005;**30**(1):69–74.

33 **Birklein F, Schmelz M**. Neuropeptides, neurogenic inflammation and complex regional pain syndrome (CRPS). Neurosci Lett 2008; **437**:199–202.

34 **Oaklander AL, Rissmiller JG, Gelman LB et al.** Evidence of focal small-fiber axonal degeneration in complex regional pain syndrome-I (reflex sympathetic dystrophy). Pain 2006;**120**:235–43.

35 **Cheng JK, Ji RR.** Intracellular signaling in primary sensory neurons and persistent pain. Neurochem Res 2008;**33**:1970–78.

36 **Couture R, Harrisson M, Vianna RM, Cloutier** F. Kinin receptors in pain and inflammation. Eur J Pharmacol 2001;**429**:161–76.

37 **Juottonen K, Gockel M, Silen T, Hurri H, Hari R, Forss N.** Altered central sensorimotor processing in patients with complex regional pain syndrome. Pain 2002;**98**:315–23.

38 **Maihofner C, Handwerker HO, Neundorfer B, Birklein F.** Patterns of cortical reorganization in complex regional pain syndrome. Neurology 2003;**61**:1707–15.

39 **Maihofner C, Handwerker HO, Neundorfer B, Birklein F.** Cortical reorganization during recovery from complex regional pain syndrome. Neurology 2004;**63**:693–701.

40 **Pleger B, Ragert P, Schwenkreis P et al.** Patterns of cortical reorganization parallel impaired tactile discrimination and pain intensity in complex regional pain syndrome. Neuroimage 2006;**32**:503–10.

41 **Pleger B, Tegenthoff M, Ragert P et al.** Sensorimotor retuning [corrected] in complex regional pain syndrome parallels pain reduction. Ann Neurol 2005;**57**:425–29.

42 **Braus DF, Krauss JK, Strobel J.** The shoulder-hand syndrome after stroke: A prospective clinical trial. Ann Neurol 1994;**36**:728–33.

43 **Christensen K, Jensen EM, Noer I.** The reflex dystrophy syndrome response to treatment with systemic corticosteroids. Acta Chir Scand 1982;**148**:653–55.

44 **Bernateck M, Rolke R, Birklein F, Treede RD, Fink M, Karst M.** Successful intravenous regional block with low-dose tumor necrosis factor-alpha antibody infliximab for treatment of complex regional pain syndrome 1. Anesth Analg 2007;**105**:1148–51.

45 **Edwards RR, Kronfli T, Haythornthwaite JA, Smith MT, McGuire L, Page GG.** Association of catastrophizing with interleukin-6 responses to acute pain. Pain 2008;**140**:135–44.

46 **Kaufmann I, Eisner C, Richter P et al.** Lymphocyte subsets and the role of TH1/TH2 balance in stressed chronic pain patients. Neuroimmunomodulation 2007;**14**:272–80.

47 **Charney DS, Woods SW, Nagy LM, Southwick SM, Krystal JH, Heninger GR.** Noradrenergic function in panic disorder. J Clin Psychiatry 1990;**51**:5–10.

48 **Harden RN, Rudin NJ, Bruehl S et al.** Increased systemic catecholamines in complex regional pain syndrome and relationship to psychological factors: A pilot study. Anesth Analg 2004;**99**:1478–85.

49 **Light KC, Kothandapani RV, Allen MT.** Enhanced cardiovascular and catecholamine responses in women with depressive symptoms. Int J Psychophys 1998;**28**:157–66.

50 **Goebel A, Barker CH, Turner-Stokes L et al.** Complex Regional Pain Syndrome in Adults: UK Guidelines for Diagnosis, Referral and Management in Primary and Secondary Care. London: RCP; 2012.

51 **Stanton-Hicks M.** Complex regional pain syndrome. J Pain Symp Manag 2006;**31**:4SS20–9.

52 **Kiefer RT, Rohr P, Ploppa A, Altemeyer KH, Schwartzman RJ.** Complete recovery from intractable complex regional pain syndrome, CRPS-type I, following anesthetic ketamine and midazolam. Pain Pract 2007;**7**(2):147–50.

53 **Kiefer RT, Rohr P, Ploppa A et al.** Efficacy of ketamine in anesthetic dosage for the treatment of refractory complex regional pain syndrome: an open-label phase II study. Pain Med 2008;**9**(8):1173–201.

54 **Koffler SP, Hampstead BM, Irani F et al.** The neurocognitive effects of 5 day anesthetic ketamine for the treatment of refractory complex regional pain syndrome. Arch Clin Neuropsychol 2007;**22**(6):719–29.

55 **Calvillo O, Racz G, Didie J et al:** Neuroaugmentation in the treatment of complex regional pain syndrome of the upper extremity. Acta Orthop Belg 1998;**64**:57–63.

56 **Robaina FJ, Dominguez MD, Diaz M et al.** Spinal cord stimulation for relief of chronic pain in vasospastic disorders of the upper limbs. Neurosurgery 1989;**24**:63–67.

57 **Oakley J, Weiner R.** Spinal cord stimulation for complex regional pain syndrome. a prospective study of 19 patients at two centers. Neuromodulation 1999;**1**:47–50.

58 **Stanton-Hicks M.** Spinal cord stimulation for the management of complex regional pain syndromes. Neuromodulation 1999;**3**:193–201.

59 **Kemler M, Gerard A, Barenose M et al.** Spinal cord stimulation in patients with chronic reflex sympathetic dystriphy. NEJM 2000;**343**:618–24.

60 **Kemler MA, De Vet HC, Barendse GA et al.** The effect of spinal cord stimulation in patients with chronic reflex sympathetic dystrophy: two years' follow-up of the randomized controlled trial. Ann Neurol 2004;**55**(1):3–18.

61 **Kemler A, Furnee CA.** Economic evaluation of spinal cord stimulation for chronic reflex sympathetic dystrophy. Neurology 2002;**59**:1203–209.

62 **Taylor RS.** Spinal cord stimulation in complex regional pain syndrome and refractory neuropathic back and leg pain/failed back surgery syndrome: results of a systematic review and meta-analysis. J Pain Symptom Manage 2006;**31**(4 Suppl):S13–19.

63 **Taylor RS, Van Buyten J-P, Buchser E.** Spinal cord stimulation for complex regional pain syndrome: A systematic review of the clinical and cost-effectiveness literature and assessment of prognostic factors. Eur J Pain 2006;**10**:91–101.

64 **Croom J, Foreman R, Chandler M, Barron K.** Cutaneous vasodilation during dorsal column stimulation is mediated by dorsal roots and CGRP. Am J Physiol 1997;**272**:H950–H957.

65 **WU M, Linderoth B, Foreman RD.** Putative mechanisms behind effects of spinal cord stimulation on vascular diseases: a review of experimental studies. Auton Neurosci 2008;**138**(1–2):9–23.

66 **Barin R, Levine J, Fields H.** Causalgia and reflex sympathetic dystrophy: does the sympathetic nervous system contribute to the generation of Pain? Muscle Nerve 1999;**22**:678–95.

Chapter 10

Spinal cord stimulation for complex regional pain syndrome II: clinical applications

Stana Bojanic and Tim McCormick

Key points

1. Correct diagnosis of CRPS is essential.
2. Multi-disciplinary management of CRPS initially involves education, pain relief, physical rehabilitation, and psychological intervention.
3. SCS should be considered in those not responding to this management.
4. SCS is effective in CRPS Type I and Type II.
5. Evidence demonstrates that SCS is a cost-effective treatment for CRPS Type I.

Introduction

Complex regional pain syndrome (CRPS) is a syndrome that usually develops after an initiating noxious event. It is not limited to the distribution of a single peripheral nerve and is disproportional to the inciting event. It is associated at some point with evidence of oedema, changes in skin blood flow, abnormal sudomotor activity in the region of the pain, or allodynia or hyperalgesia (1). However, in about 9% of cases there is no precipitating trauma at all (2). CRPS can be divided into two types based on the absence of a lesion to a major nerve (Type I) or the presence of such a lesion (Type II). Type I CRPS has previously been referred to as reflex sympathetic dystrophy. Type II CRPS has been referred to as causalgia. Diagnosis can sometimes be difficult and various sets of diagnostic criteria can be used such as the Budapest Diagnostic Criteria (Table 10.1) (3). The European incidence of CRPS is 26/100,000 person-years (4). The differential diagnoses are many and include infection, orthopaedic malfixation, joint instability, bone or soft tissue injury, compartment syndrome, thoracic outlet syndrome, and Raynaud's disease amongst others. CRPS usually affects one limb but in 7% of cases it later spreads to involve additional

Table 10.1 Diagnostic criteria for CRPS ('Budapest criteria')

Category	Sign	Symptom
1.'Sensory'	Allodynia (to light touch and/or	Hyperesthesia
	Temperature sensation and/or	does also qualify
	Joint movement) and/or	as a symptom
	Hyperalgesia (to pinprick)	
'Vasomotor'	Temperature asymmetry and\or	If you notice
	skin colour changes and/or	temperature
	skin colour asymmetry	asymmetry:
		must be >1°C
'Sudomotor/	Odema and/or sweating changes	
oedema'	and/or sweating asymmetry	
4.'Motor/	Decreased range of motion	
Trophic'	and/or motor dysfunction	
	(weakness, tremor, dystonia)	
	and/or trophic changes	
	(hair/nail/skin)	

Reproduced from Pain Medicine, 8 (4), Harden R, Bruehl S, Stanton-Hicks M, Wilson P., Proposed new diagnostic criteria for complex regional pain syndrome, p. 326–31, Copyright (2007), with permission from John Wiley & Sons Ltd.

Diagnostic criteria for CRPS ('Budapest criteria'). A–D must apply.

(A) The patient has continuing pain that is disproportionate to any inciting event.

(B) The patient has at least one sign in two or more of the categories.

(C) The patient reports at least one symptom in three or more of the categories.

(D) No other diagnosis can better explain the signs and symptoms.

limbs (5). Approximately 15% of patients with CRPS will have unrelenting pain and physical impairment 2 years after CRPS onset (6).

Clinical management of CRPS should involve a multi-disciplinary approach and may include education, physiotherapy, rehabilitation, psychological support, analgesics, referral to a pain management team, and management of skin/bone pathology (7). The aims of treatment are to reduce pain, preserve or restore function and enable patients to manage their condition and improve their quality of life (8). Spinal cord stimulation (SCS) should be considered in patients with CRPS who have not responded to these treatments.

Rationale for target selection and approach

The aim of spinal cord stimulation (SCS) in CRPS is to achieve stimulation paraesthesia covering the area of pain. The patient often describes a 'pleasant tingling sensation' or a 'pleasant warmth' in place of the pain with SCS stimulation. The SCS leads have been placed in the epidural space in locations from C1 to L5 to treat pain of the trunk and/or limb (9), depending on the indication for treatment. The aim is to stimulate the dorsal aspect of the spinal cord leading to neurophysiological and neurotransmitter effects, as described in Chapter 9.

Target levels

To stimulate the lower extremity or lower back (for axial pain), the lead placement desired is at the T9 to T12 position. Foot pain is best treated at the T12 level, while buttock pain is best treated at the T9 level (10). Above the T9 level, patients often experience nerve root irritation into the abdomen or intercostal nerves. However, these levels are not prescriptive and stimulation can vary in patient to patient at the same level. The position of the conus can vary and needs to be considered at implantation in each individual patient.

For upper limb stimulation, the lead is placed at the C3–C7 level in most cases. Vallejo et al. (11) reported occipital and supra-occipital paraesthesia with lead placements up to the C2/3 level, as well as stimulation into the upper limbs. This observation capturing the occipital regions of the head is not surprising. The greater and lesser occipital nerves emanate from the C2 root and, to a lesser extent, the C3 root, and connect in the spinal cord within the spinal nucleus of the trigeminal nerve (which become the nucleus caudalis in the cervical region) (12).

Postural effects

Postural effects have been reported relating to changes in stimulation threshold—paraesthesias were felt when in the supine position but were greatly reduced when standing or sitting (13). Cameron and Alo (14) examined these postural effects in patients in whom a percutaneous lead had been previously implanted. The mean threshold for stimulation in order to achieve paraesthesia was lowest when recumbent, whereas in three patients it was lowest while sitting. These changes in threshold with respect to posture were the result of spinal cord movement. When patients are lying on their back, their spinal cord moves ventral and therefore closer to the SCS electrodes, reducing the level of stimulation needed to reach threshold. The thickness of the CSF layer can also affect stimulation thresholds. At the thoracic level, the CSF is reduced again, further decreasing the distance between the electrode and the dorsal columns.

SCS systems

As well as considering these factors for target selection, two different SCS systems are routinely used—those allowing percutaneous placements of electrodes and those requiring an 'open' surgical approach by undertaking laminectomy/laminotomy. The percutaneous electrodes can be implanted into the epidural space via a Tuohy needle (see Fig. 10.1).

Electrode insertion via a laminectomy/laminotomy allows paddle-type leads to be implanted (see Fig. 10.2). Both systems are powered by an implantable pulse generator (IPG)

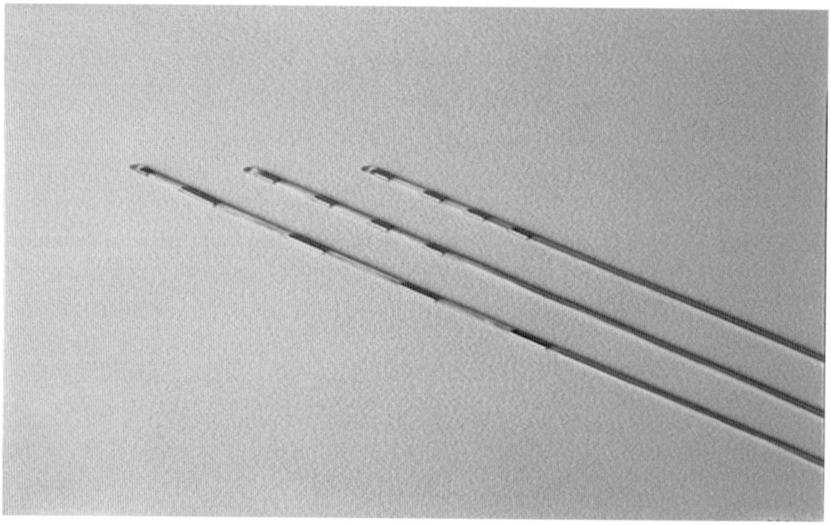

Fig. 10.1 Example of percutaneous electrodes.
Reproduced courtesy of Medtronic.

battery or an implanted radiofrequency (RF) controlled receiver. A trial period is undertaken with the electrode *in situ* in order to confirm that stimulation is of benefit and stimulation paraesthesia covers the area of pain. Considerations in choosing which system to implant can include previous spinal surgery (scarred epidural space), lead migration, local expertise, and patient preference.

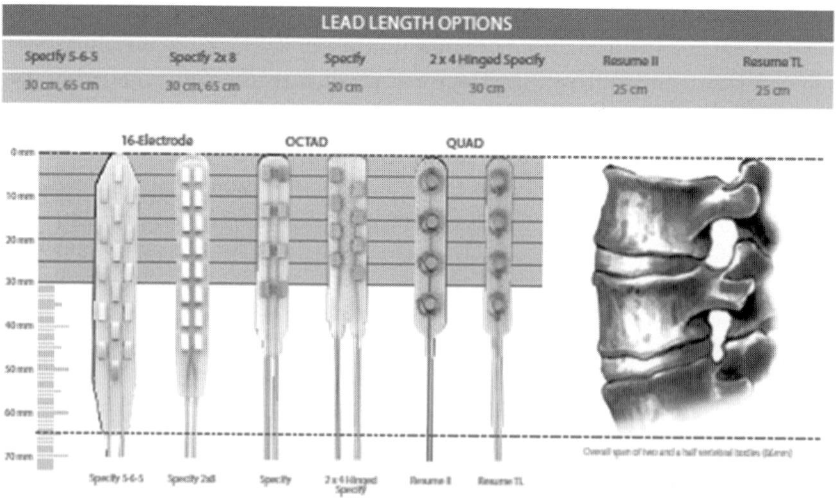

Fig. 10.2 Examples of different surgical electrodes configurations that are available and length of electrode coverage in the spine.
Reproduced courtesy of Medtronic.

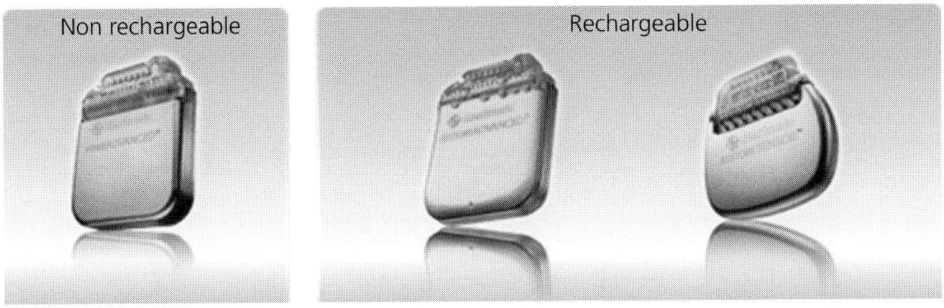

Fig. 10.3 Implantable pulse generator (IPG) batteries. Non-rechargeable and rechargeable options are available. The IPG battery sits in a sub-cutaneous pocket. The site of the pocket is agreed pre-operatively but commonly the upper buttock or abdomen is used in implants for lower limb stimulation. For upper limb stimulation, the pocket can also be sited over the thoracic area.
Reproduced courtesy of Medtronic.

There are many spinal cord stimulator systems available on the market. Electrodes can be single (such as a single percutaneous wire or a vertical four contact electrode paddle) or dual systems (using two percutaneous electrodes in parallel or surgical electrodes with two or more parallel contacts). Evidence suggests dual systems can achieve a better level of stimulation with greater clinical reliability, particularly when considering treatment of axial pain or bilateral extremity pain (15).

IPG batteries come in many shapes and sizes—the main choices being a rechargeable or non-rechargeable system (see Fig. 10.3). RF devices (an externally worn transmitter) have been used regularly in the past. However, with improved IPG technology and the introduction of the rechargeable IPG systems, these devices are not used as frequently. The IPG battery life is variable, but is usually between 2 and 8 years, depending on the pattern of use and the output required. Rechargeable devices offer increased longevity.

Indications and patient selection criteria

Current National Institute for Clinical Excellence (NICE) guidelines (16) state, 'Spinal cord stimulation is recommended as a treatment option for adults with chronic pain of neuropathic origin who:

- continue to experience chronic pain (measuring at least 50 mm on a 0–100 mm visual analogue scale) for at least 6 months despite appropriate conventional medical management, and
- who have had a successful trial of stimulation as part of the assessment in recommendation.'

Indications for SCS include CRPS Type I (17) and II (18), amongst others (see Table 10.2) (19). Patient selection is of paramount importance in establishing a successful interventional pain programme. Patients should be managed and assessed by a multi-disciplinary team prior to selection—such team members may include a consultant in pain medicine,

Table 10.2 Indications for spinal cord stimulation

Good indications for SCS (likely to respond)	Neuropathic pain in arm or leg following lumbar or cervical spine surgery (FNSS/FBSS).
	Complex regional pain syndrome (CRPS).
	Neuropathic pain secondary to peripheral nerve damage.
	Pain associated with peripheral vascular disease.
	Refractory angina pectoris (RAP).
	Brachial plexopathy: traumatic (partial, not avulsion), post-irradiation.
Intermediate indications for SCS (may respond)	Amputation pain (stump responds better than phantom pain).
	Axial pain following spinal surgery.
	Intercostal neuralgia.
	Pain associated with spinal cord damage
	(other peripheral neuropathic pain syndromes, such as those following trauma may respond).
Poor indications for SCS (rarely respond)	Central pain of non-spinal origin.
	Spinal cord injury with clinically complete loss of posterior column function.
	Perineal or anorectal pain.
Unresponsive to SCS	Complete spinal cord transection.
	Non-ischaemic nociceptive pain.
	Nerve root avulsion.

Reproduced from Appl Neurophysiol, 45, Broseta J, Roldan P, Gonalez-Darder J et al., Chronic epidural dorsal column stimulation in the treatment of causalgia pain, p. 190–194, Copyright (1982), with permission from Karger AG.

one or more consultants from other relevant specialties, such as neurosurgery or spinal surgery, a nurse specialist in pain management, a psychologist, and a physiotherapist. The preservation of topographically appropriate posterior column function seems to be necessary for SCS to be effective, but there is debate regarding which elements are necessary and to what degree.

Medical contraindications to the use of SCS include:

- uncontrolled bleeding disorder (anticoagulant therapy is a relative contraindication)
- systemic or local sepsis
- the presence of a demand cardiac pacemaker or implanted defibrillator (relative contraindication)
- immune suppression (relative contraindication).

In considering surgical insertion of a paddle electrode, there must be adequate epidural space to accommodate the electrode. A pre-operative MRI scan of the target area for electrode implant should be considered. Further laminectomy/laminotomy in patients who have already undergone spinal surgery can lead to further morbidity—such as pain around the incision/laminectomy site or instability. The surgical electrode can be fixed to the dura directly by suturing through the outer layer of the dura. However, if the inner dural layer is breached, this can lead to the development of a cerebrospinal fluid (CSF) hygroma (19).

Clinical assessment involves a careful history and examination. Referral to a psychologist is recommended to screen for mental illness, cognitive impairment, communication problems, or learning difficulties. These are not reasons to exclude a patient from SCS but these conditions may require continuing management and support. A careful pre-implant assessment should include:

- screen for coagulopathy (other routine bloods)
- screen for MRSA (plus decolonization programme, if required)
- screen for sepsis/local infection (e.g. history of recurrent urinary tract infections)
- updated medication list (need to stop anticoagulants)
- appropriate/up-to-date imaging
- other required investigations (e.g. electrocardiogram/chest X-ray)
- confirm patient information/team contact numbers
- confirm discharge plan (social support)
- check implant equipment required.

Implant procedure details

The key steps in electrode implant are the same whether a percutaneous or surgical approach is applied. An electrode is implanted into the epidural space to allow a trial period to assess stimulation. A positive trial is often defined as covering at least 80% of the area of pain and the effect of reducing the pain score by 50%. The pre-operative conditions/checklist should have been undertaken. Informed consent is taken from the patient. The site of the IPG battery should be agreed with the patient prior to the trial being undertaken. Placement of the trial lead can be carried out under local anaesthesia with minimum intravenous sedation for percutaneous electrode implant, but a general anaesthetic is usually administered when implanting a surgical paddle electrode. Prior to implant, antibiotics are given and strict aseptic technique is followed throughout. The commonest organism in SCS implant infection is *Staphylococcus aureus*—prophylactic antibiotics should, therefore, have adequate cover against this organism. Patients are positioned appropriately (usually in the prone position). The implant procedure is undertaken in sterile operating conditions. Fluoroscopic imaging is used to facilitate lead placement.

In a percutaneous implant, the electrode is inserted via a Tuohy needle placed in the para-median position, using the loss of resistance technique to confirm access to the epidural space. The electrode can be 'guided' usually in a cephalad position using fluoroscopy. Once the lead position is acceptable, an on-table trial can be undertaken to assess the pattern of stimulation achieved. This allows the electrode position to be changed to achieve optimum stimulation. Once this goal is achieved, the Tuohy needle is removed. The implanted electrode can then be used as a trial electrode, and removed completely after the trial period. The other option is to use the implanted electrode as a permanent electrode. For the latter, the electrode is then secured to the supraspinous ligament and connected to a trial wire, which is then tunnelled laterally away from the site of permanent IPG placement (site agreed pre-operatively). After a successful trial, the trial cable alone is removed, leaving the electrode *in situ* as part of the permanent implant. The IPG battery is implanted in a sub-cutaneous pocket and the electrode cables (or any extensions) tunnelled to the pocket and connected to the IPG.

For a surgical implant, a wider port of access is required to position the paddle electrode into the epidural space under direct vision. The level of the laminotomy/laminectomy is determined (assessing pre-operative imaging) and fluoroscopy used in theatre to mark this level. The author usually undertakes a laminotomy either in the mid-line or para-median, depending on the pain target area. The dura is visualized directly and the electrode inserted directly. The electrode can be secured either with an anchor or suture to the para-vertebral deep fascia. The electrode wire is then tunnelled to a lateral pocket and connected to the trial cable, which is tunnelled away from the site of the IPG battery (agreed pre-operatively). If the trial period is successful, the lateral pocket is then opened and the trial cable disconnected and removed. An IPG pocket is formed and the electrode cable (plus or minus any necessary extensions) tunnelled and connected.

Post-implant support is essential so that patients are comfortable using the patient hand-held programmer to obtain maximum benefit from their implanted system. Centres offering SCS to patients must ensure that their service is appropriately funded to support continuing system maintenance, including the inevitable need for IPG replacement in those who do not have a rechargeable system *in situ* and the possible need for lead or system revision (19). There should be access to a 24-hour support service to deal with complications, such as CSF leak or infection.

Review of clinical outcomes

Clinical effectiveness

Systematic reviews/meta-analyses examining clinical effectiveness of SCS in CRPS were undertaken by Cameron in 2004 (20) and Taylor in 2006 (21). Cameron identified 12 studies for treatment of CRPS Type I or II with SCS—224 cases in total. Successful treatment in patients in whom SCS systems were implanted for chronic pain was defined as either greater than 50% pain relief or significant reduction in visual analogue scores (VAS). Only one of the 12 studies was a prospective controlled study by Kemler in 2000 (17). The other studies examined comprised of three prospective studies without matched controls and eight retrospective studies without matched controls. When patients were grouped according to diagnosis, long-term success rates overall were 83% in the CRPS group. In the three prospective studies (19 cases) the overall success rate was 84%. In the eight retrospective studies (192 cases) the overall success rate was also 84%. Two of these studies also reported a decrease in narcotic medication intake in a mean of 80% of patients (22, 23).

Taylor identified one randomized controlled trial (17, 24), 25 case series, and one economic evaluation. In the 25 case series, there were a total of 500 patients with Type I or II CRPS. Taylor notes that the overall quality of the case series was judged to be poor, with few reporting details of the selection of patients included, potential co-interventions received (such as drug therapy), methods of outcome assessment, or losses to follow-up. On average, 67% (CI 51% to 84%) of implanted patients with CRPS, who received SCS, achieved pain relief of at least 50%.

Functional capacity was reported in three studies reviewed by Taylor using the Oswestry Questionnaire, the McGill Pain Questionnaire, or both (22, 25, 26). There was improvement across all scales and subscales following SCS implantation. In the study undertaken by Oakley in 1999 (26), the McGill–Melzack Pain Questionnaire was examined. The mean pain rating index fell from 32.97 to 19.18 after SCS implantation. Oakley also reported an improved score using the Sickness Impact Profile following SCS implantation—the overall score falling from 20.31 to 10.91 following implant (significance was not reported in the study).

Four of the case series included subgroup analyses (27–29). These analyses indicated that better outcomes were achieved with dual versus single leads (27), shorter time from first operation to implant (28), better psychological and functional status patients (29), and younger age of patients (28). A more recent retrospective study of 25 patients by Kumar et al. (30), examining SCS in CRPS Type I, concluded that best results were achieved in stage I CRPS Type I with patients under the age of 40 and those receiving SCS within 1 year of disease onset.

The type of CRPS was also felt to be a predictor of outcome of SCS success (21). On average, a greater proportion of pain relief with SCS was experienced in the case series of CRPS Type II patients (mean 69%) compared to those in the case series with Type I CRPS (mean 51%). An earlier retrospective study by Broseta (18) examining SCS in CRPS Type II showed that pain relief was 64% successful.

The randomized control trial by Kemler (17, 24) assessed the effect of spinal cord stimulation in the treatment of CRPS I. Patients were selected who had CRPS Type I restricted to one hand or foot for at least 6 months and who did not have a sustained response to standard therapy, with a mean pain intensity of at least 5 cm on a VAS. In total, 110 patients were recruited, 54 were randomized and 54 were followed. Patients were aged between 18 and 65 years. These patients were randomized (2:1) to either receive SCS plus physical therapy (n = 36) or physical therapy alone (n = 18)—control group. Both groups received a standardized programme of graded exercise designed to improve the strength, mobility, and function of the affected hand or foot. Physical therapy was administered for 30 minutes twice a week with a minimum of 2 days between sessions. Patients were treated and followed for 6 months. Twenty-four of the patients randomized to the SCS group received a permanent implant device. The outcomes assessed included pain, functional capacity, quality of life, and complications. After 6 months, patients were allowed to cross over and observational follow-up was continued. The observational part of the study has been published with a 2- (31) and 5-year follow-up (32).

In this initial study (17, 24) at 12 months, the mean change in VAS was −2.7 (+/−2.8) with SCS therapy. This compared to an increase in the control group of +0.4 (+/−1.8) and this was significant, $p<0.001$. There was no significant difference observed in functional capacity between the two groups. The SCS therapy group also reported an improvement in their health-related quality-of-life mean score (6+/−22) compared to the control group (mean 3+/−18); however, this difference was not significant.

A 2-year follow-up (31) has demonstrated that the benefits in pain outcome were maintained with a mean VAS pain improvement of −2.1 versus 0.0 in the control group, $p<0.001$. The improvement in health-related quality-of-life was also maintained. Kemler (24, 27) reports that SCS did not affect allodynia, hypoesthesia, or function. A total of 9 of the 24 SCS patients (38%) experienced 22 complications needing operations during the 2-year period after implantation. None of these complications was associated with neurological or other severe adverse sequelae.

At 5 years (32), 10 patients were excluded from the study and the analysis compared 31 patients in the SCS group compared to 13 controls. The mean pain intensity in the stimulation group was reduced from baseline by 1.7, as compared with 1.0 in the control group, $p = 0.25$. They noted similar findings at the 3-year follow-up mark. The authors concluded that long-term follow-up analysis demonstrates that the pain-alleviating effect of spinal cord stimulation in CRPS Type I diminishes with time, as compared with that in the control group, and is no longer statistically significant after 3 years.

Van Ejis (33) prospectively examined 74 patients with CRPS Type I. Six of the group were included for early SCS treatment. They reported an improvement in mean pain relief of 35% after 1 year of SCS treatment. There was no improvement in functional outcome. They raise the possibility of a randomized controlled trial for early SCS therapy in CRPS Type I but comment that the feasibility is low due to the good disease improvement with standard therapy in the first year after onset.

Cost-effectiveness

Several studies have demonstrated the cost-effectiveness of SCS for CRPS. A study undertaken by Mekhail et al. (34) compared the use of SCS and other modalities in a group of patients with CRPS (60%) and failed back surgery syndrome (FBSS—40%). They showed a substantial reduction in the overall medical costs of patients treated by SCS compared with other forms of therapy. After 3.1 years this was a net saving of $48,464 per patient.

Kemler and Fernee (35) undertook a well-conducted economic analysis of SCS based on the randomized controlled trial of Kemler (17, 24). This study examined patient and health service costs at 12-month follow-up and an extrapolation of these costs over the lifetime of a patient. Although SCS incurred high expenditures in the first year (mainly a result of the implantation procedure, which formed 83% of the expenditure), thereafter the mean annual maintenance cost for CRPS I was significantly reduced. Over a lifetime period there was a cost saving of approximately $60,800 with SCS compared with control patients. Only patients in the SCS group were noted to have an improved health-related quality of life (HRQL), corresponding to a mean cost per quality-adjusted life years (QALY) of $23,480. The study concluded that SCS significantly reduced pain intensity and improved HRQL, which was less costly after 3 years in comparison with physical therapy alone.

In 2010, Kemler et al. (36) further studied the cost-effectiveness of SCS for CRPS using a decision analytic model over a 15-year time horizon from the perspective of the UK National Health Service. They showed the incremental cost-effectiveness of SCS compared to conventional medical management (CMM) was £3562 per QALY. When the longevity of an IPG is 4 years or less, they advise that a rechargeable IPG battery is more cost-effective than a non-rechargeable IPG.

Complications

Reported complications in SCS include:

- lead migration
- dural puncture/CSF leak
- infection
- unwanted stimulation
- other hardware problems (fluid ingress into the connectors or electrode, lead breakage, disconnection, battery failure)
- other wound problems (poor healing, seroma, allergy, neuropathic scar pain)
- neurological damage (direct damage or secondary to epidural haematoma or infection—this is rare).

In Taylor's systematic review (21), eight of the studies reported at least one complication with SCS—that is a 33% complication rate (in a total of 66 patients). The majority of these complications were related to electrode issues (20% of patients), infections (4% of patients), generator issues (2% of patients), or extension cable issues (1% of patients). A further 6% of patients had other complications, such as haematomas.

Cameron (20) also notes that changes in stimulation may occur over time. These changes could be the result of cellular changes in tissue around the electrodes or temporary changes in electrode position. There are also reports of painful stimulation, as well as cases of ineffective stimulation or loss of stimulation over time.

Conclusions

CRPS is a debilitating, painful condition in a limb that can be difficult to manage. Although many patients realize an improvement in their condition with education, pain relief, physical rehabilitation, and psychological intervention, approximately 15% will have unrelenting pain and physical impairment 2 years after CRPS onset. Spinal cord stimulation appears to be an effective therapy in the management of patients with CRPS Type I and Type II. More recent follow-up in CRPS I has shown a diminishing effectiveness of SCS over time—however, 95% of these patients would repeat SCS treatment for the same result. Moreover, there is evidence to demonstrate that SCS is a cost-effective treatment for CRPS Type I.

References

1 **Merskey H, Bogduk K**. Classification of Chronic Pain: Definitions of Chronic Pain Syndromes and Definition of Pain Terms. Seattle: International Association for the Study of Pain Press; 1994.

2 **Baron R, Fields H, Janig W, Kitt C, Levine J**. National Institute of Health Workshop: reflex sympathetic dystrophy/complex regional pain syndromes-state-of-the-science. Anesth Analg 2002;**95**:1812–16.

3 **Harden R, Bruehl S, Stanton-Hicks M, Wilson P**. Proposed new diagnostic criteria for complex regional pain syndrome. Pain Med 2007;**8(4)**:326–31.

4 **de Mos M, de Bruijn A, Huygen F et al**. The incidence of complex regional pain syndrome: a population based study. Pain 2000;**88(3)**:259–66.

5 **van Rijn M, Marinus J, Putter H et al**. Spreading of complex regional pain syndrome: not a random process. J Neural Transmission 2011;**118(9)**:1303–309.

6 **Field J, Warwick D, Bannister G**. Features of algodystrophy ten years after Colles' fracture. J Hand Surg Br 1992;**17(3)**:318–20.

7 **Goebel A, Barker C, Turner-Stokes L et al**. Complex Regional Pain Syndrome in Adults: UK Guidelines for Diagnosis, Referral and Management in Primary and Secondary Care. London: RCP; 2012.

8 **Harden R**. Complex regional pain syndrome. Br J Anaesth 2001;**87(1)**:99–106.

9 **Barolat G, Ketcik B, He J**. Spinal cord stimulation for persistent pain management. In: Gildenbery PL, Tasker R (eds) Textbook of Stereotactic and Functional Neurosurgery. New York: McGraw-Hill; 1998:1519.

10 **Deer T**. The role of neuromodulation by spinal cord stimulation in chronic pain syndromes: current concepts. Tech Reg Anesth Pain Manag 1998;**2(3)**:161–7.

11 **Vallejo R, Kramer J**. Intractable neck and upper extremity pain: a case series and review of the literature. Pain Phys 2007;**10**:305–11.

12 **Taren J, Kahn E**. Anatomic pathways related to pain in face and neck. J Neurosurg 1962;**19**:116–21.

13 **Barolat G, Schwartzman R, Woo R**. Epidural spinal cord stimulation in the management of reflex sympathetic dystrophy. Stereotact Funct Neurosurg 1989;**53**:29–39.

14 **Cameron T, Alo K**. Effects of posture on stimulation parameters in SCS. Neuromodulation 1998;**1**:177–83.

15 **North R, Kidd D, Zahurak M el al**. Spinal cord stimulation for chronic, intractable pain: superiority of 'multi-channel' devices. Pain 1991;**44**:119–30.

16 National Institute for Health and Clinical Excellence. Spinal cord stimulation for chronic pain of neuropathic or ischaemic origin. November 2011. NICE technology appraisal guidance 159.

17 **Kemler M, Bararendse G, van Kleef M et al**. Spinal cord stimulation in patients with chronic reflex sympathetic dystrophy. N Engl J Med 2000;**343**:618–24.

18 **Broseta J, Roldan P, Gonalez-Darder J et al**. Chronic epidural dorsal column stimulation in the treatment of causalgia pain. Appl Neurophysiol 1982;**45**:190–94.

19 The British Pain Society. Spinal cord stimulation for the management of pain: recommendations for best clinical practice. April 2012.

20 **Cameron T**. Safety and efficacy of spinal cord stimulation for the treatment of chronic pain: a 20 year literature review. J Neurosurg (Spine) 2004;**100**:254–67.

21 **Taylor R, Van Buyten J, Buchser E**. Spinal cord stimulation for complex regional pain syndrome: a systematic review of the clinical and cost-effectiveness literature and assessment of prognostic factors. Eur J Pain 2006;**10**:91–101.

22 **Robaina F, Rodrigues J, de Vera et al**. Transcutaneous electrical nerve stimulation and spinal cord stimulation for pain relief for reflex sympathetic dystrophy. Stereotact Funct Neurosurg 1989;**52**:53–62.

23 **Sanchez-Ledesma M, Garcia-March G, Diaz-Cascajo P et al**. Spinal cord stimulation in deafferentation pain. Stereotact Funct Neurosurg 1989;**53**:40–45.

24 **Kemler M, Reulen J, Barendse G, van Kleef M, de Vet H, van den Wildenberg F**. Impact of spinal cord stimulation on sensory characteristics in complex pain syndrome type I: a randomised trial. Anesthesiology 2001;**95**:72–80.

25 **Robaina F, Dominguez M, Diaz M, Rodriguez J, de Vera J**. Spinal cord stimulation for relief of chronic pain in vasospastic disorders of the upper limbs. Neurosurgery 1989;**24**:63–67.

26 **Oakley J**. Spinal cord stimulation for the relief of pain: proceedings of a symposium during the 4th international neuromodulation society, September 1998. Neuromodulation 1999;**2**:184–87.

27 **Bennett D, Alo K, Oakley J, Feler C, Hagen J**. Spinal cord stimulation for complex regional pain syndrome I (RSD): a retrospective multicentre experience from 1995 to 1998 of 101 patients. Neuromodulation 1999;**2**:202–10.

28 **Kumar K, Toth C, Nath R**. Spinal cord stimulation for chronic pain in peripheral neuropathy. Surg Neurol 1996;**46**:363–69.

29 **Burchiel K, Brown F, Erickson R et al**. Correlates of pain relief in spinal cord stimulation recipients. In: Abstract 1335, IASP 7th World Congress on Pain, 1993.

30 **Kumar K, Rizvi S, Bnurs S**. Spinal cord stimulation is effective in management of complex regional pain syndrome I: fact or fiction. Neurosurgery 2011;**69(3)**:566–78.

31 **Kemler M, de Vet H, Barendse G, van den Wildenberg F**. The effect of spinal cord stimulation in patients with chronic reflex sympathetic dystrophy: two years' follow-up of the randomised control trial. Ann Neurol 2004;**55**:13–18.

32 **Kemler M, de Vet H, Barendse G, van den Wildenberg F, van Kleef M**. Effect of spinal cord stimulation for chronic complex regional pain syndrome Type I: five year final follow up of patients in a randomised controlled trial. J Neurosurg 2008;**108(2)**:292–98.

33 **Van Eijs F Geurts J, Van Zundert J, Faber C, Kessels A, Joosten E, van Kleef M**. Spinal cord stimulation in complex regional pain syndrome type I of less than 12 month duration. Neuromodulation 2012;**15(2)**:144–50.

34 **Mekhail N, Aeschbach A, Stanton-Hicks M**. Cost benefit analysis of neurostimulation of chronic pain. Clin J Pain 2004;**20(6)**:462–68.

35 **Kemler A, Furnee C**. Economic evaluation of spinal cord stimulation for chronic reflex sympathetic dystrophy. Neurology 2002;**59**:1203–209.

36 **Kemler M, Raphael J, Bentley A, Taylor R**. The cost effectiveness of spinal cord stimulation for complex regional pain syndrome. Value Health;**13(6)**:735–42.

Chapter 11

Trigeminal autonomic cephalalgias I: peripheral neuromodulation (occipital nerve and sphenopalatine ganglion stimulation)

Sarah Miller, Laurence Watkins, and Manjit S. Matharu

Key points

1. The trigeminal autonomic cephalalgias (TACs) are a distinct group of primary headache disorders characterized by strictly unilateral very severe and highly disabling pain that occurs in association with cranial autonomic features. The most commonly encountered in clinical practice is cluster headache.
2. Occipital nerve stimulation (ONS) has been reported to be beneficial in over 70% of patients with chronic cluster headache in open label studies and appears safe.
3. Early studies of sphenopalatine ganglion (SPG) stimulation in cluster headache are very promising
4. Severely disabled patients with chronic TACs intractable to all medical treatments should be considered for peripheral neuromodulation. The procedure and the continuing specialized post-implantation follow-up should be performed under the care of a specialist headache-led multidisciplinary team.
5. Peripheral neuromodulation is thought to exert its beneficial effects via slow neuromodulatory processes in the central pain matrix

Introduction

The trigeminal autonomic cephalalgias (TACs) are a group of primary headache disorders characterized by unilateral head pain that occurs in association with prominent ipsilateral cranial autonomic features. The TACs include cluster headache (CH), paroxysmal hemicrania (PH), short-lasting unilateral neuralgiform headache attacks with conjunctival injection and tearing (SUNCT), and its close relative, short-lasting unilateral neuralgiform headache attacks with cranial autonomic symptoms (SUNA). CH, PH, and SUNCT are currently grouped into section 3 of the revised International Classification of Headache Disorders (ICHD-II), while SUNA is described in the appendix section (1).

CH, PH, SUNCT, and SUNA are characterized by short-lasting headaches with autonomic features such as conjunctival injection, tearing, ptosis, eyelid oedema, nasal stuffiness, rhinorrhea, facial sweating or redness, and a sense of restlessness or agitation during an attack. Despite their common elements, the TACs differ in attack duration and frequency, as well as response to therapy. CH has the longest attack duration and relatively low attack frequency. PH has intermediate duration and intermediate attack frequency. SUNCT and SUNA have the shortest attack duration and the highest attack frequency. The importance of recognizing these syndromes resides in their excellent, but highly selective, response to treatment. A summary of the epidemiology, clinical features, and first-line treatment options is given in Table 11.1.

Advances in the management of headache disorders have meant that the substantial proportion of TAC patients can be effectively managed with medical treatments. However, a significant minority of these patients will develop chronic headache and prove intractable to conventional treatments. The chronic forms of the TACs can be diagnosed in patients where there are no remissions for a year or if any remission, periods last less than one month. Chronic cluster headache (CCH) is seen in 10–20% of patients, chronic paroxysmal hemicrania (CPH) in 65% (2), chronic SUNCT in 63%, and chronic SUNA in 89% of patients (3). In all cases, patients may be chronic from onset or evolve from an episodic form. These patients form a small but highly disabled group and there is a clear need for novel approaches for the management of these patients.

Neurostimulation therapies appear to offer a promising approach to intractable TACs. The peripheral targets that have been used recently include the occipital, as well as the sphenopalatine, ganglion. In this chapter, the main focus is on ONS in CCH, as this is where the bulk of literature and clinical experience lies.

Pathophysiology of trigeminal autonomic cephalalgias

The trigeminal autonomic reflex and hypothalamic activation

Any pathophysiological hypothesis for TACs must account for the three major clinical characteristics of these disorders: trigeminal distribution pain; ipsilateral autonomic features; and the distinct circadian and circannual periodicity, particularly in CH.

Table 11.1 Clinical features of the trigeminal autonomic cephalalgias

	Cluster headache	**Paroxysmal hemicrania**	**SUNCT**	**SUNA**
Sex F:M	1:2.5–7	1:1	1:1.5	Not known
Pain: **Type**	Stabbing, boring	Throbbing, boring, stabbing	Stabbing, sharp	Stabbing, sharp
Severity	Excruciating	Excruciating	Excruciating	Excruciating
Site	Orbit, temple	Orbit, temple	Orbit, temple	Orbit, temple
Attack frequency	1/alternate day –8/day	1–40/day (>5/day for more than half the time)	3–200/day	>1/day for more than half the time
Duration of attack	15–180 min	2–30 min	5–240 s	2–600 s
Autonomic features	Yes	Yes	Yes*	Yes
Migrainous features	Yes	Yes	Very rarely	Very rarely
Alcohol trigger	Yes	Occasional	No	No
Cutaneous triggers	No	No	Yes	Yes
Indometacin effect	–	+ +	–	–
Abortive treatment	Sumatriptan injection or nasal spray Oxygen	Nil	Nil	Nil
Prophylactic treatment	Verapamil Lithium Topiramate	Indometacin	Lamotrigine Oxcarbazepine Topiramate	Lamotrigine Oxcarbazepine Topiramate

*Both conjunctival injection and tearing; SUNA, short-lasting unilateral neuralgiform headache attacks with autonomic symptoms; SUNCT, short-lasting unilateral neuralgiform headache attacks with conjunctival injection and tearing.

The pain-producing innervation of the cranium projects through branches of the trigeminal and upper cervical nerves to the trigeminocervical complex, from where the nociceptive pathways project to higher centres. This suggests an integral role for the ipsilateral trigeminal nociceptive pathways in TACs. The ipsilateral autonomic features arise from cranial parasympathetic activation (lacrimation, rhinorrhoea, nasal congestion, and eyelid oedema) and sympathetic hypofunction (ptosis and meiosis). Goadsby and Lipton have, therefore, suggested that the pathophysiology of the TACs revolves around a trigeminal autonomic reflex (4). There is considerable experimental animal literature to document that stimulation of trigeminal afferents can result in cranial autonomic outflow, the trigeminal autonomic reflex (5). In fact, some degree of cranial autonomic symptomatology is a normal physiologic response to cranial nociceptive input, and patients with other headache syndromes often report these symptoms. The distinction between the TACs and other headache syndromes is the degree of cranial autonomic activation and not its presence (6).

The cranial autonomic symptoms may be more prominent in the TACs due to a central disinhibition of the trigeminal autonomic reflex (7). Supporting evidence is emerging from functional imaging studies where positron emission tomography (PET) studies in CH (8) and PH (9), and functional MRI studies in SUNCT syndrome (10), have demonstrated hypothalamic activation. The periodicity that is such a hallmark of cluster headache also points towards the posterior hypothalamic structures as important. Although hypothalamic activation is not seen in experimental trigeminal distribution head pain, there are direct hypothalamic trigeminal connections (11), which would explain its role in pain processing. There is abundant evidence for a role of the hypothalamus in mediating anti-nociceptive (12) and autonomic responses (13), including direct evidence from animal experimental studies for hypothalamic activation when intracranial pain structures are activated (14). Moreover, the hypothalamic peptides Orexin A and B can elicit pro-nociceptive and anti-nociceptive effects in the trigeminal system (15). These data have led to the formulation that the TACs are probably due to a central abnormality in hypothalamic processing with subsequent trigeminovascular and cranial autonomic activation via the superior salivatory nucleus (SSN) and trigeminal pathways.

Occipital nerve stimulation

Anatomy of the occipital nerves

The anatomy of the nerves of the occipital region has been well described (16). There are three nerves that innervate the occipital region, namely the greater, lesser, and least occipital nerves. The greater occipital nerve is a branch of the C2 spinal root. It proceeds between the inferior oblique and the semispinalis capitis muscle in a superomedial fashion. The nerve then crosses above the rectus capitis posterior major muscle and arises medial to the semispinalis capitis muscle, which it occasionally pierces. It then penetrates through the trapezius muscle to join the occipital artery (16). It provides innervations to an occipito-parietal area 6 to 8 cm wide and ascending paramedially from the subocciput to the vertex (17). The lesser occipital nerve is composed of branches of the C2 and C3 spinal roots. It runs lateral to the greater occipital nerve, crossing over the sternocleidomastoid muscle, and courses superolaterally towards the region behind and above the ear. The medial branch of the posterior division of the C3 root gives off a branch called the least occipital nerve, which pierces the trapezius and ends in the skin of the lower part of the back of the head. It lies medial to the greater occipital nerve and communicates with it.

There is an anatomical and functional overlap of trigeminal and cervical afferents throughout the trigeminocervical complex from the level of the caudal trigeminal nucleus to at least the C2 segment (18). This convergence explains how nociceptive activation at either end of this structure can result in both trigeminal and cervical distribution pain. Similarly, ONS could modulate pain not only in the territories innervated by the occipital nerves, but also areas innervated by the trigeminal nerve.

Operative techniques

ONS (see Fig. 11.1) for the treatment of medically intractable headaches was introduced by Weiner and Reed (19). ONS is typically performed with the equipment normally used for spinal cord stimulation, which includes electrodes and their leads, anchors to fasten the leads to connective tissue, and the implantable pulse generator. Cylindrical-style and paddle-style electrodes can be used. Cylindrical electrodes are thin and can be inserted through a needle, while paddle electrodes (flat and broad) are associated with a lower incidence of lead migration but require more extensive surgical dissection for placement. Electrodes can be programmed to function as either cathodes or anodes to direct the flow of current adjacent to the stimulated structure.

A stimulation trial is performed before the permanent implantation in some centres, with the view to improving selection of the candidates for a permanent stimulation. The procedure involves inserting percutaneous leads into the epidural space via a Tuohy

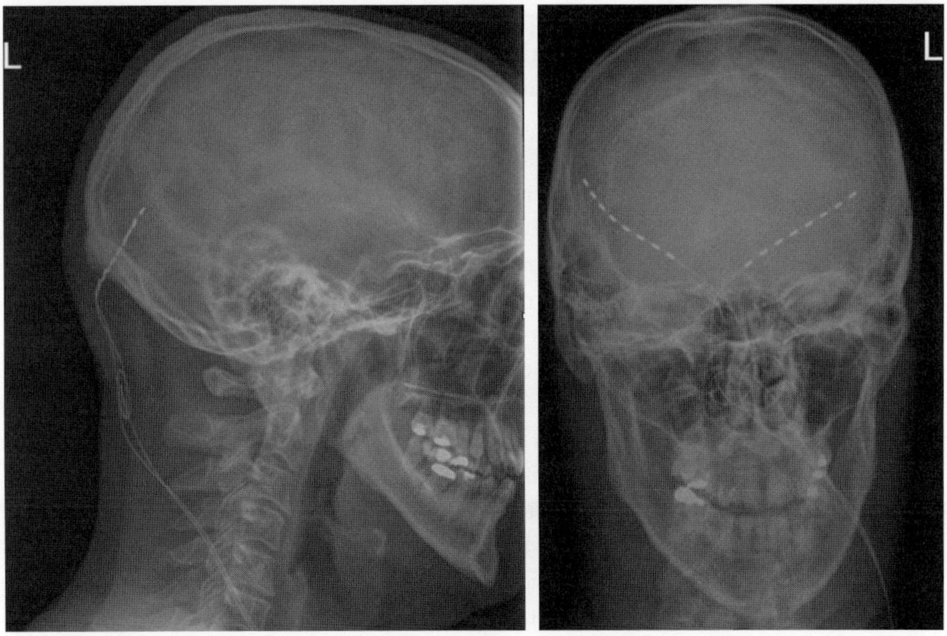

Fig. 11.1 Occipital nerve stimulator electrode placement depicted on lateral (left) and anteroposterior (right) skull radiographs.

needle and externally powering them for 5 to 7 days. If the trial is successful in terms of significant pain improvement, the patient is offered a permanent implantation. However, in primary headache syndromes, unlike in neuropathic pain, there can be a considerable delay of several weeks to months before the response emerges and, therefore, the utility of a stimulation trial in selecting patients for permanent implantation remains questionable.

The permanent implantation procedure to site the electrodes can be performed via both mid-line and retromastoid approaches. Electrodes are placed subcutaneously, superficial to the cervical muscle fascia, transverse to the affected occipital nerve trunk at the level of C1, usually using fluoroscopic guidance. The standard procedure is usually performed in two stages. The first stage, carried out under local anaesthesia with sedation, is used to test the stimulation and determine optimal placement of electrodes. The second part, which involves insertion of the rest of the ONS system, is carried out under general anaesthesia. However, a recent report of a small case series described successful placement of ONS systems entirely under general anaesthesia, while still achieving the desired occipital region stimulation (20).

The implantable pulse generator (IPG) can be located at various regions, including the buttock, mid-axillary thoracic region, or low abdomen. The battery can be non-rechargeable (with a lifespan of 2 to 5 years) or rechargeable (with a lifespan close to 10 years). The patients control the ONS with a handheld remote control by which they can turn the device on or off, besides adjusting the stimulator parameters. The stimulation parameters, including frequency, pulse width, and voltage, are adjusted such that patients experience comfortable paraesthesia in the stimulated area. Stimulation can be continuous, turned on and off as needed, or continuous with alterations in parameters as needed. There is a wide variation in the stimulation settings used with the amplitude ranging from 0.1 to 10 V, the frequency ranging from 3 to 130 Hz and pulse width ranging from 90 to 450 ms (21). Optimal stimulator settings need to be better defined since there are no data on impact of specific parameters on outcome.

Miniaturized devices are a potential new option for delivering peripheral nerve stimulation. One such device that has been used for occipital nerve stimulation is the Bion. The Bion is a rechargeable, self-contained, battery-powered, telemetrically programmable, current-controlled mini-neurostimulator with an integrated electrode and battery that are encased in a small device that can be implanted over the occipital nerves (22). Recently, Trentman and colleagues described the implantation technique and the stimulation parameters of the Bion microstimulator in nine patients with medically intractable primary headache disorders (23). Their results showed that the Bion might provide effective occipital stimulation without requiring anchoring or tunnelling of extensions to remote power sources. It may also minimize common adverse events such as lead migration. On the other hand, the microstimulator needs frequent recharging, has limited choices in terms of electrode combinations, and can become encapsulated, hence increasing the energy required to stimulate the occipital nerve. The role of these miniaturized devices in the treatment of headache syndromes remains unclear, as their efficacy and safety need to be studied further.

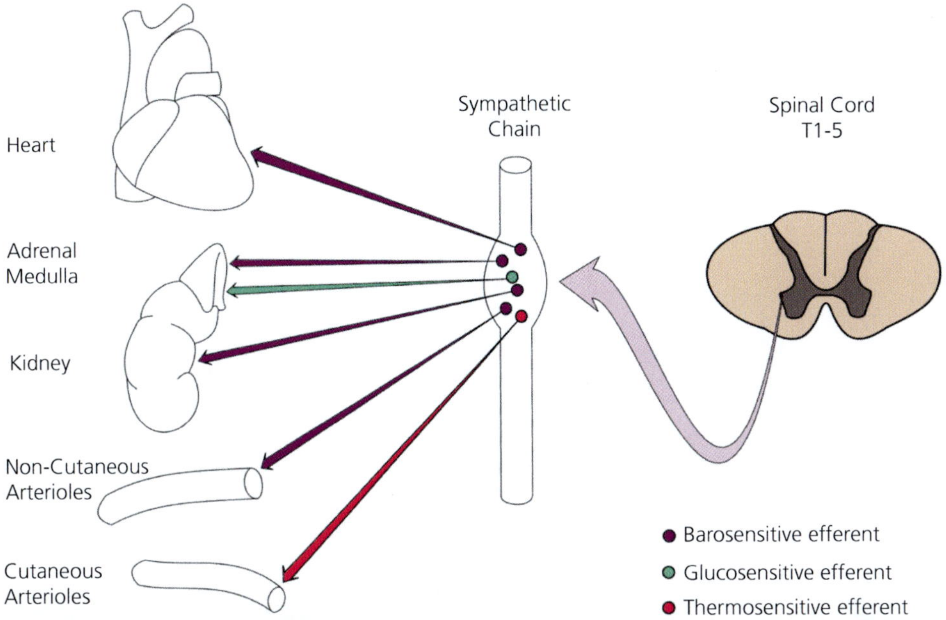

Plate 1 Schematic to demonstrate the three classes of sympathetic efferents and their end-organ targets. (See Fig. 1.4.)

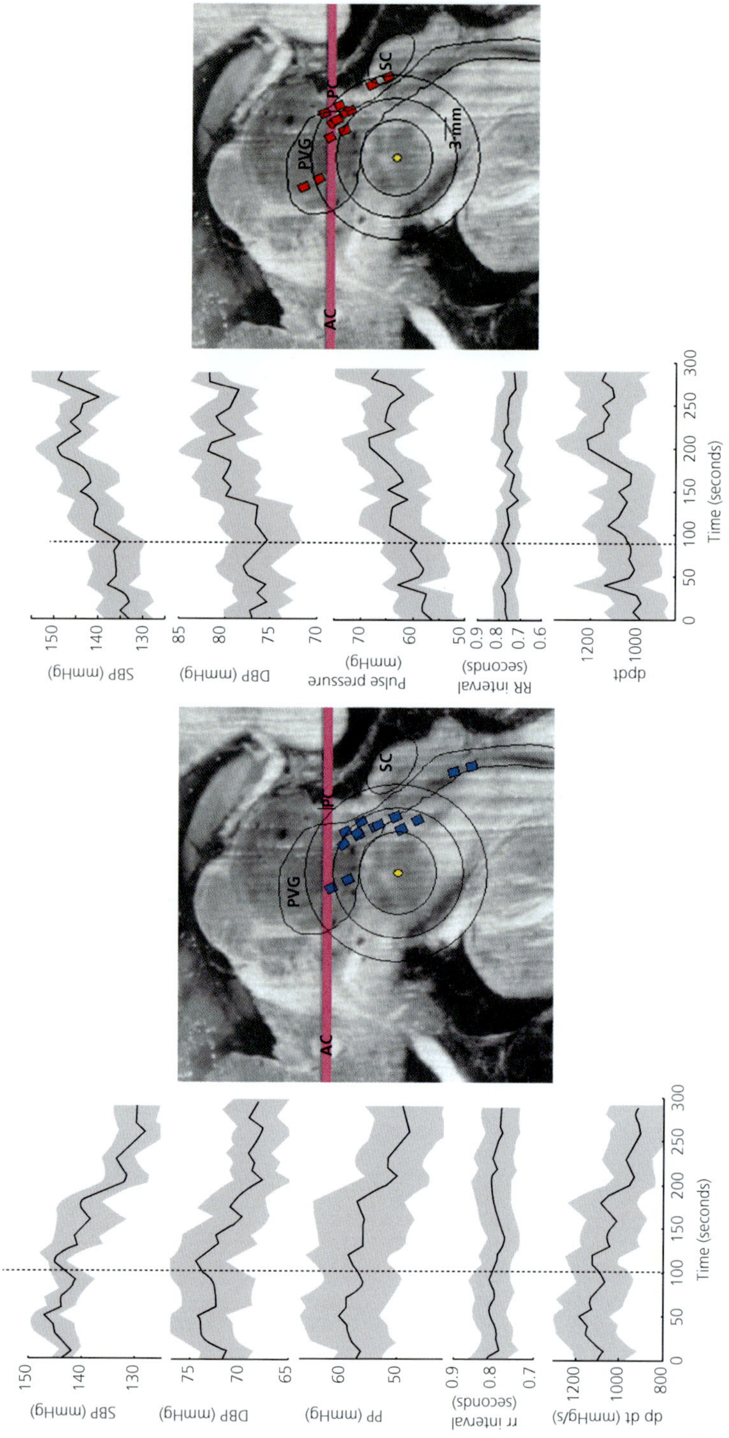

Plate 2 Mean changes in cardiovascular variables with stimulation points indicated in the central schematics. Blue squares represent the contacts of the DBS electrodes that when stimulated reduced BP and associated variables, except RR interval. The red squares indicate points that increased BP (right-hand side). Grey areas = standard error of the mean, vertical lines = start of stimulation, yellow spot = centre of red nucleus (for orientation), SC = superior colliculus, PVG = periventricular grey area, AC = anterior colliculus, PC = posterior colliculus. (See Fig. 3.2.)

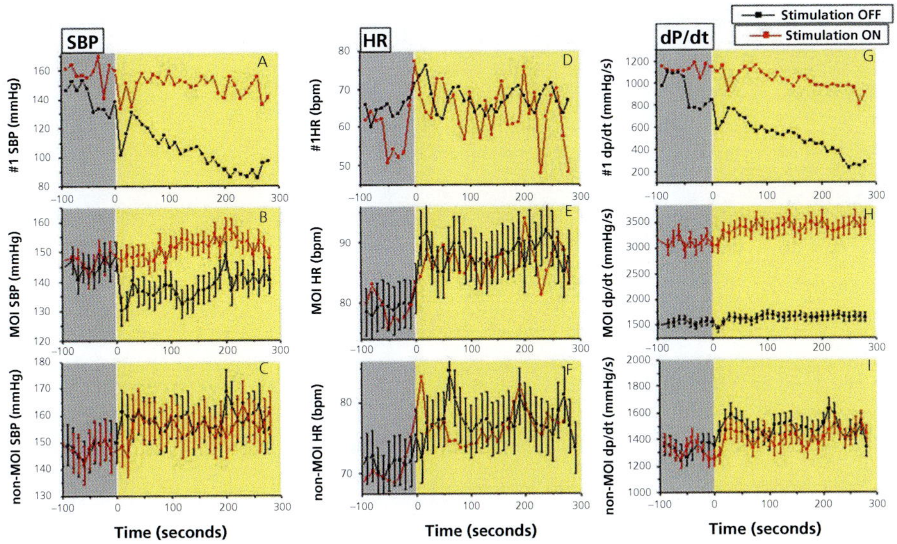

Plate 3 Modulation of BP responses to standing. (A) in a group of five asymptomatic patients undergoing DBS for pain, the usual reduction in BP on standing (black line) is reversed with PAG stimulation (red line). Grey area = patient sitting, white area = patient standing. (B) An individual patient with postural hypotension. Stimulation not only reversed the BP changes on standing but also successfully treated the clinical condition. (See Fig. 3.3.)

Reproduced from Neurosurgery, 58, Green et al., Controlling the Heart Via the Brain: A Potential New Therapy for Orthostatic Hypotension, p. 1176–1183, Copyright (2006), with permission from Wolters Kluwer Health.

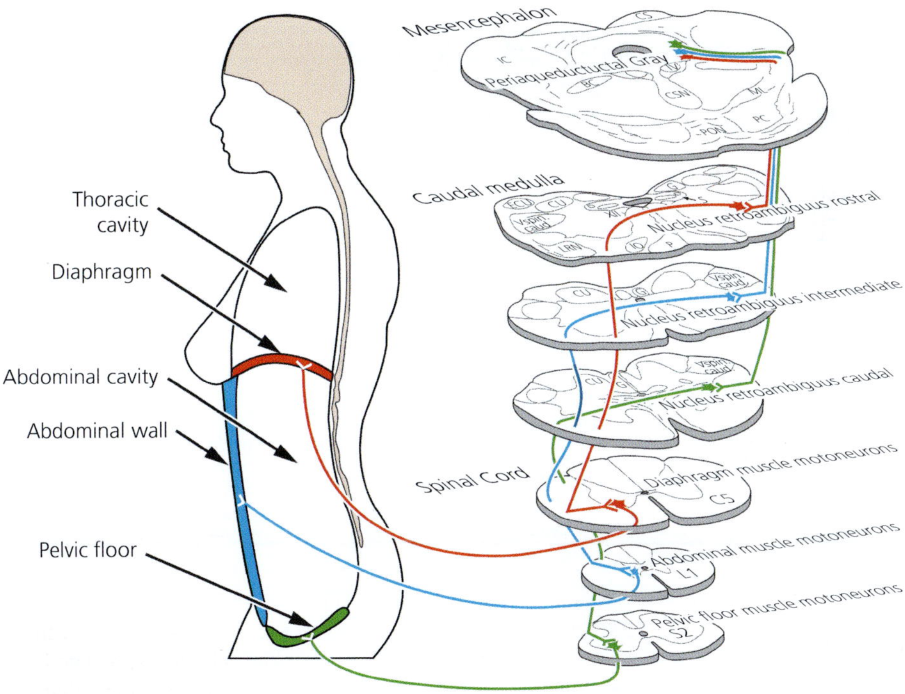

Plate 4 Diagramatic representation of supraspinal control of muscles of the abdominal cavity. (See Fig. 13.3.)

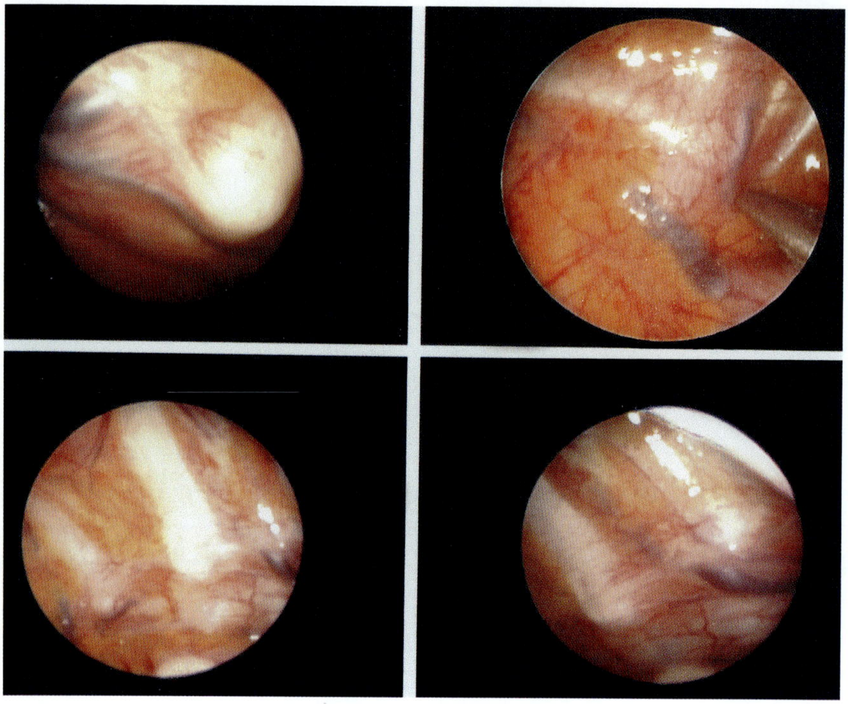

Plate 5 Endoscopic view of the left thoracic cavity. The image shows the sympathetic chain coursing over the second and third rib heads and deep to the semi-transparent parietal pleura. (See Fig. 18.1.)

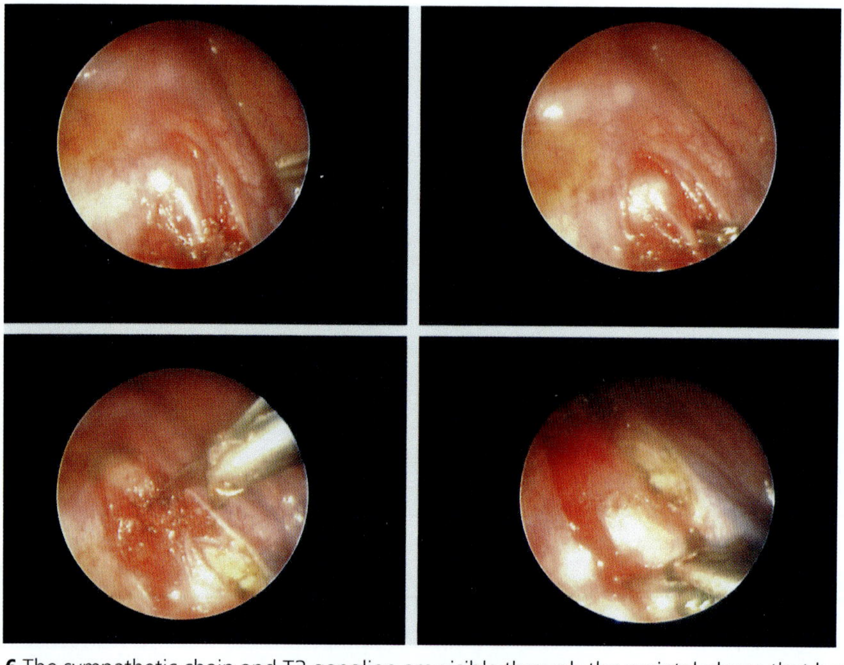

Plate 6 The sympathetic chain and T3 ganglion are visible through the parietal pleura that has been divided. The endoscopic grasper lies adjacent to the sympathetic chain below the third rib and T3 ganglion. (See Fig. 18.2.)

Evidence for efficacy of ONS in primary headache syndromes

Amongst the TACs, ONS is most commonly used in CCH and, therefore, the most extensive literature exists for this condition. For SUNCT and SUNA there is one open label case series of seven patients (24), but as yet, there are no published cases of ONS use in PH. However, unpublished experience from our centre suggests that ONS can be effective in PH as well. Table 11.2 summarizes all available published studies of ONS in the treatment of TACs (25–32).

Cluster headache

ONS appears to be effective in CCH with around 70% of intractable patients reporting an at least 50% benefit (Table 11.2).

Magis and colleagues (25) prospectively studied eight medically intractable chronic cluster headache patients treated with unilateral ONS. The mean duration of cluster headaches was 13.6 years, with a mean duration of CCH of 5.1 years. The mean stimulation parameters used were amplitude of 6.36 V (range 2.4–10 V), frequency of 66 Hz (range 40–100 Hz) and pulse width of 364 ms (range 270–450 ms). All patients had continuous stimulation. Headache diaries were completed prospectively. After a mean follow-up of 15 months (range 3–22 months), two patients were pain-free, three patients had a 90% reduction in attack frequency, two patients had improvement of around 40%, and one had no benefit. Cessation of ONS was followed within days by recurrence and increase of attacks.

Table 11.2 Evidence for occipital nerve stimulation in trigeminal autonomic cephalalgias

Trial (first author, year)	Patients (*n*)	Average follow-up (months)	Success rate (number of patients with at least 50% improvement in attack frequency)
ONS for CCH			
Magis (2007, 2011)	14	36.8	12
Burns (2007, 2009)	14	17.5	5
De Quintana-Schmidt (2010)	4	6	4
Muller (2010)	10	12	9
Fontaine (2011)	13	14.6	10
Strand (2011)	3	12	2
Brewer (2012)	5	32.6	4
Schwedt (2007)	3	20	1
TOTAL	66		47(71%)
ONS for SUNCT/SUNA			
Matharu et al (2010)	8	24	5 (63%)

ONS, occipital nerve stimulation; SUNA, short-lasting unilateral neuralgiform headache attacks with autonomic symptoms; SUNCT, short-lasting unilateral neuralgiform headache attacks with conjunctival injection and tearing.

Weekly headache frequency was reduced from 13.4 pre- to 2.8 post-ONS. Attack intensity was reduced from 2.62 to 1.47 post-ONS (scale from 1 = mildest to 4 = worst pain). All the patients who responded to ONS were able to substantially reduce their preventive drug treatments, but only one was able to stop them completely. Treatment effects from ONS were often delayed for 2 months or more after implantation. Two patients with relief of ipsilateral cluster attacks began to have the attacks on the contralateral side, which disappeared after suboccipital injections of steroids, and one patient experienced isolated painless autonomic attacks. When stimulators were turned off or batteries became depleted during the study period, the attacks worsened within days. Battery depletion occurred in half of the patients during the follow-up period. Lead displacement and electrode migration were reported in one patient each. No serious adverse effects were reported.

Burns and colleagues (27, 28) treated 14 medically intractable CCH patients using bilateral ONS. Patients had CCH for a median duration of 6 years (range 2–17 years). Patients were able to vary the stimulation parameters and a wide range of settings was used: the range for amplitude was 0–10.5 V, pulse width 60–450 ms, and frequency 3–130 Hz. Twelve patients used continuous stimulation, while two used intermittent stimulation. The median follow-up period was 17.5 months (range 4–35 months). Ten of 14 patients reported an improvement, although 11 patients recommended the treatment to other CCH patients. Three patients noticed a marked improvement of 90% or better, three reported a moderate improvement of 40–60%, and four reported a mild improvement of 20–30%. Four patients didn't notice any benefit. Improvement occurred within days to weeks for those who responded most and patients consistently reported that their attacks returned within hours to days when the device was off. One patient found that ONS helped to abort acute attacks. The mean battery life was 15 months; therefore, almost half of the patients required battery replacement. Lead migration was reported in four patients (29%). Other complications included muscle recruitment, neck stiffness, skin discomfort, superficial infection and painful paraesthesias.

Schwedt and colleagues (33) used ONS in three CCH patients. Two had unilateral and one bilateral ONS. Mean follow-up was 20 months (range 10–39 months). The efficacy of ONS was inferior compared to the other studies, albeit that this is a very small series. The headache frequency remained unchanged in two patients and increased in the third, while severity decreased in two patients (VRS 8/10 to 5/10 and 8/10 to 3.5/10) and remained unchanged in one. Lead migration was confirmed as the main adverse events also in these patients.

Brewer and colleagues (34) treated five intractable cluster patients with ONS. All patients underwent a trial stimulation period and bilateral implants were only used if headaches were bilateral. Mean follow-up was 32.6 months (range 5–163 months). Four patients reported a more than 50% benefit and one reported no benefit at all. Four patients required lead revision procedures, one with multiple revisions but no other adverse events were listed in this group.

De Quintana-Schmidt (29) reported four patients with intractable CCH who underwent ONS. All implants were bilateral with octopolar electrodes. At 6 months follow-up there was a 56% (range 25–95%) reduction in attack frequency, 49% (range 20–60%) reduction in attack intensity, and 64% (range 0–88%) reduction in attack duration. All patients stated they would recommend the procedure to others and no post-operative complications were observed.

Fontaine and colleagues (31) carried out ONS on 13 CCH sufferers. After a mean follow-up period of 14.6 months, 10 patients reported more than a 50% improvement in their headaches and were classed as responders. The authors reported a 68% reduction in mean attack frequency and a 49% reduction in mean attack intensity. Eight patients were able to stop their preventative medication completely.

Strand's feasibility study of ONS in CCH (32) consisted of three patients who had suffered intractable CCH for a mean period of 14.3 years and who underwent insertion of a unilateral Bion device. Only one patient reported a response (more than 50% reduction in attack frequency) by 3 months. At the end of the 12-month study period, all three patients reported ongoing benefit with two recording more than 50% reduction in attack frequency. Adverse events were limited to neck stiffness and battery depletion.

Though the published open-label studies report encouraging results of ONS in CCH, they have also highlighted some issues regarding the design of the trials, patient selection, and the assessment of the outcome. In the prospective pilot study of CCH patients by Magis and colleagues (25), the average attacks per day was quite low and the follow-up after the operation was very short for some of the patients. In the retrospective study of eight CCH subjects (27), there was a discrepancy between patient estimation of benefits and objective improvement. This led Leone and colleagues (35) to make recommendations about the criteria for the use of neurostimulation in primary headaches. They suggested the following: patients should have daily or almost daily attacks over 2 years; all reasonable drugs must be tried at sufficient doses for sufficient time, unless contraindicated; an adequate length of post-implant follow-up is required (at least 1 year); a psychological assessment is required before the surgery; patients should keep a prospective headache diary (frequency, severity, and duration of headache attacks, and analgesic consumption); and, quality of life measurements and the self-assessment of pain are required.

SUNCT and SUNA Matharu and colleagues (24) reported the outcome of seven medically intractable SUNCT (short-lasting unilateral neuralgiform headache attacks with conjunctival injection and tearing) and one SUNA (short-lasting neuralgiform headache attacks with autonomic symptoms) patients treated with bilateral ONS. These patients failed to respond to at least five of the following preventive treatments: lamotrigine, topiramate, gabapentin, pregabalin, carbamazepine, oxcarbazepine, mexiletine, and melatonin. At a median follow-up of 24 months (range 4–29), four patients reported a substantial improvement (95–100%), one reported moderate benefit (50%), and one patient reported a temporary marked benefit (50%) for 6 months followed by recurrence of headache at the pre-ONS baseline, and one failed to respond. The onset of the benefit was rapid (within 2 weeks) with attacks recurring rapidly when the stimulator was switched off or malfunctioned. One patient developed hemicrania continua 1 month after implantation and was successfully treated with indomethacin. No major adverse events were reported.

Sphenopalatine ganglion stimulation

Anatomical basis of the autonomic phenomena in trigeminal autonomic cephalalgias

The autonomic features of TACs are characterized by a parasympathetic discharge (lacrimation, conjunctival injection, and nasal secretion, nasal congestion, and facial sweating) and sympathetic deficit (ptosis and miosis) on the side ipsilateral to the pain during the acute attacks.

The parasympathetic fibres originate in the superior salivatory nucleus, which has a functional brainstem connection to the trigeminal nucleus caudalis (36). The fibres traverse the facial nerve and the greater superficial petrosal nerve to join the vidian nerve (the greater superficial petrosal nerve and greater deep petrosal nerve join to form the vidian nerve) and synapse in the sphenopalatine ganglion. Postganglionic fibres loop back as orbital rami to the cavernous sinus and internal carotid artery, where they form a plexus with sympathetic and trigeminal fibres (ophthalmic and maxillary division fibres), before advancing to provide vasomotor and secretomotor innervation to the cerebral blood vessels and the lacrimal and nasal mucosal glands, respectively. The activation of this trigeminal parasympathetic reflex provides the anatomic basis for the expression of first-division trigeminal pain and ipsilateral cranial autonomic symptoms that occur during cluster attacks.

The sympathetic outflow is influenced by important nuclei in the hypothalamus, midbrain, and brainstem, and descends through the cervical spinal cord, where axons synapse in the intermediolateral cell mass. From the thoracic and upper lumbar spinal segments, myelinated axons emerge in the white rami and synapse in the paravertebral ganglia. Sympathetic fibres innervating the cranial structures arise from the superior cervical ganglion and course along the internal carotid artery, through the cavernous sinus to the long ciliary nerve which innervates the dilator pupillae. Some fibres follow the external carotid artery and innervate Muller's muscle of the eyelid, and the blood vessels and sweat glands of the face, except for sweating of the medial aspect of the forehead, which follows the internal carotid artery. Pharmacological investigation of the pupillary abnormalities in CH suggests that the dysfunction is confined to postganglionic sympathetic fibres (37–39).

A pathophysiological model that integrates the parasympathetic hyperactivity and sympathetic deficit in TACs has been proposed (40). Activation of the trigeminal parasympathetic reflex contributes to cranial parasympathetic symptoms and local vasodilatation during attacks of TACs. This vasodilatation or oedema in the wall of the internal carotid artery may compromise sympathetic fibres, producing transient or permanent signs of ocular sympathetic deficit.

Evidence for sphenopalatine ganglion stimulation in chronic cluster headache

The sphenopalatine ganglion (SPG) is an extracranial structure lying in the pterygopalatine fossa (PPF), containing parasympathetic and sympathetic elements. Due to the direct and indirect connections it has to the somatic and visceral nerve structures of the face, and to the trigeminovasular system, the superior salivatory nucleus (SSN), and the hypothalamus, it has been theorized as being an important part of the pathophysiology of cluster headache and, therefore, chosen as a therapeutic target.

Local anaesthetic blockade or lesioning of the SPG has been employed to treat CH, though any improvement was at best transient (41). However, a recent prospective, randomized blinded multicentre study was employed to test the efficacy and safety of SPG stimulation (see Fig. 11.2) as an acute treatment for CCH (42). Altogether 28 patients with CCH underwent unilateral SPG stimulator insertion with a miniaturized implantable device with an integral lead containing six electrodes. The lead extended from the neurostimulator body to the SPG within the PPF. A handheld device was then used to control the implanted neurostimulator. The stimulator was placed under general anaesthetic using a minimally invasive, trans-oral, gingival buccal technique. All patients underwent a parasinus CT to aid positioning. The SPG stimulator was implanted so that the stimulating

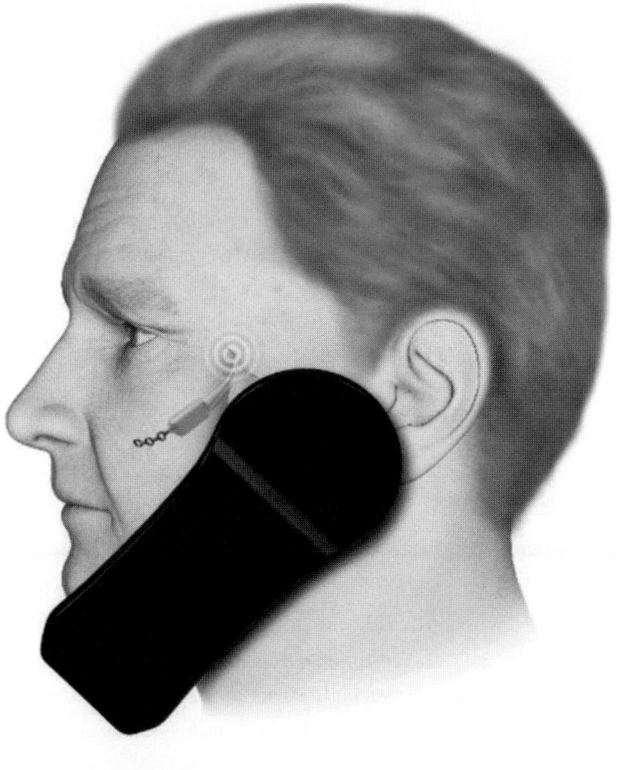

Fig. 11.2 Sphenopalatine ganglion stimulation in use: during an attack of cluster headache, the patient holds the handset to the cheek to activate the stimulator.
Reproduced courtesy of ATI Technologies.

electrodes on the integral lead were positioned within the PPF proximal to the SPG, with the body of the stimulator positioned on the lateral-posterior maxilla medial to the zygoma and anchored to the zygomatic process of the maxilla using the integral fixation plate. The position of the stimulator was checked immediately post-operatively with X-ray.

The SPG stimulator was used as an acute treatment, with the patients activating their stimulator on-demand during an attack. Each attack was randomly treated with full, sub-perception or sham stimulation. The primary endpoint was pain relief at 15 minutes following SPG stimulation. Pain relief was achieved in 67.1% of full stimulation-treated attacks compared to 7.4% of sham treated, and 7.3% of sub-perception treated attacks ($p < 0.0001$). Interestingly, although used as an acute treatment, 43% of patients reported a greater than 50% reduction in attack frequency implying the stimulation was having a prophylactic effect.

Safety of peripheral neurostimulation

ONS is a relatively safe procedure with no reports of any serious adverse events. There is one report of the development of hemicrania continua (HC) 1 month after an ONS implant in a SUNCT patient; it remains unclear whether the ONS implant was causal in the development of HC or that this is merely coincidental (43). Other adverse events reported in ONS include lead migration, lead site pain, myofascial incision site pain, neck stiffness, discharged battery, battery site pain, and contact dermatitis. Jasper and Hayek (44) have reviewed the safety of ONS. They report that lead migration occurred frequently with percutaneous cylindrical leads, being described in 26% of patients, but occur in only 6% of patients implanted with paddle-type leads. Recent development of anchoring techniques will likely reduce cylindrical lead migration. Battery failure due to depletion is an expected event requiring IPG replacement and, therefore, should not be considered a complication. However, rapid battery depletion (less than 1 year) is reported and highlights the need of less expensive and longer lasting power sources, especially for patients who require high voltage and frequency to control the pain (21). The increased use of rechargeable devices will obviate this in clinical practice.

In SPG stimulation, 81% of patients reported transient sensory disturbances within the maxillary nerve regions, which resolved in the majority within 3 months (33). Other adverse effects reported included lead misplacement in two patients, lead migration in two patients, and two infections requiring antibiotic use.

Mechanism of action of peripheral neurostimulation

The mechanisms by which peripheral neurostimulation mediates the anti-nociceptive effect is poorly understood. To date all work has focused on ONS and, therefore, this is the literature reviewed here. Several sites of action within the peripheral and central nervous systems have been proposed, including the peripheral nerve, spinal segmental level, and supraspinal levels. It is likely that peripheral neurostimulation exerts its effect by multiple mechanisms and that these mechanisms may differ in the various headache and pain syndromes.

Direct effects of neurostimulation on peripheral nerve fibre excitability have been described, including transient slowing of conduction velocity, increase in electrical threshold, and decrease in response probability (45). However, ONS did not significantly modify pain thresholds in CCH (25), which argues against a diffuse analgesic effect.

A widely accepted theory for the anti-nociceptive effect of neurostimulation is the Gate Control Theory of pain, which proposes that the activation of large-diameter afferent nerve fibres act in the spinal dorsal horn to inhibit onward transmission in small-diameter primary afferent nociceptive fibres, thereby preventing the nociceptive signals from reaching the higher neural centres and being interpreted as pain (46, 47). Indeed, a number of physiological studies have confirmed that afferent activity set up by peripheral neurostimulation blocks nociceptive transmission in the spinal cord (48–50). The explanation for the anti-nociceptive effect of spinal cord stimulation (SCS) according to the Gate Control Theory is that nociceptive input from the periphery could be inhibited at the first dorsal horn relay by stimulation-induced antidromic activation of collaterals of large dorsal column fibres projecting onto the same spinal segment (51–53). However, the gate theory does not adequately explain some of the animal and human experimental data and, therefore, several additional mechanisms of action for neurostimulation have been postulated. Some of the theories proposed include: activation of supraspinal mechanisms; alteration of putative neurotransmitter levels; and blockade of sympathetic mechanisms (54–56).

The involvement of supraspinal sensory pathways is a requisite for the orthodromic transmission of the activation resulting from neurostimulation. The key issues are whether the ascending and descending pain pathways are involved in mediating an anti-nociceptive effect and, if so, then which supraspinal structures are involved. Anti-nociception in animal models produced by sensory afferent stimulation is reduced by spinal transection, thus implicating the involvement of supraspinal mechanisms (57, 58). Similarly, with spinal cord stimulation it has been argued that the inhibitory effects on nociceptive transmission in the spinal dorsal horn cannot be entirely attributed to antidromic activation of the dorsal columns because they persist after dorsal column transection caudal to the stimulating electrode (59). Furthermore, on the basis of animal studies, various supraspinal structures have been proposed as candidates for mediating the anti-nociceptive effect, including the periaqueductal grey (PAG) (60) and thalamus (61).

One PET study investigated the effect of spinal cord stimulation in patients with refractory angina pectoris (62). The study was performed when the patients were not in pain and, therefore, the regional cerebral blood flow (rCBF) changes reflect the effects of spinal cord stimulation solely. During stimulation, activation was noted in the PAG, dorsomedial, and the pulvinar nuclei of the thalamus, prefrontal cortex, medial temporal gyrus, posterior caudate nuclei, and posterior cingulate cortex, while a relative decrease in rCBF was observed in the insulae and anterior cingulate cortex. Furthermore, a functional magnetic resonance imaging (fMRI) study in three patients with chronic pain syndromes showed primary and secondary somatosensory cortex and anterior cingulate cortex activation with spinal cord stimulation (63).

A further PET study has investigated the brain structures modulated by ONS in chronic migraine (64). Eight patients with a marked beneficial response to bilateral ONS were studied in three states: during stimulation when patient was pain-free; during pain with the ONS switched off; and during partial stimulation and varying levels of pain and paraesthesia. Stimulation suppressed the headache within 30 minutes and pain recurred within 20 minutes of switching off the device. Stimulation evoked local paraesthesia, the presence of which was a criterion of pain relief. There were significant changes in regional cerebral blood flow in the dorsal rostral pons, anterior cingulate cortex and cuneus correlated to pain scores, and in the anterior cingulate cortex and left pulvinar correlated to stimulation-induced paraesthesia scores.

The activation pattern in the dorsal rostral pons in this study is highly suggestive of a role for this structure in the pathophysiology of chronic migraine. However, this brainstem region may also be a locus for neuromodulation by ONS. The PAG has long been proposed as a candidate for mediating the anti-nociceptive effects of neurostimulation. Stiller and colleagues (60) performed micro-dialysis studies on transmitter release in the PAG of rats receiving SCS. They observed that SCS affected a decrease of gamma-aminobutyric acid (GABA) levels but not of serotonin or substance P. As GABA-neurones in the PAG exert a tonic depressive effect on the activity in descending pain inhibitory pathways, the authors proposed that a decreased GABA level in this region following repeated SCS might indicate an increased pain inhibition.

Magis and colleagues (65) studied 10 ONS-treated medically intractable CCH and 39 drug-free healthy volunteers (HV) using 18-fluorodeoxyglucose (FDG) PET. The ten CCH patients underwent an 18 FDG-PET scan after ONS, at delays varying between 0 and 30 months. All were scanned with ongoing ONS and with the stimulator switched off. After 6–30 months of ONS, three patients were pain-free and four had a ≥90% reduction of attack frequency (responders). In all patients compared to controls, several areas of the pain matrix showed hypermetabolism, including the ipsilateral hypothalamus, midbrain, and ipsilateral lower pons. All normalized after ONS, except for the hypothalamus. Switching the stimulator on or off had little influence on brain glucose metabolism. The perigenual anterior cingulate cortex (PACC) was hyperactive in ONS responders compared to non-responders.

These results may support the hypothesis that ONS exerts its beneficial effects via slow neuromodulatory processes in the central pain matrix. The finding of a possible selective perigenual AAC in responders raises the possibility that ONS activates descending pain control systems in a top-down manner and restores equilibrium in anti-nociceptive opioidergic pathways. The study also reported persistent hypermetabolism of the ipsilateral posterior hypothalamus outside of an attack, which might be a hallmark of CH and also explains why attacks rapidly recur after interruption of ONS.

Conclusions

Peripheral neuromodulation, especially ONS, has emerged as a promising treatment modality for medically intractable TACs, including cluster headache and SUNCT/SUNA. It has already improved quality of life for some and gives future hope to many more. However, the ultimate confirmation of the utility of a new therapeutic modality should come from randomized, double-blind, placebo-controlled trials. This poses a special problem in designing blinded studies of treatment with stimulation, since there is no placebo equivalent for the paraesthesia that accompanies stimulation. Any credible sham device would, therefore, be required to produce a discernible stimulus, which could then be criticized for providing neurostimulation. Nonetheless, it is possible to work around this challenging problem with particular trial designs such as that utilized in the ONSTIM trial (66). Further large-scale controlled trials are required to differentiate the neuromodulatory effects from the non-specific effects, such as placebo response, regression to the mean, and spontaneous improvement.

Ideally, results from controlled trials should be available before widespread open-label use of ONS can be recommended, though it might be several years before these studies are available. Given the highly challenging nature of the management of medically intractable headache syndromes, most of which are very disabling, and taken together with the promising efficacy data for ONS, it seems reasonable to cautiously proceed with the open-label use of this procedure, preferably in tertiary referral settings. Patients who are considered for ONS should satisfy the following criteria: clearly established headache diagnosis using IHS classification criteria with a careful workup, including brain imaging,

Table 11.3 Criteria for the use of peripheral neurostimulation in primary headache

◆ Patient must meet the IHS criteria for trigeminal autonomic cephalalgia (1)
◆ Patients should have had daily or near daily attacks for at least 2 years prior to stimulation
◆ Patients should have been under the care of the referring headache specialist team for at least 1 year
◆ All reasonable drugs must have been tried at the correct doses and for sufficient durations unless contraindicated
◆ All patients should have a psychological assessment prior to surgery
◆ All co-existent conditions should be identified and treated where possible prior to surgery (e.g. depression, medication overuse)
◆ Patients (and doctors) must have a realistic expectation of the surgical outcome
◆ Patients should be followed-up by the referring specialist for at least 1 year
◆ Prospective headache diaries recording headache attack frequency, severity and duration as well as analgesia intake must be kept
◆ Appropriate quality of life measures, disability scores and self-assessments must be kept by the patient prior and post-operatively
◆ Where possible, the neurostimulator should only be switched off for efficacy assessment, ideally in a double-blind fashion.
◆ A clear record of adverse events is kept

Adapted from Lancet Neurol, 6 (4), Leone M, Franzini A, Cecchini AP, Broggi G, Bussone G., Stimulation of occipital nerve for drug-resistant chronic cluster headache, p. 289–91, Copyright (2007), with permission from Elsevier.

lumbar puncture, and indometacin tests, where appropriate; medically intractable as defined by the consensus statements (67), which suggests failure of a minimum of four classes of preventive treatments in cluster headache; and, the patient is severely disabled by the headache syndrome. In addition, we recommend that the criteria suggested by Leone and colleagues (35) should be fulfilled (Table 11.3).

With regard to future prospects, it would be helpful to have predictors of success with ONS. Occipital nerve blocks do not appear to be correlated with response (68). It is likely that large-scale studies will be required to tease out these predictors. The role of the surgical technique used, including the anchoring method, electrode type, and optimal stimulation parameters, are all variables that require further exploration. Finally, the mode of action of ONS is poorly understood and further studies are required to elucidate the underlying mechanisms by which the anti-nociceptive effect is exerted.

References

1 Headache Classification Subcommittee of the International Headache Society. The International Classification of Headache Disorders, 2nd edn. Cephalalgia 2004;**24**(Suppl 1):1–160.

2 **Cittadini E, Matharu MS, Goadsby PJ**. Paroxysmal hemicrania: a prospective clinical study of 31 cases. Brain 2008 Apr;**131**(Pt 4):1142–55. PubMed PMID: 18252775. Epub 2008/02/07. eng.

3 **Cohen AS, Matharu MS, Goadsby PJ**. Short-lasting unilateral neuralgiform headache attacks with conjunctival injection and tearing (SUNCT) or cranial autonomic features (SUNA)—a prospective clinical study of SUNCT and SUNA. Brain 2006 Oct;**129**(Pt 10):2746–60. PubMed PMID: 16905753.

4 **Goadsby PJ, Schoenen J, Ferrari MD, Silberstein SD, Dodick D**. Towards a definition of intractable headache for use in clinical practice and trials. Cephalalgia 2006;**26**:1168–70.

5 **May A, Goadsby PJ**. The trigeminovascular system in humans: pathophysiologic implications for primary headache syndromes of the neural influences on the cerebral circulation. J Cerebr Blood F Met: official journal of the International Society of Cerebral Blood Flow and Metabolism 1999 Feb;**19**(2):115–27. PubMed PMID: 10027765.

6 **Goadsby PJ, Matharu MS, Boes CJ**. SUNCT syndrome or trigeminal neuralgia with lacrimation. Cephalalgia 2001 Mar;**21**(2):82–83. PubMed PMID: 11422087.

7 **Leone M, Bussone G**. Pathophysiology of trigeminal autonomic cephalalgias. Lancet Neurol 2009 Aug;**8**(8):755–64. PubMed PMID: 19608101.

8 **May A, Bahra A, Büchel C et al**. Hypothalamic activation in cluster headache attacks. Lancet 1998;**352**:275–78.

9 **Matharu MS, Cohen AS, Frackowiak RS, Goadsby PJ**. Posterior hypothalamic activation in paroxysmal hemicrania. Ann Neurol 2006 Mar;**59**(3):535–45. PubMed PMID: 16489610.

10 **Cohen AS**. Short-lasting unilateral neuralgiform headache attacks with conjunctival injection and tearing. Cephalalgia 2007 Jul;**27**(7):824–32. PubMed PMID: 17598764.

11 **Malick A, Burstein R**. Cells of origin of the trigeminohypothalamic tract in the rat. J Comp Neurol 1998 Oct 12;**400**(1):125–44. PubMed PMID: 9762871.

12 **Dafny N, Dong WQ, Prieto-Gomez C, Reyes-Vazquez C, Stanford J, Qiao JT**. Lateral hypothalamus: site involved in pain modulation. Neuroscience 1996 Jan;**70**(2):449–60. PubMed PMID: 8848153.

13 **Lumb BM, Lovick TA**. The rostral hypothalamus: an area for the integration of autonomic and sensory responsiveness. J Neurophysiol 1993 Oct;**70**(4):1570–77. PubMed PMID: 8283214.

14 **Benjamin L, Levy MJ, Lasalandra MP et al.** Hypothalamic activation after stimulation of the superior sagittal sinus in the cat: a Fos study. Neurobiol Dis 2004 Aug;**16**(3):500–505. PubMed PMID: 15262261.

15 **Bartsch T, Levy MJ, Knight YE, Goadsby PJ.** Differential modulation of nociceptive dural input to [hypocretin] orexin A and B receptor activation in the posterior hypothalamic area. Pain 2004 Jun;**109**(3):367–78. PubMed PMID: 15157698.

16 **Natsis K, Baraliakos X, Appell HJ, Tsikaras P, Gigis I, Koebke J.** The course of the greater occipital nerve in the suboccipital region: a proposal for setting landmarks for local anesthesia in patients with occipital neuralgia. Clin Anat 2006 May;**19**(4):332–36. PubMed PMID: 16258972.

17 **Poletti CE.** C2 and C3 pain dermatomes in man. Cephalalgia 1991 Jul;**11**(3):155–59. PubMed PMID: 1889073.

18 **Kerr FW, Olafson RA.** Trigeminal and cervical volleys. Convergence on single units in the spinal gray at C-1 and C-2. Arch Neurol 1961 Aug;**5**:171–78. PubMed PMID: 13752662.

19 **Weiner R, Reed KL.** Peripheral neurostimulation for control of intractable occipital neuralgia. Neuromodulation 1999;**2**(3):217–21.

20 **Trentman TL, Zimmerman RS, Dodick DW, Dormer CL, Vargas BB.** Occipital nerve stimulator placement under general anesthesia: initial experience with 5 cases and review of the literature. J Neurosurg Anesthesiol 2010 Apr;**22**(2):158–62. PubMed PMID: 19816202. Epub 2009/10/10. eng.

21 **Trentman TL, Zimmerman RS.** Occipital nerve stimulation: technical and surgical aspects of implantation. Headache 2008 Feb;**48**(2):319–27. PubMed PMID: 18234049. Epub 2008/02/01. eng.

22 **Schwedt TJ, Dodick DW, Trentman TL, Zimmerman RS.** Occipital nerve stimulation for chronic cluster headache and hemicrania continua: pain relief and persistence of autonomic features. Cephalalgia 2006 Aug;**26**(8):1025–27. PubMed PMID: 16886942. Epub 2006/08/05. eng.

23 **Trentman TL, Rosenfeld DM, Vargas BB, Schwedt TJ, Zimmerman RS, Dodick DW.** Greater occipital nerve stimulation via the Bion microstimulator: implantation technique and stimulation parameters. Clinical trial: NCT00205894. Pain Physician 2009 May/Jun;**12**(3):621–28. PubMed PMID: 19461827.

24 **Matharu M, Watkins L, Shanahan P.** Treatment of medically intractable SUNCT and SUNA with occipital nerve stimulation. J Neurol Neurosurg Psychiatry 2010;**81**(11):e51–2.

25 **Magis D, Allena M, Bolla M, De Pasqua V, Remacle JM, Schoenen J.** Occipital nerve stimulation for drug-resistant chronic cluster headache: a prospective pilot study. Lancet Neurol 2007 Apr;**6**(4):314–21. PubMed PMID: 17362835. Epub 2007/03/17. eng.

26 **Magis D, Gerardy PY, Remacle JM, Schoenen J.** Sustained effectiveness of occipital nerve stimulation in drug-resistant chronic cluster headache. Headache 2011 Sept;**51**(8):1191–201. PubMed PMID: 21848953. Epub 2011/08/19. eng.

27 **Burns B, Watkins L, Goadsby PJ.** Treatment of medically intractable cluster headache by occipital nerve stimulation: long-term follow-up of eight patients. Lancet 2007 Mar 31;**369**(9567):1099–106. PubMed PMID: 17398309. Epub 2007/04/03. eng.

28 **Burns B, Watkins L, Goadsby PJ.** Treatment of intractable chronic cluster headache by occipital nerve stimulation in 14 patients. Neurology 2009 Jan 27;**72**(4):341–45. PubMed PMID: 19171831. Epub 2009/01/28. eng.

29 **de Quintana-Schmidt C, Casajuana-Garreta E, Molet-Teixido J et al.** [Stimulation of the occipital nerve in the treatment of drug-resistant cluster headache]. Revista de Neurologia 2010 Jul 1;**51**(1):19–26. PubMed PMID: 20568064. Epub 2010/06/23. Estimulacion del nervio occipital para la cefalea en racimos refractaria al tratamiento farmacologico. spa.

30 **Muller OM, Gaul C, Katsarava Z, Sure U, Diener HC, Gasser T.** [Bilateral occipital nerve stimulation for the treatment of chronic cluster headache: case series and initiation of a prospective study]. Fortschritte der Neurologie-Psychiatrie 2010 Dec;**78**(12):709–14. PubMed PMID:

21136339. Epub 2010/12/08. Beidseitige Nervus-occipitalis-Stimulation zur Behandlung des therapierefraktaren chronischen Cluster-Kopfschmerzes: eigene Fallserie und Initiierung einer prospektiven Studie. ger.

31 **Fontaine D, Christophe Sol J, Raoul S et al.** Treatment of refractory chronic cluster headache by chronic occipital nerve stimulation. Cephalalgia 2011 Jul;**31**(10):1101–105. PubMed PMID: 21727143. Epub 2011/07/06. eng.

32 **Strand NH, Trentman TL, Vargas BB, Dodick DW.** Occipital nerve stimulation with the Bion(R) microstimulator for the treatment of medically refractory chronic cluster headache. Pain Physician 2011 Sept/Oct;**14**(5):435–40. PubMed PMID: 21927047. Epub 2011/09/20. eng.

33 **Schwedt TJ, Dodick DW, Hentz J, Trentman TL, Zimmerman RS.** Occipital nerve stimulation for chronic headache—long-term safety and efficacy. Cephalalgia 2007 Feb;**27**(2):153–7. PubMed PMID: 17257236. Epub 2007/01/30. eng.

34 **Brewer AC, Trentman TL, Ivancic MG et al.** Long-Term Outcome in Occipital Nerve Stimulation Patients With Medically Intractable Primary Headache Disorders. Neuromodulation 2012 Aug;**16**(6):557–62.

35 **Leone M, Franzini A, Cecchini AP, Broggi G, Bussone G.** Stimulation of occipital nerve for drug-resistant chronic cluster headache. Lancet Neurol 2007 Apr;**6**(4):289–91. PubMed PMID: 17362827. Epub 2007/03/17. eng.

36 **Knight YE, Classey JD, Lasalandra MP et al.** Patterns of fos expression in the rostral medulla and caudal pons evoked by noxious craniovascular stimulation and periaqueductal gray stimulation in the cat. Brain Res 2005 May 31;**1045**(1–2):1–11. PubMed PMID: 15910757.

37 **Drummond PD.** Autonomic disturbances in cluster headache. Brain 1988 Oct;**111** (Pt 5):1199–209. PubMed PMID: 3179690.

38 **Fanciullacci M, Pietrini U, Gatto G, Boccuni M, Sicuteri F.** Latent dysautonomic pupillary lateralization in cluster headache. A pupillometric study. Cephalalgia 1982 Sept;**2**(3):135–44. PubMed PMID: 6897524.

39 **Salvesen R, Sand T, Sjaastad O.** Cluster headache: combined assessment with pupillometry and evaporimetry. Cephalalgia 1988 Sept;**8**(3):211–18. PubMed PMID: 3197101.

40 **Drummond PD.** Sweating and vascular responses in the face: normal regulation and dysfunction in migraine, cluster headache and harlequin syndrome. Clin Auton Res 1994 Oct;**4**(5):273–85. PubMed PMID: 7888747.

41 **Oomen KP, van Wijck AJ, Hordijk GJ, de Ru JA.** Effects of radiofrequency thermocoagulation of the sphenopalatine ganglion on headache and facial pain: correlation with diagnosis. J Orofac Pain 2012 Winter;**26**(1):59–64. PubMed PMID: 22292141. Epub 2012/02/01. eng.

42 **Schoenen J, Jensen RH, Lanteri-Minet M et al.** Stimulation of the sphenopalatine ganglion (SPG) for cluster headache treatment. Pathway CH-1: A randomized, sham-controlled study. Cephalalgia 2013 Jan 11;**0**(0):1–15. PubMed PMID: 23314784. Epub 2013/01/15. Eng.

43 **Shanahan P, Watkins L, Matharu MS.** Treatment of medically intractable short-lasting unilateral neuralgiform headache attacks with conjunctival injection and tearing (SUNCT) and short-lasting unilateral neuralgiform headache attacks with autonomic symptoms (SUNA) with occipital nerve stimulation (ONS) in 6 patients. Cephalagia 2009;**29**(Suppl. 1):150.

44 **Jasper JF, Hayek SM.** Implanted occipital nerve stimulators. Pain Physician 2008 Mar/Apr;**11**(2):187–200. PubMed PMID: 18354711. Epub 2008/03/21. eng.

45 **Ignelzi RJ, Nyquist JK.** Excitability changes in peripheral nerve fibers after repetitive electrical stimulation. Implications in pain modulation. J Neurosurg 1979 Dec;**51**(6):824–33. PubMed PMID: 315452. Epub 1979/12/01. eng.

46 **Melzack R, Wall PD.** Pain mechanisms: a new theory. Science 1965;**150**(699):971–79.

47 **Wall PD**. The gate control theory of pain mechanisms. A re-examination and re-statement. Brain 1978;**101**(1):1–18.

48 **Woolf CJ, Wall PD**. Chronic peripheral nerve section diminishes the primary afferent A-fibre mediated inhibition of rat dorsal horn neurones. Brain Res 1982;**242**(1):77–85.

49 **Chung JM, Lee KH, Hori Y, Endo K, Willis WD**. Factors influencing peripheral nerve stimulation produced inhibition of primate spinothalamic tract cells. Pain 1984;**19**(3):277–93.

50 **Garrison DW, Foreman RD**. Effects of transcutaneous electrical nerve stimulation (TENS) on spontaneous and noxiously evoked dorsal horn cell activity in cats with transected spinal cords. Neurosci Lett 1996;**216**(2):125–28.

51 **Hillman P, Wall PD**. Inhibitory and excitatory factors influencing the receptive fields of lamina 5 spinal cord cells. Exp Brain Res 1969;**9**(4):284–306.

52 **Foreman RD, Applebaum AE, Beall JE, Trevino DL, Willis WD**. Responses of primate spinothalamic tract neurons to electrical stimulation of hindlimb peripheral nerves. J Neurophysiol 1975;**38**(1):132–45.

53 **Dubuisson D**. Effect of dorsal-column stimulation on gelatinosa and marginal neurons of cat spinal cord. J Neurosurg 1989;**70**(2):257–65.

54 **Hansson P, Lundeberg T**. Transcutaneous electrical nerve stimulation, vibration and acupuncture as pain-relieving measures. In: Melzack R, Wall PD (eds) Textbook of Pain. New York: Churchill Livingstone; 1999:1341–51.

55 **Krames E**. Spinal cord stimulation: indications, mechanism of action, and efficacy. Curr Rev Pain 1999;**3**(6):419–26.

56 **Linderoth B, Meyerson BA**. Spinal cord stimulation: mechanism of action. In: Burchiel K (ed.) Surgical Management of Pain. New York: Thieme; 2002:505–26.

57 **Chung JM, Fang ZR, Hori Y, Lee KH, Willis WD**. Prolonged inhibition of primate spinothalamic tract cells by peripheral nerve stimulation. Pain 1984;**19**(3):259–75.

58 **Woolf CJ, Mitchell D, Barrett GD**. Antinociceptive effect of peripheral segmental electrical stimulation in the rat. Pain 1980;**8**(2):237–52.

59 **Saade NE, Tabet MS, Banna NR, Atweh SF, Jabbur SJ**. Inhibition of nociceptive evoked activity in spinal neurons through a dorsal column-brainstem-spinal loop. Brain Res 1985;**339**(1):115–18.

60 **Stiller CO, Linderoth B, O'Connor WT et al.** Repeated spinal cord stimulation decreases the extracellular level of gamma-aminobutyric acid in the periaqueductal gray matter of freely moving rats. Brain Res 1995;**699**(2):231–41.

61 **Nyquist JK, Greenhoot JH**. Responses evoked from the thalamic centrum medianum by painful input: suppression by dorsal funiculus conditioning. Exp Neurol 1973;**39**(2):215–22.

62 **Hautvast RW, Ter Horst GJ, DeJong BM et al.** Relative changes in regional cerebral blood flow during spinal cord stimulation in patients with refractory angina pectoris. Eur J Neurosci 1997;**9**(6):1178–83.

63 **Kiriakopoulos ET, Tasker RR, Nicosia S, Wood ML, Mikulis DJ**. Functional magnetic resonance imaging: a potential tool for the evaluation of spinal cord stimulation: technical case report. Neurosurgery 1997;**41**(2):501–04.

64 **Matharu MS, Bartsch T, Ward N, Frackowiak RS, Weiner R, Goadsby PJ**. Central neuromodulation in chronic migraine patients with suboccipital stimulators: a PET study. Brain 2004;**127**:220–30.

65 **Magis D, Bruno MA, Fumal A et al.** Central modulation in cluster headache patients treated with occipital nerve stimulation: an FDG-PET study. BMC Neurol 2011;**11**:25. PubMed PMID: 21349186. Pubmed Central PMCID: 3056751. Epub 2011/02/26. eng.

66 **Saper JR, Dodick DW, Silberstein SD, McCarville S, Sun M, Goadsby PJ**. Occipital nerve stimulation for the treatment of intractable chronic migraine headache: ONSTIM feasibility study. Cephalalgia 2011 Feb;**31**(3):271–85. PubMed PMID: 20861241. Pubmed Central PMCID: PMC3057439. Epub 2010/09/24. eng.

67 **Goadsby PJ, Schoenen J, Ferrari MD, Silberstein SD, Dodick D**. Towards a definition of intractable headache for use in clinical practice and trials. Cephalalgia 2006 Sept;**26**(9):1168–70. PubMed PMID: 16919073.

68 **Schwedt TJ, Dodick DW, Trentman TL, Zimmerman RS**. Response to occipital nerve block is not useful in predicting efficacy of occipital nerve stimulation. Cephalalgia 2007 Mar;**27**(3):271–74. PubMed PMID: 17381559. Epub 2007/03/27. eng.

Chapter 12

Trigeminal autonomic cephalalgias II: deep-brain stimulation of the posterior hypothalamus for chronic cluster headache

Giuseppe Messina, Roberto Cordella, Michele Rizzi, Massimo Leone, and Angelo Franzini

Key points

1. The hypothalamus is a small, still crucial diencephalic structure involved in the integration of different homeostatic and vegetative functions.
2. The main and clearest hypothalamic connections are with the amygdala, hippocampus, and retina.
3. Posterior hypothalamus (pHyp) contains different types of cells with regard to released neurotransmitters.
4. High-frequency stimulation of pHyp has been shown to be a promising therapeutic modality for trigeminal autonomic cephalalgias (TACs).
5. The existence of the trigemino-cervical complex and the supposed existence of the trigemino-hypothalamic tract in humans could explain occipital nerve stimulation (ONS) efficacy in TACs

Introduction

The hypothalamus lies at the base of the diencephalon beneath the thalamus from which it is separated by the hypothalamic sulcus. The rostral boundary is taken to be at the level of the lamina terminalis, while the caudal end is at the level of the mammillary bodies (1).

Modern studies have demonstrated that the hypothalamus functions to integrate autonomic response and endocrine functions with behaviour, especially with behaviour related to the basic homeostatic requirements of everyday life (2). It serves this integrative function by regulating some pivotal physiological functions:

- blood pressure and electrolytic composition;
- body temperature;
- energy metabolism;
- reproduction;
- emergency response to stress.

Although the hypothalamus is a small part of the whole central nervous system (CNS), it is packed with a complex array of cell groups and fibre pathways. It can be divided into three anatomical regions: anterior, middle, and posterior. These three regions are associated with different group of nuclei or groups of cell bodies (1, 2). Main connections and networks are well defined (3, 4), while others are more diffuse and harder to define. Amongst the afferent fibres that have been identified, the hippocampo-hypothalamic fibres, the amygdalo-hypothalamic fibres, brainstem reticular afferents, and the retino-hypothalamic afferents are of particular note (1). Recently, it has been suggested that the posterior hypothalamus is involved in the pathogenesis of trigeminal autonomic cephalalgias due to neuroimaging evidence of its activation during pain attacks (5). These data led to the introduction of new therapeutic procedures aimed at inhibition of the hypothalamic pathological activation (6) for alleviating symptoms of such diseases.

Anatomy and physiology of the posterior hypothalamus

The posterior nucleus of the hypothalamus (pHyp), also named the posterior hypothalamic area, is located above the mammillary bodies at both sides of the third ventricle. The pHyp contains a homogeneous population of small- to medium-sized cells, with occasional large neurones scattered throughout the rostrocaudal extent of the nucleus. Cell-packing density is low relative to neighbouring hypothalamic structures, and fibre tracks course through and around the pHyp along its rostrocaudal extent (3). A chemoarchitectural analysis has shown four main cell types: the majority of pHyp cells are glutamatergic, followed by melanin-concentrating hormone cells, tyrosine hydroxylase cells, and hypocretins cells. GABAergic cells, neuropeptide Y cells, enkephalin cells, serotoninergic, and dopaminergic neurones are also present. The most important neurotransmitters produced by pHyp neurones are the orexins, also called hypocretins, the common names given to a pair of highly excitatory neuropeptide hormones; despite being produced by a very small population of cells in the lateral and posterior hypothalamus, they send projections throughout the brain.

Major fibre tracks, cell morphology, and packing-density differences of adjacent structures demarcate the boundaries of the pHyp dorsally (thalamus, fasciculus retroflexus, and periaqueductal grey), ventrally (dorsal premammillary nucleus, dorsomedial tuberomammillary nucleus, and supramammillary decussation), caudally (periaqueductal grey and mesencephalic reticular formation), and laterally (lateral hypothalamic area, zona incerta, fornix, and mammillothalamic tracks). The periventricular hypothalamic nucleus and fibre systems separate the pHyp from the ependyma of the third ventricle. The rostral border of pHyp appears to extend as a uniform structure rostrally to the level of the dorsal hypothalamic nucleus (3). The pHyp receives afferents from cortical, subcortical, and brainstem structures involved in autonomic regulation. These include the insular cortex, septal nuclei, amygdala, subiculum, bed nucleus of stria terminalis, central grey, parabrachial nucleus, nucleus of the solitary tract, and brainstem reticular nuclei. In addition the pHyp receives inputs from structures such as the cingulate, frontal, parietal, and insular cortices (3, 7). In older literature, the posterior hypothalamus has been mentioned as a controlling centre for the sympathetic system and consciousness. The posterior hypothalamic area was once also reported to show cell loss in a case of Cushing's disease (8). Extensive descending projections, as described in the rat, may serve a role in these functions (9). Experimental findings in rats have pointed out that the posterior hypothalamus also receives spino-hypothalamic inputs, probably involving somatosensory and visceral sensory information (8).

The posterior hypothalamus has been linked to the control of behavioural states (10, 11). Early studies have demonstrated that experimental lesions of the pHyp induced long-lasting somnolence in monkeys and rats (12–15). Moreover muscimol injections in the posterior hypothalamus in animal models have reinforced the idea of the importance of the pHyp in maintaining arousal (10, 16). Single-unit recordings, performed in animal models, have reported that during wakefulness cats' posterior hypothalamic neurones spontaneously discharge at around 25 spikes/second. During slow-wave sleep (SWS) the firing rate decreases to around 15 Hz (17) with a tonic discharge pattern; in anesthetized rats it is around 13 Hz (18)

Karplus and Kreidl (19) have extensively examined the effect of posterior hypothalamic stimulation to cardiorespiratory and behavioural responses. These authors described changes in cardiopulmonary functions and behavioural alteration following pHyp lesions. Subsequent studies have reported the increase in mean arterial blood pressure, heart and respiratory rates, and escape/defence behaviour following the electrical (20) and chemical stimulation of the pHyp, through glutamate (21), acetylcholine agonists (22, 23), or neuropeptide Y (24–26), and GABA antagonists (27, 28). Single-unit recordings were sampled both *in vivo* and *in vitro* within the pHyp of spontaneously hypertensive rats (18). The authors compared the neuronal firing rate between a group of rats with free access to a running wheel (exercise hypertensive rats) and a group with no access to the running wheel (no exercise hypertensive rats). In the *in vivo* experiments, the average firing rate for the exercise group was lower (8.5 Hz) compared to the no-exercise group (13.7 Hz). These results were also confirmed *in vitro*, although the overall firing rate was lower compared to the *in vivo* experiments. All of the units have shown no rhythmic firing patterns. These findings suggest that pHyp maintains behavioural and sympathetic activation characteristic of escape/defence behaviour. It has been suggested that the role of the pHyp in defence behaviour and its associated physiological correlates is related to its involvement in the maintenance of arousal (3).

pHyp is also involved in the generation of large-amplitude, sinusoidal electrical oscillations, the theta (θ) oscillations (4–7 Hz), in the hippocampus of awake behaving rats, and in rats undergoing REM sleep episodes. pHyp is part of a neuronal network, along with the oral pontine reticular formation, supramammillary nucleus, medial septum, and diagonal band of Broca (29). In particular, the role of pHyp in tonic modulation of neuronal activity in the medial septum during hippocampal theta activity has been shown (30, 31). In addition, this nucleus receives descending inhibitory inputs from the medial septum during theta oscillations in the hippocampus. This suggests that pHyp neurones are important in modulating theta rhythms, and in turn may be modulated by hippocampal activity through the inhibitory projections from the lateral septum (4). The existence of topographically organized projections from the hippocampus to the lateral septum has in fact been demonstrated (3). Single-unit discharge has been recorded from the rats' pHyp, during hippocampal theta oscillations elicited from stimulation of the reticular nucleus pontis oralis (4). All pHyp neurones were classified as tonic theta-ON, namely an increased tonic discharge rate during the elicited hippocampal theta. The authors also reported bursting discharge in neurones located within the supramammillary and the medial mammillary nuclei.

Besides the role in the control of behavioural states, experimental findings in rats have shown that two distinct fibre tracts convey sensory information from the skin surface to the posterior hypothalamus, namely the trigemino-hypothalamic tract and the reticulo-hypothalamic tract. The former conveys nociceptive inputs only from the facio-cephalic region to the hypothalamus; the latter conveys sensory inputs from both cephalic and extra-cephalic regions (32). It is important to mention that the trigemino-hypothalamic pathway displays receptive fields only from the contralateral side, while the reticulo-hypothalamic pathway displays more complex receptive fields, comprising both sides of the body. In humans, electrical stimulation of this nucleus has evoked cognitive responses (anxiety/phobia), but not vegetative modifications such as blood pressure changes (6). An older report (33) has described that the high-voltage stimulation of the posterior area of the hypothalamus evoked an increase in heart rate, blood pressure, pupillary dilatation, and EEG de-synchronization.

In the last decade there has been a resurgence of attention on the posterior area of the hypothalamus as the target for the placement of deep-brain stimulation (DBS) leads in the treatment of disorders such as trigeminal autonomic cephalalgias (TACs), aggressive behaviour, and epilepsy (6, 34).

Posterior hypothalamus chronic high-frequency stimulation and cluster headache

Chronic cluster headache (CCH), short unilateral neuralgiform headache with conjunctival injection and tearing (SUNCT), along with the chronic paroxysmal hemicrania (CPH), constitute trigeminal autonomic cephalagias (TACs). These syndromes are characterized by a sudden and fast onset of unilateral pain sited around the eye, temple, and superior portion of the cheeks (35). The TACs differ for attack duration and frequency, as well as for response to therapy. CCH has the longest duration and relatively low frequency; CPH has intermediate duration and frequency; SUNCT has the shortest duration and the highest frequency (36). All these syndromes are described, as the most unpleasant form of pain experienced by human beings and it is often accompanied by autonomic symptoms. In fact, the clinically differentiating factor for TACs, as a group, is the prominence of cranial autonomic activation, such as lacrimation, conjunctival injection, eyelid oedema, or rhinorrhoea (37).

It has been suggested that TACs should be referred to as 'neurovascular headaches' (38), in which the vascular change that is seen in the cranial circulation is driven by the trigeminal autonomic reflex (trigeminal facial nuclei). Stimulation of the trigeminal ganglion in cats (39) or monkeys (40) leads to a decrease in carotid resistance, which increases flow and facial temperature, mostly through a reflex mechanism. The afferent limb of this reflex is the trigeminal nerve, and the efferent is the facial/greater superficial petrosal nerve (parasympathetic) dilator pathway (38). The trigeminal neural innervation of the cerebral circulation is somatotopically selective. In humans, painful stimulation through the administration of capsaicin produces dilatation of the internal carotid artery when administered into the skin innervated by the first (ophthalmic) division of the trigeminal nerve (41). However, when capsaicin is injected into the skin innervated by the third (mandibular) division, or into the leg, there is no response in the ipsilateral carotid artery, despite the experience of pain (42).

The circadian timing, with two significant peaks of bouts in July and January (43), along with the alterations in plasma melatonin, cortisol, testosterone, gonadotropins, prolactin, growth hormone, and thyrotropin have been documented in TACs (44). Taken together, these results strongly suggest a hypothalamic involvement in TACs pathophysiology.

In recent years, the knowledge of TACs' central mechanisms has greatly improved due to new neuroimaging data. Recently, neuroimaging techniques have shown the activation of the ipsilateral, to the painful side, posterior hypothalamus during CCH (41, 45), SUNCT (46), and paroxysmal hemicrania (47) attacks. This activation may be specific in these patients since it is not reported in other painful conditions, such as migraine. Moreover, the pHyp is activated in nitroglycerin-evoked TACs bouts, and is not activated when the subjects were pain-free (41).

The evidence that TACs bouts do not disappear after multiple retrogasserian thermorizotomies supports the central origin of this pain (48, 49). Trigeminal thermorizotomy is the radiofrequency lesion, through the use of heat, of that part of the trigeminal nerve, which is the cause of pain. In 2003, Franzini et al. (6) implanted deep-brain stimulation electrodes in the posterior hypothalamic area of patients suffering from chronic cluster headache. This had been the first time that an anatomical target for placing a stimulating electrode was chosen by functional neuroimaging data (PET), which had shown an hyperactivation of the posterior hypothalamic area during cluster headache pain attacks. The clinical results in the mid- and long-term periods have shown the efficacy of this procedure (48, 50). Subsequently, other authors have confirmed these results in CCH (51–55).

Surgical methodology of posterior hypothalamus DBS

The planning procedure is performed with a Leksell head frame (Eleckta) with the patient under local or general anaesthesia, depending on the pre-operative conditions.

Pre-operative volumetric magnetic resonance (MR) images (with Gadolinium and T2-weighted sets) are obtained for precisely defining the location of anterior and posterior commissures (AC, PC) and midbrain structures below the commissural plane (mammillary bodies and red nucleus). MR images are then merged with computer tomography (CT) scans obtained under stereotactic conditions immediately after positioning the head frame. The merged images are then co-registered to obtain AC, PC, and mid-commissural point (MCP)-related coordinates in the value of millimetres.

The pHyp coordinates (with reference to the MCP) are the following: 2 mm lateral, 3 mm posterior, and 5 mm inferior to the commissural plane. Micro-recording is first performed at the target with detection of single-neurone activity. Several reports about intrinsic pHyp spontaneous activity exist, discharge frequency being detected at values ranging from 13 to 24 Hz (34); in trigeminal autonomic cephalalgias, these recordings revealed tonic, low-frequency, and non-oscillatory patterns of discharge (56).

After the stereotactic procedure, bilateral (Soletra, Medtronic, Inc.) or dual-channel unilateral (Kinetra, Medtronic, Inc.) internal pulse generators (IPGs) are positioned into sub-clavicular sub-cutaneous pockets and connected to the electrodes. Post-operative CT is routinely performed to evaluate the position of the electrodes and the absence of surgical complications. We adopted a new anatomical landmark that was named interpeduncular point (IPP), to address the issue of a possible positioning error when only relying on MCP as a reference system. IPP is localized at the apex of the interpeduncular cistern 8 mm below the AC–PC plane at the level of the maximum diameter of the mammillary bodies (Fig. 12.1). The resulting 'corrected' target coordinates are 2 mm lateral to the mid-line,

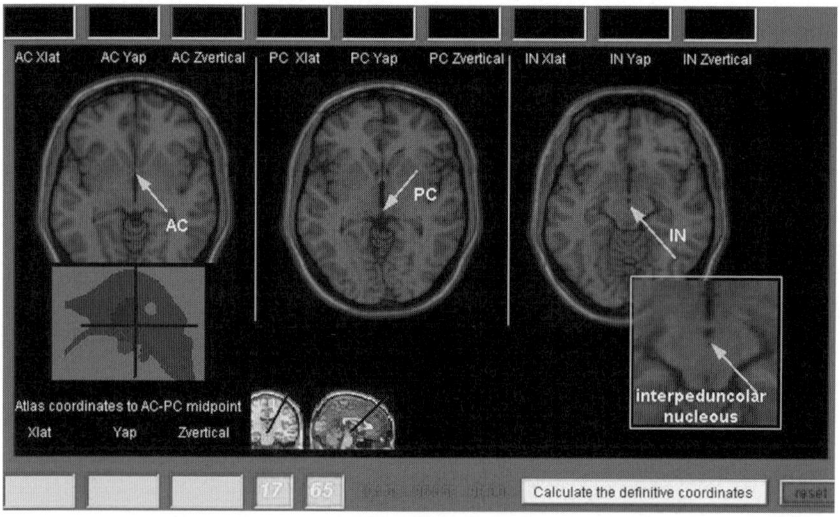

Fig. 12.1 Front page of the software used to calculate the stereotactic coordinates of the target (X;Y;Z). The software has been developed at the Department of Neurosurgery of the Fondazione IRCCS Istituto Neurologico 'C. Besta' in Milan. Axial slices showing the anterior commissure (AC), posterior commissure (PC), and the interpeduncular nucleus (IN).

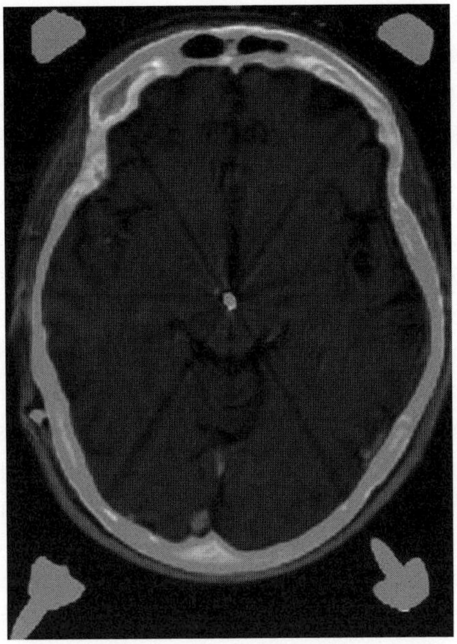

Fig. 12.2 Post-operative neuroimage with computerized tomographic and magnetic resonance images showing the localization of deep brain electrode's tip at the inferior portion of the posterior hypothalamic area.

2 mm posterior to the IPP (instead of 3 mm posterior to the MCP), and 5 mm below the AC–PC plane (Fig. 12.2).

Long-term results of posterior hypothalamic stimulation in chronic cluster headache patients

Since 2001 at our Institute, 19 patients were submitted to DBS for chronic cluster headache refractory to conservative therapies. Long-term follow-up (6–12 years) is available only for 17 of them because one patient died of septic shock, unrelated to DBS, 29 months after surgery (at such follow-up time, he was anyway free of pain) and one patient had been followed for only 2 years (decrease of pain bouts had been observed in this case: from 16/day to about 4/day). Of 17 patients, 12 (70%) presented stable improvement: 6 of these patients are pain-free, whereas the remaining 6 do not present with daily attacks any more, though episodic bouts (with long remission periods) still occur. It is noteworthy that 5 of these latter patients had the pulse generators turned off for a median of 3 years. Of 17 patients, 5 did not present any improvement after DBS (57).

Conclusions

The posterior hypothalamus, which lies dorsal to mammillary bodies, has been implicated in the pathogenesis of chronic cluster headache following structural and functional (5) data in patients suffering from this disease. The concept of the involvement of this anatomical region in such pathology has been reinforced by the observation of an increased blood flow in the insular lobe, frontal lobe, and anterior cingulate cortex following pHyp stimulation; these structures are thought to play an important role in the maintenance and development of chronicity of pain (58), maybe through synaptic long-term potentiation mechanisms involving glutamate receptors. Although chronicity and drug-refractoriness of some CCH patients could be explained by such processes, it is still not clear the reason why some patients are responders to pHyp DBS and some are not; no predictive clinical and neuroimaging factors exist up to now.

It is noteworthy that the implementation of occipital nerve stimulation (ONS) as first-line treatment for CCH patients (because of its less invasive nature and lower rate of surgical-related risks) has in part limited surgical indications to pHyp DBS; at our Institution this procedure is, in fact, reserved for CCH patients who do not respond to ONS (about 40% of CCH patients treated by ONS). The use of occipital nerve stimulation for the treatment of this pathology is justified by the existence of the trigemino-cervical complex (59), a nuclear structure comprising trigeminal nucleus caudalis and grey matter extending to the C2 spinal segment. Functional and anatomical correlations between pHyp and trigemino-cervical complex have not been elucidated yet, so it is difficult to draw any conclusion about the anatomic substrates that could potentially indicate a shared guideline on which patients could benefit from either procedure.

Advances in correlations between functional neuroimaging studies and clinical outcomes in CCH patients will shed some light onto the physiopathological phenomena that underlie these discrepancies, thus leading us to more specific and clinically oriented procedures.

References

1 **Greenstein B, Greenstein A**. Color Atlas of Neuroscience, Neuroanatomy and Neurophysiology. Thieme Stuttgart: New York; 2000.

2 **Iversen S, Kupfermann I, Kandel ER**. Emotional states and feelings. In: Kandel ER, Schwartz JH, Jessell TM (eds), Principles of Neural Science (4th edn). McGraw-Hill: New York; 2000.

3 **Abrahamson EE, Moore RY**. The posterior hypothalamic area: chemoarchitecture and afferent connections. Brain Res 2001; **889**:1–22.

4 **Kirk IJ, Oddie SD, Konopacki J, Bland BH**. Evidence for differential control of posterior hypothalamic, supramammillary, and medial mammillary theta-related cellular discharge by ascending and descending pathways. J Neurosci 1996;**16**:5547–54.

5 **May A, Bahra A, Buchel C, Frackowiak KJ, Goadsby P**. Hypothalamic activation in cluster headache attacks. Lancet 1998;**352**:275–78.

6 **Franzini A, Ferroli P, Leone M, Broggi G**. Stimulation of the posterior hypothalamus for treatment of chronic intractable cluster headaches: first reported series. Neurosurgery 2003;**52**(5):1095–101.

7 **Cavdar S, Onat F, Aker R, Sehirli U, San T, Yananli HR**. The afferent connections of the posterior hypothalamic nucleus in the rat using horseradish peroxidase. J Anat 2001;**198**:463–72.

8 **Swaab DF**. The Human Hypothalamus: Basic and Clinical Aspects. Elsevier: Amsterdam; 2003.

9 **Vertes RP, Crane AM**. Descending projections of the posterior nucleus of the hypothalamus: Phaseolus vulgaris leucoagglutinin analysis in the rat. J Comp Neurol 1996;**374**(4):607–31.

10 **Lin JS, Sakay K, Vanni-Mercier G, Jouvet M**. A critical role of the posterior hypothalamus in the mechanisms of wakefulness determined by microinjection of muscimol in freely moving cats. Brain Res 1989;**479**:225–40.

11 **Sallanon M, Denoyer M, Kitahama K, Aubert C, Gay N, Jouvet M.** Long-lasting insomnia induced by preoptic neuron lesions and its transient reversal by muscimol injection into the posterior hypothalamus in the cat. Neuroscience 1989;**32**:669–83.

12 **Davison C, Demuth EL.** Disturbances in sleep mechanism: a clinicopathalogic study. III. Lesions at the diencephalic level (hypothalamus). Arch Neurol Psychiat 1946;**55**:111–25.

13 **Fulton JF, Bailey P.** Tumors in the region of the third ventricle: their diagnosis and relation to pathological sleep. J Nerv Ment Dis 1929;**69**:1–25.

14 **Nauta WJH.** Hypothalamic regulation of sleep in rats: an experimental study. J Neurophysiol 1946;**9**:285–316.

15 **Ranson SW.** Somnolence caused by hypothalamic lesions in the monkey. Arch Neurol Psychiat 1939;**41**:1–23.

16 **Vanni-Mercier G, Sakai K, Jouvet M.** Specific neurons for wakefulness in the posterior hypothalamus in the ca. CR Acad Sci III-VIE 1984;**III** 298:195–200.

17 **Parè D, Smith Y, Parent A, Steriade M.** Neuronal activity of identified posterior hypothalamic neurons projecting to the brainstem peribrachial area of the cat. Neurosci Lett 1989;**107**:145–50.

18 **Beatty JA, Kramer JM, Plowey ED, Waldrop TG.** Physical exercise decreases neuronal activity in the posterior hypothalamic area of spontaneously hypertensive rats. J Appl Physiol 2005;**98**:572–78.

19 **Karplus JP, Kreidl A.** Gehirn und sympathicus. II. Ein sympathicus-zentrum im zwischenhirn, Pflügers Archiv European. J Physiol 1910;**135**:401–16.

20 **Lammers JH, Kruk MR, Meelis W, van der Poel AM.** Hypothalamic substrates for brain stimulation-induced patterns of locomotion and escape jumps in the rat. Brain Res 1988;**449**:294–310.

21 **Ohta H, Nakamura S, Watanabe S, Ueki S.** Effect of L-glutamate, injected into the posterior hypothalamus, on blood pressure and heart rate in unanesthetized and unrestrained rats. Neuropharmacology 1985;**24**:445–51.

22 **Martin JR.** Mechanisms of the cardiovascular response to posterior hypothalamic nucleus administration of carbachol. J Cardiovasc Pharmacol 1996;**27**:891–900.

23 **Martin JR.** Evidence of systemic neuropeptide Y release after carbachol administration into the posterior hypothalamic nucleus. J Cardiovasc Pharmacol 1996;**28**:447–57.

24 **Martin JR. Beinfeld MC, Westfall TC.** Blood pressure increases after injection of neuropeptide Y into posterior hypothalamic nucleus. Am J Physiol 1988;**254**:H879–88.

25 **Martin JR, Knuepfer MM, Beinfeld MC, Westfall TC.** Mechanism of pressor response to posterior hypothalamic injection of neuropeptide Y. Am J Physiol 1989;**257**:H791–98.

26 **Martin JR, Knuepfer MM, Westfall TC.** Hemodynamic effects of posterior hypothalamic injection of neuropeptide Y in awake rats. Am J Physiol 1991;**261**:H814–24.

27 **DiMicco JA, Abshire VM.** Evidence for GABAergic inhibition of a hypothalamic sympathoexcitatory mechanism in anesthetized rats. Brain Res 1987;**402**:1–10.

28 **Shekhar A, DiMicco JA.** Defense reaction elicited by injection of GABA antagonists and synthesis inhibitors into the posterior hypothalamus in rats. Neuropharmacology 1987;**26**:407–17.

29 **Vertes RP, Kocsis B.** Brainstem-diencephalo-septohippocampal systems controlling the theta rhythm of the hippocampus. Neuroscience 1997;**81**:893–926.

30 **Bland BH, Colom LV, Ford RD.** Responses of septal u-on and u-off cells to activation of the dorsomedial-posterior hypothalamic region. Brain Res Bull 1990;**24**:71–79.

31 **Oddie SD, Bland BH, Colom LV, Vertes RP.** The midline posterior hypothalamic region comprises a critical part of the ascending brainstem hippocampal synchronizing pathway. Hippocampus 1994;**4**:454–73.

32 **Malik A, Strassman AM, Burnstein R**. Trigeminohypothalamic and retinohypothalamic tract neurons in the upper cervical spinal cord and caudal medulla of the rat. J Neurophysiol 2000;**84**(4):2078–112.

33 **Sano K, Mayanagi Y, Sekino H, Ogashiwa M, Ishijima B**. Results of stimulation and destruction of the posterior hypothalamus in man. J Neurosurg 1970;(33):689–707.

34 **Franzini A, Messina G, Cordella R, Marras C, Broggi G**. Deep brain stimulation of the posteromedial hypothalamus: indications, long-term results, and neurophysiological considerations. Neurosurg Focus. 2010 Aug;**29**(2):E13.

35 **Headache Classification Committee of the international headache Society**. The international classification of headache disorders, second edition. Cephalalgia 2004;**24**(Suppl. 1):8–160.

36 **Cohen AS, Matharu MS, Goadsby PJ**. Trigeminal autonomic cephalalgias: current and future treatments. Headache 2007 Jun;**47**(6):969–80.

37 **May A, Leone M**. Update on cluster headache. Curr Opin Neurol 2003;**16**:333–40.

38 **Goadsby PJ**. Pathophysiology of cluster headache: a trigeminal autonomic cephalalgia. Lancet Neurol 2002;**1**:251–57.

39 **Lambert GA, Bogduk N, Goadsby PJ, Duckworth JW, lance JW**. Decreased carotid arterial resistance in cats in response to trigeminal stimulation. J Neurosurg 1984;**61**:307–15.

40 **Goadsby PJ, Lambert GA, Lance JW**. Stimulation of the trigeminal ganglion increases flow in the extracerebral but not the cerebral circulation of the monkey. Brain Res 1986;**381**:63–67.

41 **May A, Kaube H, Büchel C et al**. Experimental cranial pain elicited by capsaicin: a PET study. Pain 1998;**74**(1):61–66.

42 **Pareja JA, Antonaci F, Vincent M**. The hemicrania continua diagnosis. Cephalalgia 2001;**21**:940–46.

43 **Kudrow L**. The cyclic relationship of natural illumination to cluster period frequency. Cephalalgia 1987;**7**(suppl. 6):76–78.

44 **Leone M, Bussone G**. A review of hormonal findings in cluster headache. Evidence for hypothalamic involvement. Cephalalgia 1993;**13**(5):309–17.

45 **Sprenger T, Boecker H, Toelle TR, Bussone G, May A, Leone M**. Specific hypothalamic activation during a spontaneous cluster headache attack. Neurology 2004;**3**(62):516–17.

46 **Sprenger T, Valet M, Platzer S, Pfaffenrath V, Steude U, Tolle TR**. SUNCT: bilateral hypothalamic activation during headache attacks and resolving of symptoms after trigeminal decompression. Pain 2005;**113**(3);422–26.

47 **Matharu MS, Cohen AS, Frackowiak RS, Goadsby PJ**. Posterior hypothalamic activation in paroxysmal hemicrania. Ann Neurol 2006;**59**(3):535–45.

48 **Leone M, Franzini A, Broggi G, May A, Bussane G**. Long-term follow-up of bilateral hypothalamic stimulation for intractable cluster headache. Brain 2004;**127**:2259–64.

49 **Matharu MS, Goadsby P J**. Persistence of attacks of cluster headache after trigeminal nerve root section. Brain 2002;**125**:976–84.

50 **Leone M, Franzini A, Felisati G et al**. Deep brain stimulation and cluster headache. Neurol Sci 2005;**26**(Suppl. 2):s138–39.

51 **Bartsch T, Pinsker MO, Rasche D et al**. Hypothalamic deep brainstimulation for cluster headache: experience from a new multicase series. Cephalalgia 2008 Mar;**28**(3):285–95.

52 **Brittain JS, Green AL, Jenkinson N et al**. Local field potentials reveal a distinctive neural signature of cluster headache in the hypothalamus. Cephalalgia 2009 Nov;**29**(11):1165–73.

53 **Fontaine D, Lazorthes Y, Mertens P et al**. Safety and efficacy of deep brain stimulation in refractory cluster headache: a randomized placebo-controlled double-blind trial followed by a 1-year open extension. J Headache Pain 2010 Feb;**11**(1):23–31.

54 **Schoenen J, Di Clemente L, Vandenheede M et al.** Hypothalamic stimulation in chronic cluster headache: a pilot study of efficacy and mode of action. Brain 2005;**128**(Pt. 4):940–47.

55 **Sillay KA, Sani S, Starr PA.** Deep brain stimulation for medically intractablecluster headache. Neurobiol Dis 2010 Jun;**38**(3):361–68.

56 **Cordella R, Carella F, Leone M et al.** Spontaneous neuronal activity of the posterior hypothalamus in trigeminal autonomic cephalalgias. Neurol Sci 2007;**28**(2):93–95.

57 **Leone M, Franzini A, Proietti Cecchini A, Bussone G.** Success, failure, and putative mechanisms in hypothalamic stimulation for drug-resistant chronic cluster headache. Pain 2013;**154**(1):89–94.

58 **May A, Leone M, Boecker H et al.** Hypothalamic deep brain stimulation in positron emission tomography. J Neurosci 2006;**26**(13):3589–93.

59 **Piovesan EJ, Kowacs PA, Oshinsky ML.** Convergence of cervical and trigeminalsensory afferents. Curr Pain Headache Rep 2003 Oct;**7**(5):377–83.

Chapter 13

The central nervous system in control of continence and sexual functions

Thelma Lovick and Gert Holstege

Key points

1 Micturition, defecation, parturition, and ejaculation may all be considered as voiding activities that show common features.

2 Activation of parallel spinal–midbrain–pontine–spinal loops, involving the periaqueductal grey (PAG), the pontine organ stimulating centre (POSC), and pelvic floor stimulating centre (PFSC) are a basic requirement for voiding.

3 Normally, these reflex pathways are locked in storage mode.

4 Descending influences from higher centres and cross-talk between the pathways ensures that voiding of individual organs takes place only at an appropriate time.

5 Laterality exists within circuitry the pathways controlling different organs.

Introduction

Within the abdominal cavity, four hollow organs can be considered as storage vessels, in the broadest sense. These are the bladder for storage of urine, the rectum for storage of faeces, the uterus to accommodate the growing foetus in females, and the epididymis in males for storage of sperm. Periodically, these vessels expel their contents into the external environment in the form of micturition, defecation, parturition, or ejaculation, respectively. Voiding occurs only when specific sets of physiological conditions and social criteria have been fulfilled. In humans and other highly socialized animals these conditions are met fully only when the individual perceives him/herself to be in a safe and socially appropriate situation. Failure to exert appropriate control of voiding has significant impact on the quality of life.

Each of the storage organs, i.e. bladder, rectum, uterus, and epididymis, is under the control of the sympathetic and parasympathetic branches of the so-called autonomic nervous system, which, fortunately, is not completely autonomous at all. In addition, somatic nerves control the striated muscles of the pelvic floor, including the external urethral and anal sphincters. The spinal cord appears to contain the synaptic machinery to integrate a crude approximation of voiding. However, under normal circumstances, the spinal circuits are critically dependent on descending influences from the brain. The brain uses the physiological switches 'go' or 'don't go', whose status is determined by a combination of factors in the external and internal environments, to control each voiding event.

In this chapter we will review the organization of the neural control of these pelvic voiding organs, focusing on supraspinal control. We will highlight the remarkable parallels (and some differences) between them and also explore interactions between the systems.

Micturition

Bladder afferents and efferents

The innervation and spinal organization of control of the lower urinary tract (LUT) has been the subject of several comprehensive reviews (1, 2) and will, therefore, be considered only briefly.

The LUT comprises the detrusor muscle or urinary bladder, which serves as the reservoir for urine, and the urethra, which is the outlet via which urine is expelled into the external environment. As urine drains into the bladder from the ureters, the smooth muscle wall relaxes to accommodate the increasing volume. At the same time, increased afferent activity in the pelvic and hypogastric nerves reflexively induces tonic contraction of the smooth muscles of the internal urethral sphincter. This sympathetically mediated 'guarding reflex' ensures that continence is maintained during filling. When bladder volume and bladder wall tension reach a certain level, the guarding reflex is subsumed by the requirement to void. The act of micturition involves contraction of the detrusor and relaxation of the external urethral sphincter, and is mediated by sacral autonomic and somatic nerves. Microstimulation of inhibitory inter-neurones in the dorsal grey commissure at S1 resulted in a phasic inhibition of external urethral sphincter activity (3).

Spinal–midbrain–spinal loop

The integrated response is critically dependent on activation of a spinal–midbrain–spinal cord loop. Mechano-sensitive Aδ afferents, which signal stretch and pressure, travel mainly through the hypogastric and pelvic nerves to terminate in Gert's nucleus, a group of neurones in the lateral funiculus of the upper sacral cord, just lateral to the dorsal horn, which in turn projects rostrally to terminate bilaterally in the central part of the periaqueductal grey (PAG) (2, 4, 5) (Fig. 13.1, left).

Pathophysiological states, such as bladder over-distension or infection, are detected by nociceptive C-fibre afferents, which terminate on inter-neurones in an area in or near the dorsal commissure, extending laterally through laminae I and II into lamina V in the

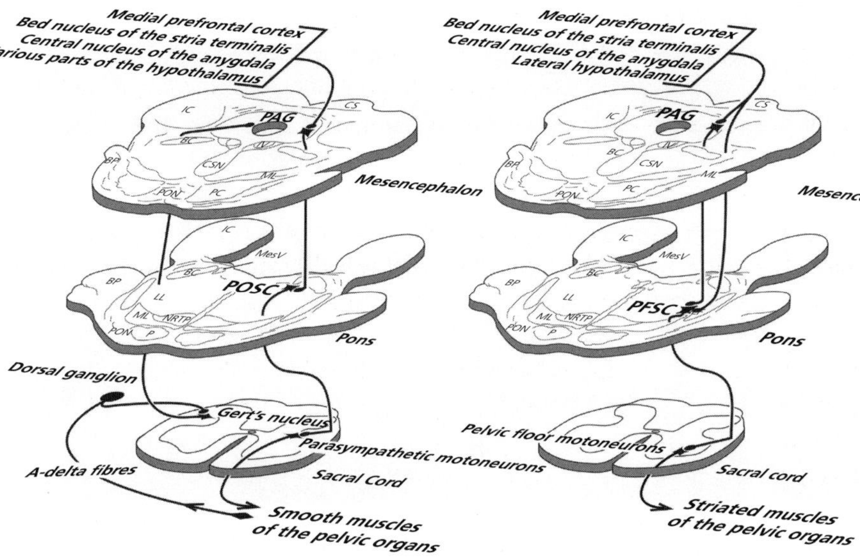

Fig. 13.1 Spinal–midbrain–spinal loop controlling voiding. Left side: afferent input from pelvic organs ascends to the PAG, which in turn activates descending projections to the pelvic organ stimulating centre (POSC) that controls muscles of voiding. Right side: a separate nucleus the pelvic floor stimulating centre (PFSC) controls the muscles of the pelvic floor.

lateral edge of the dorsal horn. Axons from these inter-neurones ascend in the contralateral spinothalamic tract to terminate in the dorsomedial, lateral, and ventrolateral PAG, as well as in the mediodorsal thalamic nucleus and lateral ventral posterolateral thalamic nuclei.

The functional integrity of the PAG is essential for voiding to take place. Lesions, or functional inactivation of this region, lead to urinary retention in humans and animals (6, 7). Successful micturition is accompanied by a decrease in extracellular GABA in the PAG, which presumably reflects a lifting of inhibitory tone on transmission through the region (8).

Neurones in the lateral, ventrolateral, and, to a lesser extent, dorsomedial PAG send dense projections to the dorsal tegmentum of the pons to a region previously known as the pontine micturition centre, M-region, or Barrington's nucleus (9, 10, 11). More recently, this region has been renamed the pelvic organ stimulating centre (POSC), to more accurately reflect its involvement in pelvic voiding activities in general, not just micturition (2, 12). Chemical and electrical stimulation of the POSC engages three groups of spinal neurones to produce, respectively, contraction of the bladder (13), and relaxation of the internal (14) and external urethral sphincters (15, 16) (Fig. 13.1, left). PET-scan studies in men and women (Fig. 13.2, top left) also showed that this cell group appeared to be activated during micturition, but interestingly only on the right side of the brain (17, 18). A similar right-sided activation in this region has been reported during micturition in rats (19). Beckel

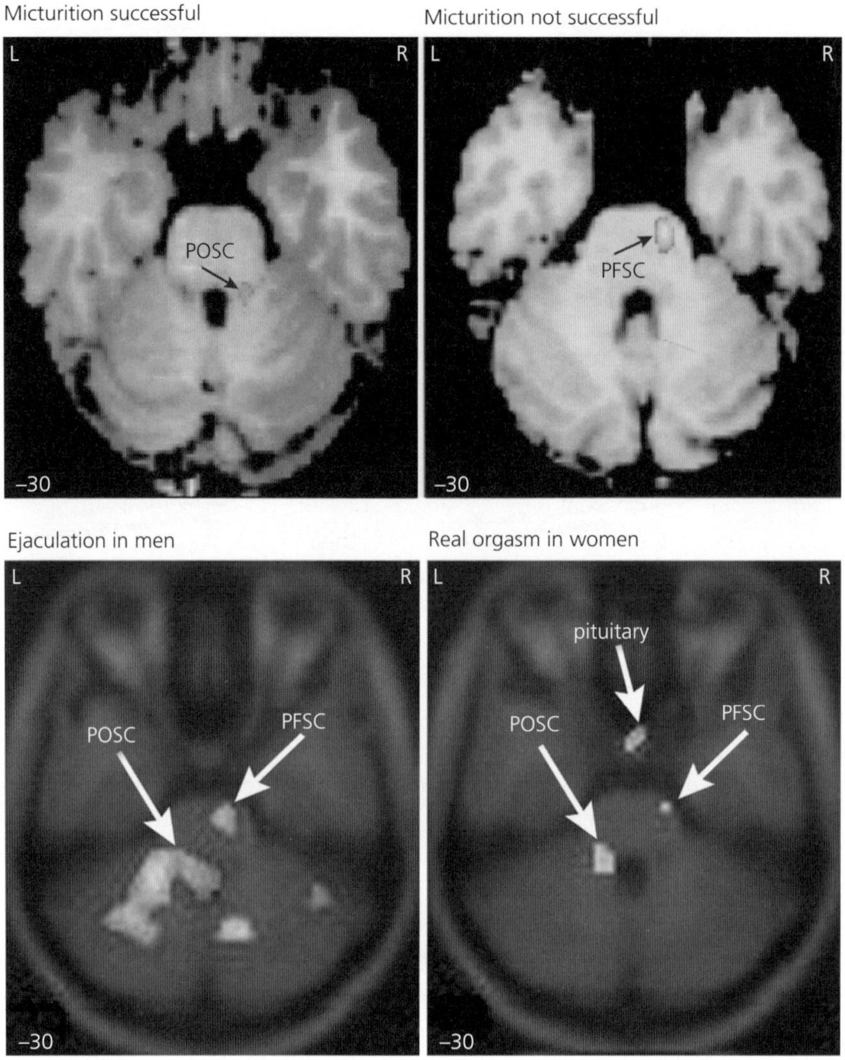

Fig. 13.2 Top: PET-scans in women show activation of the pelvic organ stimulating centre (POSC) on the right side during successful micturition but activation of the pelvic floor stimulating centre (PFSC) in the 50% of subjects who were not able to 'let go' and micturate. Bottom: ejaculation in men the POSC adjoining regions in the cerebellum was activated on the left side, whilst the PFSC was activated on the right side. A similar but less intense activation was seen during orgasm in women. Note in women, but not in men, the pituitary was activated too.

and Holstege (2) have suggested that the POSC contains the neural 'switch' that turns on different forms of voiding, whilst the PAG can be considered the hand that 'throws' the switch in the POSC.

Forebrain control—role of the emotional motor system

In humans and many socialized animals, micturition can be deferred, even when the bladder is full, until the individual finds himself or herself in a safe and socially acceptable environment, such as a bathroom or litter tray. Afferent input to the PAG from spinal levels is transmitted to higher centres of the brain involved in emotion and decision-making, such as the medial orbitofrontal cortex, hypothalamus, amygdala, and bed nucleus of the stria terminalis. In humans, the anterior portion of the anterior cingulate gyrus becomes active during voiding, whilst a smaller more posterior portion is activated during filling (5). The medial prefrontal cortex is recognized for its involvement in decision-making in a social context, based on the social situation (20). In all likelihood, it is in the prefrontal cortex that the decisions to 'go' or 'not go' are made. In rats and primates, the prefrontal cortex sends a dense projection to the ventrolateral PAG (Fig. 13.1, left) (21, 22). If connections between the medial orbitofrontal cortex to the PAG are interrupted, the message: 'no micturition now' no longer arrives in the PAG. In this case, the message from Gert's nucleus that bladder pressure is increasing is sufficient for the PAG to activate the POSC to initiate a void. In all likelihood, the reason that over-active bladder (OAB) or urge-incontinence ('a sudden compelling desire to pass urine that is difficult to defer' (23)) is such a frequent disease in the elderly is the multitude of small lesions in their brains interrupting the pathways from the medial prefrontal cortex to the PAG (24, 25).

Defecation

Rectal afferents and efferents

The distal colon and rectum act as the storage organs for the alimentary tract. Unlike the bladder, which fills continuously with urine draining from the ureters, the waste products of digestion are propelled only periodically into the rectum (26). The distension of the rectum by faecal matter stimulates mechano-sensitive afferent A∂ fibre input to the sacral cord, which, under appropriate conditions, i.e. when the individual is in a safe and socially acceptable environment, triggers defecation. Co-ordinated activity of smooth and striated muscles of the rectum and anal sphincters, reinforced by contraction of the abdominal wall, culminates in expulsion of the rectal contents. Contraction of the abdominal muscles and the diaphragm, by means of a Valsalva manoeuvre, assists with defecation to a variable extent by increasing the intrapelvic (and hence rectal) pressure (26–28).

In rats, motoneurones innervating the external anal sphincter (EAS) are located at L6 in a distinct dorsomedial nucleus, while those innervating the external urethral sphincter (EUS) are located in a separate ventrolateral cell group (29). Tonic activity in the sphincter maintains continence between voids. Interestingly, the basal frequency of the spinal oscillator driving the EAS during inter-voiding periods is only half that of the EUS (30). The difference in basal frequency may reflect the different electrophysiological properties and fibre-type profiles of these two muscles (26). Microstimulation in the sacral cord can induce relaxation of the EAS (31), presumably by activating inhibitory inter-neurones similar to those that inhibit contraction of the EUS during micturition (3).

Spinal–midbrain–spinal loop

Compared to micturition, considerably less is known about the supraspinal integration of defecation. However, as this field of research develops, striking similarities between the control systems of these two voiding activities are beginning to emerge, as well as evidence for interactions between the systems that control micturition, ejaculation, and parturition.

Normal defecation in humans is impossible or at best severely compromised after spinal cord transection above sacral levels. Studies in rats have revealed that, as for micturition, neurones in the PAG and POSC are involved in defecation. The PAG is activated by non-noxious distal colonic distension (32). Electrical stimulation in the PAG and wider midbrain area can disrupt both defecation and micturition (33), presumably by disrupting the patterning of activity in the circuitry that initiates voiding. In the POSC, which receives afferent input from the PAG, at least three neuronal populations have been identified in the rat: those that were linked, respectively, to control of either bladder or distal bowel (34), and another population responsive to distension of both bladder and distal colon (35). The latter suggests that a degree of interaction between these voiding activities may occur at pontine levels. Interestingly, the stomach, another hollow storage organ but one not associated with voiding under physiological conditions, showed little representation in the POSC (35). This highlights the specificity of the POSC in the control of voiding functions. It is worth mentioning that in the rat, unlike the cat (36) and probably humans, the POSC receives direct spinal inputs, which could potentially short-circuit the spinal–PAG–POSC connection. However, the fact remains that even in the rat, the functional integrity of the PAG is essential for micturition and, by analogy, for defecation too (Fig. 13.1 left).

Forebrain control—role of the emotional motor system

At present there is very little information from human or animal studies relating to forebrain involvement in the act of defecation. In humans, fMRI studies have shown that the urge to defecate (rather than the act of defecation itself) in response to rectal distension was associated with activation of the anterior cingulate gyrus and the insula bilaterally. Further activation could be seen bilaterally in the anterior and medial core of the thalamus, as well as in the supplemental motor cortex (Brodmann area 6), together with minor deactivation of the posterior cingulate gyrus (Brodmann area 23/31) and in the prefrontal region (Brodmann area 9/10) (37).

Ejaculation

Our current understanding of the neurophysiological and neuroanatomical organization of ejaculation has been derived mainly from studies on rat models. The epididymis, an elongated organ on the posterior surface of the testis, forms the convoluted end of the vas deferens and stores sperm as they mature. Unlike other voiding events, ejaculation is not initiated in response to sensory information signalling distension of the hollow viscus where the sperm is stored but rather, from penile afferents relaying information to the central nervous system primarily via the dorsal penile nerve (38). Ejaculation consists of an emission phase when sperm is 'matured' and an expulsion phase in which seminal fluid containing sperm is ejected rapidly via the urethra. The process is mediated via the synchronized activity of the sympathetic, parasympathetic, and somatic nerves (39).

During the emission phase, contractions of the seminal vesicles, prostate, and vas deferens facilitate transfer of their respective contents into the prostatic urethra to mix with sperm to form the seminal fluid. At the same time, the bladder neck contracts to prevent the backflow of sperm into the bladder (39). During the expulsion phase, a sequence of intense sympathetic bursting activity in the vas deferens' nerve (a branch of the hypogastric nerve) induces rhythmic contractions and expulsion of seminal fluid (40). In addition, powerful rhythmic contractions of the striated bulbospongiosus muscle, supplemented by contraction of the ischiocavernosus and urethralis muscles, propel the semen through the urethra (41).

Spinal afferents and efferents

In spinal animals, ejaculation can be evoked by intra-spinal stimulation below the level of transection (40) or in spinally transected men by prolonged intense penile stimulation (42). This implies that the spinal cord contains some kind of spinal generator for ejaculation. A group of inter-neurones located dorsal to the central canal at L3–L4, subsequently identified as spinothalamic tract neurones (43), function as a spinal ejaculation pattern generator. These cells integrate sensory inputs related to the summation of sexual activity prior to ejaculation and coordinate the sympathetic, parasympathetic, and motor outflow to the genitalia. However, despite an intact spinal reflex arc, ejaculation is severely impaired, or in most cases impossible, in men with spinal injuries cranial to T10 (44, 45). Indeed, sexual dysfunction is a major concern for such patients (46). As with micturition and defecation, the involvement of a spinal–midbrain–spinal loop, the excitability of which is regulated by forebrain influences, appears critical for normal function (47, 48).

Spinal–midbrain–spinal loop

Studies using trans-synaptic viral tracing in rats have revealed a pathway from the caudal ventrolateral PAG and the POSC to motoneurons innervating the bulbospongiosus muscle (49). A similar projection to the clitoris and vagina has been identified in females (50). In a recent PET imaging study in humans, ejaculation was associated with activation of a discrete region on the left side in the pontine tegmentum, which appears to correspond to the POSC (Fig. 13.2, bottom left) (12). A similar region on the left side was activated during orgasm in women (Fig. 13.2, bottom right). These findings suggest that the same region of the dorsolateral pontine tegmentum that controls other voiding activities, such as micturition and defecation, is involved in ejaculation as well.

Pelvic floor stimulating centre

Interestingly, during ejaculation and female orgasm in humans, another cell group ventral to the POSC was activated on the right side (Fig. 13.2, bottom) (12). Cells in the equivalent region in cats have direct access to Onuf's nucleus in the sacral cord, which contains the somatic motoneurones of the pudendal nerve (51–54) (Fig. 13.1, right) (55, 56). Electrical stimulation of this cell group evoked contraction of the pelvic floor and increased pressure in the urethra (9). This ventral cell group acts as a pelvic floor stimulating centre (PFSC), which induces contraction of the pelvic floor during ejaculation and orgasm in women. The PFSC was also activated on the right side in humans who were asked to micturate whilst lying in a PET-scanner, but who, for emotional reasons, failed to void and kept their pelvic floor contracted (17, 18) (Fig. 13.2, top right).

Forebrain control—role of the emotional motor system

As with micturition or defecation, a host of psychosocial factors impact on whether sexual activity culminating in ejaculation can take place. Ejaculation is preceded by sexual arousal and is accompanied by the powerful emotional experience termed orgasm. In animals too, ejaculation/orgasm is a highly positively reinforcing experience (57). In humans, ejaculation is associated with de-activation of anxiety related cortical and subcortical regions, to a much greater extent than for other voiding activities, perhaps reflecting the much higher emotional reward compared to micturition or defecation.

It is almost impossible to dissect the physiological (ejaculation) from the emotional (orgasm) components using animal models. However, imaging studies in humans are starting to provide information related to the circuitry that is specifically involved in the ejaculation phase of sexual activity. The first studies of Holstege and co-workers, using PET to image ejaculation, revealed widespread forebrain and mesencephalic activation (58, 59). One technical difficulty associated with that study was the artefact introduced by head movements. More recently, by re-analysing the data on a frame-by-frame basis, in order to remove this source of artefact, Holstege and Huynh (60) showed that the principal event during ejaculation in men and orgasm in women was strong *de-activation* mainly on the left side in extended regions of the parietal, prefrontal, medial orbitofrontal, and temporal cortex. In contrast, activation was confined mainly to the insula in men and the somatomotor and somatosensory cortex in women. This suggests that, much like micturition and defecation, the ejaculation circuitry is also normally locked in 'no go' mode due to inhibitory forebrain influences. Only when the level of afferent stimulation is high enough, and social and safety conditions are right, does a release phenomenon occur, which allows this voiding activity take place.

Parturition

The expulsion of the foetus or parturition is initiated by an increase in secretion of oxytocin by the pituitary gland, under the control of the supraoptic hypothalamic nucleus. In its absence there is significant prolongation of parturition (61). However, during the last stage of parturition, when the pressure in the vagina increases, the crucial foetus-expulsion reflex is initiated.

Spinal afferents and efferents

Increased uterine contractions induced by raised oxytocin levels excite A∂ afferent fibres in the uterine wall. These fibres, together with those of bladder and distal colon, travel via the pelvic nerve to enter the sacral cord, where they terminate in Gert's nucleus (62). This nucleus, in turn, via direct, long, ascending pathways (4), not only informs the PAG about the pressure in bladder and distal colon, but also about the pressure in the cervix. In the case of parturition in rats, the mechanical stimulation of the upper vagina and cervix results in an increase of the intra-abdominal pressure, induced by contractions of the abdominal muscles and the diaphragm, and an inhibition of respiratory movements (63). Notably, after bilateral, but not unilateral, section of the pelvic nerves, no foetus-expulsion reflex takes place (63).

Spinal–midbrain–spinal loop

At present, there is no information available regarding functional activation of supraspinal pathways during parturition. However, by analogy with evacuation of the bladder and bowel, where stretch initiates contraction of the hollow viscus and relaxation of sphincters that normally maintain continence, we propose the following.

A∂ afferents from the uterus activate the PAG, which, via its direct projection to the POSC, reflexively activates those cells that project to the spinal parasympathetic motoneurones innervating the upper part of the uterus in order to increase the inter-uterine pressure. In order to facilitate expulsion of the foetus, other neurones in the POSC initiate relaxation of the cervix, similar to the POSC-evoked inhibition of the internal urethral sphincter during micturition (Fig. 13.1, left). At the same time, the PAG inhibits those neurones in the PFSC that project to the motoneurones in Onuf's nucleus, which innervate the pelvic floor muscles surrounding the vagina (Fig. 13.1, right) to facilitate passage of the foetus through the pelvic floor. To supplement these actions, activation of the descending pathway from the PAG to the nucleus retroambiguus (NRA) may also engage premotor inter-neurones innervating all the muscles involved in increasing thoracic and abdominal pressure, such as the pharynx, larynx, diaphragm, internal intercostal, abdominal muscles, and pelvic floor (Fig. 13.3).

Forebrain control—role of the emotional motor system

Similar to micturition, defecation, and ejaculation, the decision whether or not to excite or inhibit cells in the POSC, PFSC, and NRA not only depends on the incoming information from Gert's nucleus (Fig. 13.1, left), but also from the information from the prefrontal and cingulate cortices, which have strong access to the PAG (21, 22). The prefrontal and cingulate cortices in humans determine whether or not the situation is appropriate for parturition to take place. As in ejaculation, it is quite well possible that neurones in the pre-optic

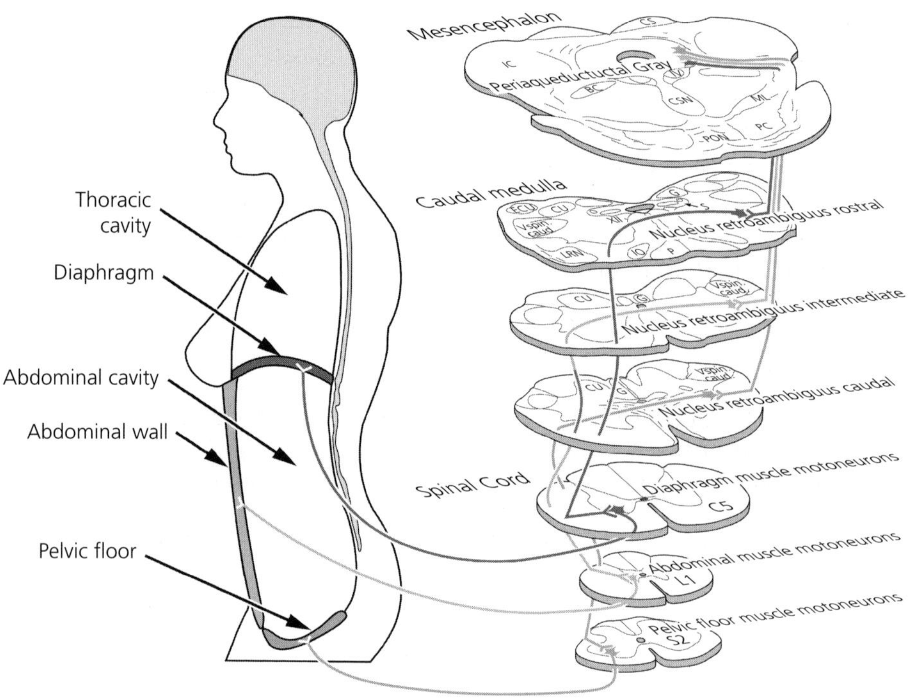

Fig. 13.3 Diagramatic representation of supraspinal control of muscles of the abdominal cavity. (See Plate 4.)

region of the hypothalamus, that have direct access to the POSC (Fig. 13.3) (51), may also play a role in this reflex. However, the extent to which voluntary control can over-ride hormonal influences during parturition is not known.

Conclusions

A common feature in the control of micturition, defecation, parturition, and ejaculation is a basic spinal–midbrain–pontine–spinal loop, involving the PAG, the POSC, and the PFSC. Within this loop, organ-specific cells control different voiding activities. Normally the circuitry is locked in storage mode and in socialized animals, voiding only takes place once a certain set of social conditions has been fulfilled. The complex social mores associated with voiding cannot be modelled readily in animals. However, studies in non-human primates indicate that the orbital and medial prefrontal cortices integrate sensory and motor aspects of visceral functions. Is it safe and socially acceptable for me to void now? (64). The medial network sends dense projections to the PAG (Fig. 13.1, left) (21), which may disinhibit the voiding circuits, enabling the POSC and PFSC to switch from the storage to the voiding mode. The presence of multimodal cells (34) at the level of the PAG and POSC/PFSC suggest that cross-talk between the circuits ensures that only the spinal circuitry controlling the appropriate organ is stimulated.

An interesting finding is the laterality of the brain's involvement in different voiding functions. At forebrain levels, ejaculation was associated with right-sided activation, whilst widespread de-activation was present on the left (60). Although still a contentious issue, there is evidence for laterality in forebrain processing of emotions (65). Arguably, ejaculation is associated with a much higher level of emotional arousal than micturition and defecation. At pontine levels, ejaculation-related activation was left-sided, whilst micturition was represented on the right side (12, 17, 18). These features may be important in diagnostic tools in assessing lesions that result in voiding dysfunction.

References

1 **Fowler CJ, Griffiths D, De Groat WC**. The neural control of micturition. Nature Reviews Neuroscience 2008;**9**:453–66.

2 **Beckel JM, Holstege G**. The lower urinary tract. In: Paxinos G (ed.) The Rat Nervous System. Sydney, Tokyo: Academic Press; 2015;247–63.

3 **Blok BF, Van Maarseveen JT, Holstege G**. Electrical stimulation of the sacral dorsal gray commissure evokes relaxation of the external urethral sphincter in the cat. Neuroscience Letters 1998;**249**:68–70.

4 **Vanderhorst VG, Mouton LJ, Blok BF et al**. Distinct cell groups in the lumbosacral cord of the cat project to different areas in the periaqueductal gray. Journal of Comparative Neurology 1996;**376**:361–85.

5 **Athwal BS, Berkley KJ, Hussain I et al**. Brain responses to changes in bladder volume and urge to void in healthy men. Brain 2001;**124**:369–77.

6 **Yaguchi H, Soma H, Miyazaki Y et al**. A case of acute urinary retention caused by periaqueductal grey lesion. Journal of Neurology, Neurosurgery and Psychiatry 2004;**75**:1202–203.

7 **Stone E, Coote JH, Allard J et al**. GABAergic control of micturition within the periaqueductal grey matter of the male rat. Journal of Physiology 2011;**589**:2065–78.

8 **Kitta T, Matsumoto M, Tanaka H et al**. GABAergic mechanism mediated via D receptors in the rat periaqueductal gray participates in the micturition reflex: an in vivo microdialysis study. European Journal of Neuroscience 2008;**27**:3216–25.

9 **Holstege G, Griffiths D, De Wall H et al**. Anatomical and physiological observations on supraspinal control of bladder and urethral sphincter muscles in the cat. Journal of Comparative Neurology 1986;**250**:449–61.

10 **Blok BF, Holstege G**. The neuronal control of micturition and its relation to the emotional motor system. Progress in Brain Research 1996;**107**:113–26.

11 **Barrington FJF**. The effect of lesions of the hind- and mid-brain on micturition in the cat. Experimental Physiology 1925;**15**:81–102.

12 **Huynh HK, Willemsen A, Lovick TA et al**. Pontine control of ejaculation and female orgasm. Journal of Sexual Medicine 2013;10:3038–48.

13 **Keast JR**. Visualization and immunohistochemical characterization of sympathetic and parasympathetic neurons in the male rat major pelvic ganglion. Neuroscience 1995;**66**:655–62.

14 **Sugaya K, Matsuyama K, Takakusaki K et al**. Electrical and chemical stimulations of the pontine micturition center. Neuroscience Letters 1987;**80**:197–201.

15 **Blok BF, Van Maarseveen JT, Holstege G**. Electrical stimulation of the sacral dorsal gray commissure evokes relaxation of the external urethral sphincter in the cat. Neuroscience Letters 1998;**249**:68–70.

16 **Sie JA, Blok BF, De Weerd H et al.** Ultrastructural evidence for direct projections from the pontine micturition center to glycine-immunoreactive neurons in the sacral dorsal gray commissure in the cat. Journal of Comparative Neurology 2001;**429**:631–37.

17 **Blok BF, Willemsen AT, Holstege G.** A PET study on brain control of micturition in humans. Brain 1997;**120 (Pt 1)**:111–21.

18 **Blok BF, Sturms LM, Holstege G.** Brain activation during micturition in women. Brain 1998;**121 (Pt 11)**:2033–42.

19 **Tai C, Wang J, Jin T et al.** Brain switch for reflex micturition control detected by FMRI in rats. Journal of Neurophysiology 2009;**102**:2719–30.

20 **Adolphs R.** Social cognition and the human brain. Trends in Cognitive Science 1999;**3**:469–79.

21 **An X, Bandler R, Ongur D et al.** Prefrontal cortical projections to longitudinal columns in the midbrain periaqueductal gray in macaque monkeys. Journal of Comparative Neurology 1998;**401**:455–79.

22 **Floyd NS, Price JL, Ferry AT et al.** Orbitomedial prefrontal cortical projections to distinct longitudinal columns of the periaqueductal gray in the rat. Journal of Comparative Neurology 2000;**422**:556–78.

23 **Abrams P, Cardozo L, Fall M et al.** The standardisation of terminology of lower urinary tract function: report from the Standardisation Sub-committee of the International Continence Society. Neurourology and Urodynamics 2002;**21**:167–78.

24 **Perneczky R, Diehl-Schmid J, Forstl H et al.** Urinary incontinence and its functional anatomy in frontotemporal lobar degenerations. European Journal of Nuclear Medicine and Molecular Imaging 2008;**35**:605–10.

25 **Griffiths DJ, Tadic SD, Schaefer W et al.** Cerebral control of the lower urinary tract: how age-related changes might predispose to urge incontinence. Neuroimage 2009:**47**:981–86.

26 **Brookes SJ, Dinning PG, Gladman MA.** Neuroanatomy and physiology of colorectal function and defaecation: from basic science to human clinical studies. Neurogastroenterology and Motility 2009;**21(Suppl. 2)**:9–19.

27 **Bharucha AE.** Pelvic floor: anatomy and function. Neurogastroenterology and Motility 2006;**18**:507–19.

28 **Palit S, Lunniss PJ, Scott SM.** The physiology of human defecation. Digestive Diseases and Sciences 2012;**57**:1445–64.

29 **Schroder HD.** Organization of the motoneurons innervating the pelvic muscles of the male rat. Journal of Comparative Neurology 1980;**192**:567–87.

30 **Buffini M, O'halloran KD, O'herlihy C et al.** Comparison of the motor discharge to the voluntary sphincters of continence in the rat. Neurogastroenterology and Motility 2012;**24**:e175–84.

31 **Tai C, Booth AM, De Groat WC et al.** Colon and anal sphincter contractions evoked by microstimulation of the sacral spinal cord in cats. Brain Research 2001;**889**:38–48.

32 **Mönnikes H, Ruter J, Konig M et al.** Differential induction of c-fos expression in brain nuclei by noxious and non-noxious colonic distension: role of afferent C-fibers and 5-HT3 receptors. Brain Research 2003;**966**:253–64.

33 **Fukuda H, Koga T.** Midbrain stimulation inhibits the micturition, defecation and rhythmic straining reflexes elicited by activation of sacral vesical and rectal afferents in the dog. Experimental Brain Research 1991;**83**:303–16.

34 **Rouzade-Dominguez ML, Pernar L, Beck S et al.** Convergent responses of Barrington's nucleus neurons to pelvic visceral stimuli in the rat: a juxtacellular labelling study. European Journal of Neuroscience 2003;**18**:3325–34.

35 **Rouzade-Dominguez ML, Miselis R, Valentino RJ.** Central representation of bladder and colon revealed by dual transsynaptic tracing in the rat: substrates for pelvic visceral coordination. European Journal of Neuroscience 2003;**18**:3311–24.

36 **Blok BF, De Weerd H, Holstege G.** Ultrastructural evidence for a paucity of projections from the lumbosacral cord to the pontine micturition center or M-region in the cat: a new concept for the organization of the micturition reflex with the periaqueductal gray as central relay. Journal of Comparative Neurology 1995;**359**:300–09.

37 **Bittorf B, Ringler R, Forster C et al.** Cerebral representation of the anorectum using functional magnetic resonance imaging. British Journal of Surgery 2006;**93**:1251–57.

38 **Giuliano F.** Neurophysiology of erection and ejaculation. Journal of Sexual Medicine 2011;**8(Suppl. 4)**:310–15.

39 **Giuliano F, Clement P.** Neuroanatomy and physiology of ejaculation. Annual Review of Sex Research 2005;**16**:190–216.

40 **Stafford SA, Tang K, Coote JH.** Sympathetic genital responses induced by p-chloroamphetamine in anaesthetized female rats. Neuroscience 2006;**138**:725–32.

41 **Carro-Juarez M, Rodriguez-Manzo G.** The spinal pattern generator for ejaculation. Brain Research Reviews 2008;**58**:106–20.

42 **Sonksen J, Biering-Sorensen F, Kristensen JK.** Ejaculation induced by penile vibratory stimulation in men with spinal cord injuries. The importance of the vibratory amplitude. Paraplegia 1994;**32**:651–60.

43 **Truitt WA, Coolen LM.** Identification of a potential ejaculation generator in the spinal cord. Science 2002;**297**:1566–69.

44 **Sachs BD, Bitran D.** Spinal block reveals roles for brain and spinal cord in the mediation of reflexive penile erections in rats. Brain Research 1990;**528**:99–108.

45 **Seftel AD, Oates RD, Krane RJ.** Disturbed sexual function in patients with spinal cord disease. Neurologic Clinics 1991;**9**:757–78.

46 **Anderson KD.** Targeting recovery: priorities of the spinal cord-injured population. Journal of Neurotrauma 2004;**21**:1371–83.

47 **Kaplan JM, Hao JX, Sodersten P.** Apomorphine induces ejaculation in chronic decerebrate rats. Neuroscience Letters 1991;**129**:205–08.

48 **Marson L.** Lesions of the periaqueductal gray block the medial preoptic area-induced activation of the urethrogenital reflex in male rats. Neuroscience Letters 2004;**367**:278–82.

49 **Tang Y, Rampin O, Giuliano F et al.** Spinal and brain circuits to motoneurons of the bulbospongiosus muscle: retrograde transneuronal tracing with rabies virus. Journal of Comparative Neurology 1999;**414**:167–92.

50 **Marson L, Murphy AZ.** Identification of neural circuits involved in female genital responses in the rat: a dual virus and anterograde tracing study. American Journal of Physiology, Regulatory Integrative and Comparative Physiology 2006;**291**:R419–28.

51 **Holstege G.** Some anatomical observations on the projections from the hypothalamus to brainstem and spinal cord: an HRP and autoradiographic tracing study in the cat. Journal of Comparative Neurology 1987;**260**:98–126.

52 **Holstege G, Kerstens L, Moes MC et al.** Evidence for a periaqueductal gray-nucleus retroambiguus-spinal cord pathway in the rat. Neuroscience 1997;**80**:587–98.

53 **Pullen AH.** Quantitative synaptology of feline motoneurones to external anal sphincter muscle. Journal of Comparative Neurology 1988;**269**:414–24.

54 **Sato M, Mizuno N, Konishi A.** Localization of motoneurons innervating perineal muscles: a HRP study in cat. Brain Research 1978;**140**:149–54.

55 **Holstege G, Kuypers HG, Boer RC.** Anatomical evidence for direct brain stem projections to the somatic motoneuronal cell groups and autonomic preganglionic cell groups in cat spinal cord. Brain Research 1979;**171**:329–33.

56 **Holstege G, Kuypers HG.** The anatomy of brain stem pathways to the spinal cord in cat. A labeled amino acid tracing study. Progress in Brain Research 1982;**57**:145–75.

57 **Pfaus JG, Kippin TE, Centeno S.** Conditioning and sexual behavior: a review. Hormones and Behavior 2001;**40**:291–321.

58 **Holstege G, Georgiadis JR, Paans AM et al.** Brain activation during human male ejaculation. Journal of Neuroscience 2003;**23**:9185–93.

59 **Georgiadis JR, Kortekaas R, Kuipers R et al.** Regional cerebral blood flow changes associated with clitorally induced orgasm in healthy women. European Journal of Neuroscience 2006;**24**:3305–16.

60 **Holstege G, Huynh HK.** Brain circuits for mating behavior in cats and brain activations and de-activations during sexual stimulation and ejaculation and orgasm in humans. Hormones and Behavior 2011;**59**:702–07.

61 **Luckman SM, Antonijevic I, Leng G et al.** The maintenance of normal parturition in the rat requires neurohypophysial oxytocin. Journal of Neuroendocrinology 1993;**5**:7–12.

62 **Kawatani M, Takeshige C, De Groat WC.** Central distribution of afferent pathways from the uterus of the cat. Journal of Comparative Neurology 1990;**302**:294–304.

63 **Higuchi T, Uchide K, Honda K et al.** Pelvic neurectomy abolishes the fetus-expulsion reflex and induces dystocia in the rat. Experimental Neurology 1987;**96**:443–55.

64 **Price JL.** Prefrontal cortical networks related to visceral function and mood. Annals of the New York Academy of Sciences 1999;**877**:383–96.

65 **Miller GA, Crocker LD, Spielberg JM et al.** Issues in localization of brain function: The case of lateralized frontal cortex in cognition, emotion, and psychopathology. Frontres in Integrative Neuroscience 2013;**7**:2.

Chapter 14

Pudendal nerve stimulation

Philip E. V. Van Kerrebroeck and Martijn A. C. Smits

Key points

1 The pudendal nerve is a major contributor to bladder afferent regulation.
2 Pudendal nerve can be accessed at the ischial spine by a posterior approach.
3 Electrical stimulation of the pudendal nerve is possible with a percutaneously placed tined lead electrode.
4 Neuromodulation of the lower urinary tract is possible with electrical stimulation of the pudendal nerve.
5 Neuromodulation of the lower urinary tract by electrical stimulation of the pudendal nerve can produce better results than sacral nerve stimulation.

Introduction

Sacral neurostimulation (SNS) is a minimally invasive treatment option for symptoms of over-active bladder (OAB) when non-invasive therapies, such as behavioural modification, pelvic floor rehabilitation, and pharmacological therapy, have failed. The efficacy of SNS in patients with idiopathic OAB has been shown in clinical trials, with a reported long-term success rate of approximately 70% (1, 2) and a 5-year patient satisfaction of up to 90% (3). The largest systematic review evaluating SNS for neurogenic lower urinary tract dysfunction calculated an overall success rate of 68% (4). It follows from these data that in spite of its potential, SNS still offers no solution to the problems of a considerable number of patients with symptoms of (neurogenic) over-active bladder.

Sacral neuromodulation consists of implantation of a tined electrode in the S3 sacral foramen with subsequent connection to an implantable pulse generator. The working mechanism of SNS is unclear, but it is indicated that electrical stimulation of the S3 sacral nerve root leads to modulation of the afferent signals and micturition reflex pathways in the central nervous system (5). One limitation of the selection of S3 is that only one of the pathways inducing the inhibitory reflex is stimulated.

The pudendal nerve originates from S2, S3, and S4 sacral nerve roots. Therefore, selection of the pudendal nerve, as a site for stimulation, provides afferent stimulation of S2, S3, and S4 nerve roots. Since more afferents are stimulated with direct PNS than with SNS, chronic pudendal nerve stimulation may be an alternative option in patients in whom SNS fails (6).

The pudendal nerve

The pudendal nerve (PN) is a peripheral nerve, and consists mainly of afferent sensory fibres from sacral nerve roots S1, S2, and S3. Human cadaveric studies have shown that 50% of the pudendal nerves contain nerve fibres originating from the roots S2, S3, and S4, 40% only from S2 and S3, and 10% from S3 and S4 only (7). Consequently, the PN is a major contributor to bladder afferent regulation and hence bladder function. Pudendal nerve entrapment often leads to significant voiding dysfunction, including urinary incontinence and detrusor over-activity (8–10).

Anatomy of the pudendal nerve

The PN originates in the sacral plexus and derives its fibres from the ventral rami of second, third, and fourth sacral nerves (S2, S3, and S4). The nerve also gets contributions from the adjacent roots of S1 and S5 (7). The pudendal nerve roots emerge from the anterior sacral foramina containing both somatic and autonomic fibres. The PN, together with the internal pudendal artery, exits the pelvis through the greater sciatic foramen, travelling anterior to the piriformis muscle and posterior to the coccygeal muscle and the sacrospinous ligament. At this point the PN winds posteriorly around the ischial spine, medial to the pudendal vessels and deep to the sacrotuberous ligament in the biligamentary tunnel. It swings anteriorly through the lesser sciatic foramen and the Alcock's canal to enter the perineum. Here the PN terminally branches into the dorsal genital nerve, the inferior rectal nerve, and the perineal nerve (7, 11). The dorsal genital nerve eventually runs through the suspensory ligament to the dorsum of the penis or clitoris. The inferior rectal nerve extends motor branches to the levator ani muscle and the external anal sphincter, and sensory branches to the perianal region and the scrotum. Alongside these branches to the scrotum runs the scrotal branch of the perineal nerve into the common scrotal branch, which enervates the scrotal skin. The other branches of the perineal nerve, the bulbocavernosus branch and the medial urethral sphincter branch, runs down to the striated urethral sphincter (11, 12).

Pudendal nerve stimulation

Stimulation of nerve fibres can be achieved by implanting an electrode close to the nerve. The initial nerve localization and implanting techniques used were initially complex and have recently been replaced by minimally invasive, percutaneous approaches. The percutaneous procedures can be performed with use of the quadripolar tined lead that is also used for SNS, connected to an implantable pulse generator. Using the combination of this tined lead and an implantable pulse generator gives the opportunity for a staged implant procedure. During the first stage the lead is implanted adjacent to the PN and connected to an external stimulator. When during the testing period the stimulation is successful, the second stage consists of implanting an implantable pulse generator.

An alternative to this 'electrode' system is a lead-less mini-neurostimulator with integrated electrodes, which can be implanted at its target location (Alcock's canal) (6).

Surgical access to the pudendal nerve

The anatomy of the PN and its branches enables the implantation of an electrode at several sites. At the ischial spine, the PN is a relatively isolated structure and stimulation at this site theoretically diminishes the risk of unwanted activation of S2 motor fibres to the sciatic nerve (13). The PN can be accessed percutaneous for stimulation at the ischial spine by a posterior or perineal approach for insertion of the electrode. With the perineal approach, the PN can also be reached at the Alcock's canal (14).

When implanting an electrode by the posterior approach at the ischial spine, the ischial spine can be located by palpating the lower margin of the sacrotuberous ligament where it forms an angle with the ischial tuberosity (14–16). The electrode can also be inserted perpendicular at the intersection of a horizontal line from the greater trochanter and a vertical line from the ischial tuberosity tip (using fluoroscopy) (13, 14).

The perineal approach is performed by insertion of the electrode perpendicularly to the perineum between the ischial tuberosity and the anus. A finger is placed into the rectum or the vagina to prevent puncturing the bowel or vagina and then used to guide the needle to the ischial spine or Alcock's canal (6, 17, 18).

EMG recordings for ensuring correct electrode placement

Since the outcome of PNS depends on the proximity of the electrode to the nerve (19), it has been suggested that at the time of the development of the percutaneous placement techniques, that placement of the electrode needs electrophysiological confirmation. Anal sphincter electromyography (EMG) and measurement of amplitude and latency during acute stimulation have been used (17). In practice, the positioning of the electrode based on EMG recordings appears to be difficult. A recent study combining clinical results with cadaver studies has shown that the electrode can also be positioned satisfactorily without EMG confirmation. The authors conclude that lead placement can be based on evidence of visible and palpable sphincter contraction (13).

Dorsal genital nerve stimulation

As an alternative method to direct stimulation of the PN, stimulation of nerve branches originating from the PN can be used. For this purpose, the dorsal genital nerve (DGN) has been used as a peripheral stimulation site of the PN. The DGN can be accessed either using surface electrodes, as part of the DGN is localized superficially to the skin outside the pelvis, or with an electrode inserted more proximal along the tract of the DGN. In addition to using sensory function of the nerve to locate the stimulus in the glans penis or the clitoris, electrodes can be positioned near the DGN using the genito-anal reflex (20).

Mechanism of action

Stimulation of the PN is different from SNS, as it provides afferent stimulation not only of the S3 sacral nerve root, but also of the S2 and S4 roots. Both forms of stimulation, however, seem to rely on the same neurophysiological mechanisms. The working mechanism of stimulation of sacral nerve roots is not fully understood. In over-active bladder, neurostimulation is supposed to act by inhibiting bladder afferent activity through its action on somatic afferent pathways, and hence blocking abnormal sensory input to spinal cord and brain. Neurostimulation may also block inter-neurone transmission of bladder sensory input and can directly inhibit bladder preganglionic neurones of bladder efferent pathways as well (5, 21).

Experimental studies

The modulatory effects of pudendal nerve stimulation have been studied in normal and spinal animals, and important aspects of the spinal mechanism of action have been identified. These mechanisms rely on spinal interaction between somatic afferent fibres of the pudendal nerve and autonomic pathways controlling the bladder and bladder neck (22–26). Projection of pudendal pathways into spinal sympathetic and sacral parasympathetic systems has been found in several animal experiments, but also in humans (27–29).

Clinical results

The number of published studies and the experience with PNS are limited compared to SNS. In a single blinded crossover trial, 30 patients randomly received a test with SNS and PNS (both tined quadripolar lead) by the perineal approach for OAB and urinary retention (10%). The overall reduction in symptoms was 63% for PNS and 46% for SNS. PNS was chosen as a superior lead in 79.2% of patients (16). Another study evaluating the success of PNS with a percutaneous nerve evaluation test included 14 female patients with idiopathic OAB. Six patients (42%) responded positively (>50% improvement urodynamic parameters) and received permanent PNS with a leadless mini-neurostimulator (6). One of the first relevant clinical studies on the effect of PNS with use of intermittent (weekly) needle stimulation, was performed in a heterogeneous group of patients with idiopathic and neurogenic detrusor over-activity (n = 29). These authors succeeded to show a significant increase in functional bladder capacity in all patients and a 30% decrease of frequency in 11 patients (18). There is only one other study that has evaluated the effect of PNS in patients with neurogenic OAB. In this study test stimulation has been performed with a tined quadripolar lead in 15 patients. Eight patients regained continence during the test phase and two patients improved by more than 88%. Two patients reduced the number of incontinence episodes by 50% and three patients had no improvement (17).

Clinical experience with DGN

Studies using stimulation of the DGN have been performed in acute and experimental settings, without long-term chronic trials. Only 1 larger study using continuous stimulation during 1 week is available. Of 21 female patients with urgency incontinence 55% showed an increase in cystometric capacity and 47% experienced a greater than 50% reduction in incontinence episodes (30).

Other indications

As with SNS, the effect of PNS has also been evaluated for other (urological) indications. In a small (21 patients) prospective, single blind, randomized crossover trial of SNS versus PNS for bladder pain syndrome, 77% of patients had a significant improvement in the outcome of pain questionnaires and received a permanent implant. PNS was chosen as the better method of stimulation in 77% (31). In one study, the effect of PNS on non-obstructive urinary retention was evaluated in three patients as part of a study mixed with patients suffering OAB (16). Faecal incontinence is currently being evaluated as a novel indication for PNS. One study showed a success rate of 70%, considering a more than 50% symptom reduction as success (13). This indicates that patients suffering from OAB in combination with faecal incontinence, not responding to SNS for both problems, could be candidates for PNS.

Conclusions

Pudendal nerve stimulation (PNS) is considered an interesting alternative form of electrical stimulation for the treatment of over-active bladder (OAB) when non-invasive therapies have failed. As the pudendal nerve (PN) contains afferent fibres of S2, S3, and S4 nerve roots, more afferents are stimulated with PNS than with sacral nerve stimulation (SNS), and therefore may be an alternative option in patients in whom SNS fails. Anatomically, the PN can be approached in different ways and clinical research indicates better overall results with PNS than with SNS. However, only a limited number of permanent implantations has been performed and long-term results are lacking. Therefore, further research has to clarify the exact place of PNS in the treatment of lower urinary tract dysfunction.

References

1 **van Kerrebroeck PE, van Voskuilen AC, Heesakkers JP et al.** Results of sacral neuromodulation therapy for urinary voiding dysfunction: outcomes of a prospective, worldwide clinical study. J Urol 2007;**178**(5):2029–34. Epub 2007/09/18.

2 **Marcelissen TA, Leong RK, de Bie RA, van Kerrebroeck PE, de Wachter SG.** Long-term results of sacral neuromodulation with the tined lead procedure. J Urol 2010;**184**(5):1997–2000. Epub 2010/09/21.

3 **Leong RK, Marcelissen TA, Nieman FH, De Bie RA, Van Kerrebroeck PE, De Wachter SG.** Satisfaction and patient experience with sacral neuromodulation: results of a single center sample survey. J Urol 2011;**185**(2):588–92. Epub 2010/12/21.

4 **Kessler TM, La Framboise D, Trelle S et al.** Sacral neuromodulation for neurogenic lower urinary tract dysfunction: systematic review and meta-analysis. Eur Urol 2010;**58**(6):865–74. Epub 2010/10/12.

5 **Blok BF, Groen J, Bosch JL, Veltman DJ, Lammertsma AA.** Different brain effects during chronic and acute sacral neuromodulation in urge incontinent patients with implanted neurostimulators. BJU Int 2006;**98**(6):1238–43. Epub 2006/10/13.

6 **Groen J, Amiel C, Bosch JL.** Chronic pudendal nerve neuromodulation in women with idiopathic refractory detrusor overactivity incontinence: results of a pilot study with a novel minimally invasive implantable mini-stimulator. Neurourol Urodynam 2005;**24**(3):226–30. Epub 2005/04/13.

7 **Mahakkanukrauh P, Surin P, Vaidhayakarn P.** Anatomical study of the pudendal nerve adjacent to the sacrospinous ligament. Clin Anat 2005;**18**(3):200–205. Epub 2005/03/16.

8 **Popeney C, Ansell V, Renney K.** Pudendal entrapment as an etiology of chronic perineal pain: Diagnosis and treatment. Neurourol Urodynam 2007;**26**(6):820–27. Epub 2007/05/08.

9 **Beco J, Climov D, Bex M.** Pudendal nerve decompression in perineology: a case series. BMC Surg 2004;**4**:15. Epub 2004/11/02.

10 **Burks FN, Bui DT, Peters KM.** Neuromodulation and the neurogenic bladder. Urol Clin N Am 2010;**37**(4):559–65. Epub 2010/10/20.

11 **Schraffordt SE, Tjandra JJ, Eizenberg N, Dwyer PL.** Anatomy of the pudendal nerve and its terminal branches: a cadaver study. ANZ J Surg 2004;**74**(1–2):23–26. Epub 2004/01/17.

12 **Shafik A, Doss S.** Surgical anatomy of the somatic terminal innervation to the anal and urethral sphincters: role in anal and urethral surgery. J Urol 1999;**161**(1):85–89. Epub 1999/02/26.

13 **George AT, Dudding TC, Nicholls RJ, Vaizey CJ.** A new minimally invasive technique for pudendal nerve stimulation. Colorectal Dis: the official journal of the Association of Coloproctology of Great Britain and Ireland 2012;**14**(1):98–103. Epub 2010/11/09.

14 **Martens FM, Heesakkers JP, Rijkhoff NJ.** Surgical access for electrical stimulation of the pudendal and dorsal genital nerves in the overactive bladder: a review. J Urol 2011;**186**(3):798–804. Epub 2011/07/27.

15 **Schmidt RA.** Technique of pudendal nerve localization for block or stimulation. J Urol 1989;**142**(6):1528–31. Epub 1989/12/01.

16 **Peters KM, Feber KM, Bennett RC.** Sacral versus pudendal nerve stimulation for voiding dysfunction: a prospective, single-blinded, randomized, crossover trial. Neurourol Urodynam 2005;**24**(7):643–47. Epub 2005/09/24.

17 **Spinelli M, Malaguti S, Giardiello G, Lazzeri M, Tarantola J, Van Den Hombergh U.** A new minimally invasive procedure for pudendal nerve stimulation to treat neurogenic bladder: description of the method and preliminary data. Neurourol Urodynam 2005;**24**(4):305–09. Epub 2005/06/25.

18 **Ohlsson BL, Fall M, Frankenberg-Sommar S.** Effects of external and direct pudendal nerve maximal electrical stimulation in the treatment of the uninhibited overactive bladder. Brit J Urol 1989;**64**(4):374–80. Epub 1989/10/01.

19 **Ranck JB, Jr.** Which elements are excited in electrical stimulation of mammalian central nervous system: a review. Brain Res 1975;**98**(3):417–40. Epub 1975/12/01.

20 **Martens FM, Heesakkers JP, Rijkhoff NJ.** Minimal invasive electrode implantation for conditional stimulation of the dorsal genital nerve in neurogenic detrusor overactivity. Spinal Cord 2011;**49**(4):566–72. Epub 2010/10/06.

21 **Elkelini MS, Abuzgaya A, Hassouna MM.** Mechanisms of action of sacral neuromodulation. Int Urogynecol J 2010;**21**(Suppl 2):S439–46. Epub 2010/10/26.

22 **Boggs JW, Wenzel BJ, Gustafson KJ, Grill WM.** Frequency-dependent selection of reflexes by pudendal afferents in the cat. J Physiol 2006;**577**(Pt 1):115–26. Epub 2006/09/02.

23 **Boggs JW, Wenzel BJ, Gustafson KJ, Grill WM.** Bladder emptying by intermittent electrical stimulation of the pudendal nerve. J Neural Eng 2006;**3**(1):43–51. Epub 2006/03/03.

24 **Tai C, Wang J, Chancellor MB, Roppolo JR, de Groat WC.** Influence of temperature on pudendal nerve block induced by high frequency biphasic electrical current. J Urology 2008;**180**(3):1173–78. Epub 2008/07/22.

25 **Yoo PB, Woock JP, Grill WM.** Bladder activation by selective stimulation of pudendal nerve afferents in the cat. Exp Neurol 2008;**212**(1):218–25. Epub 2008/05/27.

26 **Woock JP, Yoo PB, Grill WM.** Mechanisms of reflex bladder activation by pudendal afferents. Am J Reg I 2011;**300**(2):R398–407. Epub 2010/11/12.

27 **Reitz A, Schmid DM, Curt A, Knapp PA, Schurch B.** Afferent fibers of the pudendal nerve modulate sympathetic neurons controlling the bladder neck. Neurourol Urodynam 2003;**22**(6):597–601. Epub 2003/09/03.

28 **Reitz A, Gobeaux N, Mozer P, Delmas V, Richard F, Chartier-Kastler E.** Topographic anatomy of a new posterior approach to the pudendal nerve for stimulation. Eur Urol 2007;**51**(5):1350–55; discussion 5–6. Epub 2006/10/31.

29 **Yoo PB, Klein SM, Grafstein NH et al.** Pudendal nerve stimulation evokes reflex bladder contractions in persons with chronic spinal cord injury. Neurourol Urodynam 2007;**26**(7):1020–23. Epub 2007/05/08.

30 **Goldman HB, Amundsen CL, Mangel J et al.** Dorsal genital nerve stimulation for the treatment of overactive bladder symptoms. Neurourol Urodynam 2008;**27**(6):499–503. Epub 2007/12/20.

31 **Peters KM, Feber KM, Bennett RC.** A prospective, single-blind, randomized crossover trial of sacral vs pudendal nerve stimulation for interstitial cystitis. BJU Int 2007;**100**(4):835–39. Epub 2007/09/08.

Chapter 15

Sacral nerve stimulation for lower urinary tract dysfunction

Philip E. V. Van Kerrebroeck
and Tom A. T. Marcelissen

Key points

1. Lower urinary tract dysfunction (LUTD) consists of the over-active bladder syndrome (OAB) and non-obstructive urinary retention (NOUR), and is an important medical problem.
2. A conservative approach often fails to treat LUTD.
3. The micturition cycle involves spinal cord reflexes and brain networks that can be modulated by electrical stimulation of the S3 sacral nerve (SNS).
4. SNS with an implanted electrode and pulse generator results in an excellent symptomatic relief in the majority of patients with LUTD.
5. Side-effects and complication of SNS are limited.

Introduction

Electrical stimulation of sacral nerves that innervate most organs and structures of the pelvis, including the bladder, urethra, and urethral sphincter, as well as the pelvic floor muscles, has become an important therapeutic tool in the treatment of lower urinary tract dysfunction (LUTD). With low-amplitude stimulation of the sacral nerves, below the threshold for pain, a neuromodulation effect is realized that allows control of lower urinary tract reflexes. Sacral neuromodulation (SNM) offers an alternative treatment for patients with LUTD with symptoms refractory to conservative treatment, including pharmacotherapy, pelvic floor re-education, and clean intermittent self-catheterization (1–3). SNM is based on the application of electrical currents to the sacral nerves in order to modulate reflexes involved in lower urinary tract control. Initially, more invasive surgical procedures, such as bladder augmentation or urinary diversion, have been advocated for patients with refractory symptoms. However, these procedures have variable success rates and have been associated with significant morbidity and risk. Therefore, SNM must be considered prior to more invasive surgery (4).

SNM was developed in the early 1980s and now has become a well-established treatment modality. S3 sacral nerve neuromodulation received approval by the US Food and Drug Administration (FDA) for the treatment of urgency incontinence in 1997 and for urgency/frequency and non-obstructive urinary retention in 1999. The efficacy of SNM treatment has been shown in clinical trials, with a reported 5-year success rate of approximately 70% (5).

Historical overview

The first application of the use of electrical currents in medicine dates back to AD 46, when Scribonius Largus, a Roman physician, recorded the use of torpedo fish for treatment of headaches and gout in his *Compositiones Medicae* (6). The concept of electrical stimulation of the bladder started in 1878. The Danish surgeon Saxtorph reported on the use of intravesical electrostimulation in patients with acontractile bladder and complete urinary retention (7). A specially designed catheter was inserted transurethrally with a metal electrode inside and a neutral electrode placed suprapubically. In 1959 this technique was again used by Katona, who described a technique of intraluminal electrotherapy for various disorders of the gastrointestinal tract (8). He also applied this treatment in newborns with meningomyelocoele to enhance detrusor reflexes. Since then, intravesical electrostimulation has been researched by others with inconsistent results (9, 10).

With the growing experience of direct bladder stimulation, alternative methods, such as stimulation of the spinal cord and pelvic nerves, have been evaluated. A study by Nashold et al. reported successful implantation of a neural prosthesis in the sacral segment of the spinal cord (11). In order to achieve greater coordination, stimulation was directed at the sacral micturition centre. The first implants were used to activate voiding in patients with spinal cord injury. However, simultaneous activation of the detrusor, as well as the urethral sphincter, prevented adequate success. It was Jonas and Tanagho who further evaluated this prosthesis, and found that voiding was possible in patients with spinal cord lesions at the end of each stimulus due to an earlier decline in urethral sphincter pressure (12). Ultimately, Tanagho and Schmidt demonstrated that stimulation of the third sacral root (S3) generally modulates detrusor and sphincter activity and could stabilize the whole micturition reflex mechanism in patients with over-activity of the lower urinary tract. With an implantable stimulator connected to an electrode positioned in the sacral foramen, the S3 root can be stimulated continuously (Fig. 15.1) (13, 14). Due to technological advancements, the technique has now become minimally-invasive and easy to perform. Currently, this therapy has been successfully used for more than 20 years.

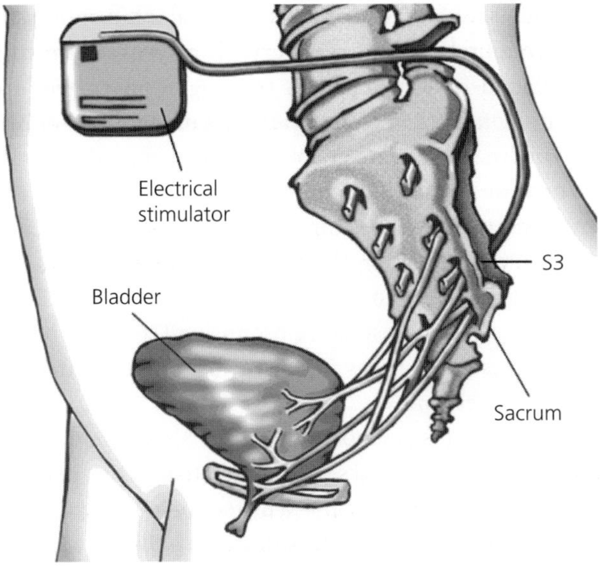

Fig. 15.1 Stimulation of the third sacral nerve root (S3) with an implantable neurostimulator.

Indications

Sacral neuromodulation is an established treatment for patients with various chronic bladder disorders that have failed to respond to traditional treatments. Although SNM currently only has FDA approval for over-active bladder and urinary retention, clinical benefit has been observed for various other chronic pelvic floor disorders, including faecal incontinence, chronic pelvic pain, and interstitial cystitis.

Over-active bladder

Over-active bladder (OAB) syndrome involves a group of symptoms, including frequency, urgency, and leakage immediately preceded by urgency (15). Bladder over-activity can occur with urine incontinence (OAB wet) or without (OAB dry).

Epidemiological data from Europe and in the US estimated an OAB prevalence of approximately 16–17% in the adult population, of which a third (predominantly women) have complaints of urgency urinary incontinence (16, 17). OAB is a distressing syndrome and has a significant negative impact on quality of life (18–20). The cause of OAB is often idiopathic. It can also be neurogenic, involving the central nervous system, the peripheral nervous system, or the end organ itself. Myogenic changes of the bladder are also important in the aetiology, particularly in the elderly (21). Often, a combination of these factors accounts for the development of OAB.

Before considering treatment, a proper clinical evaluation should be performed in order to rule out underlying causes, such as infections, malignancies, or anatomical obstruction. This includes a voiding diary, urinalysis, physical examination, and urodynamic evaluation. Conservative management is usually advocated as an initial intervention since it carries minimal risks (22, 23). Behavioural and lifestyle interventions are recommended as first-line treatment, followed by bladder and pelvic floor training or pharmacological treatment with antimuscarinic drugs. Often, these conservative treatments do not result in a sufficient relief of symptoms, with many patients unable to tolerate the side-effects of antimuscarinic drugs (24, 25). When conservative treatments fail after 8–12 weeks, alternative therapies can be considered (15). At present, minimally invasive techniques available include SNM, posterior tibial nerve stimulation (PTNS), and intravesical injections with botulinum toxin (BTX). Although BTX is not currently approved by the FDA for the treatment of idiopathic OAB, the long-term results are promising (26–28). The most common adverse events are post-void residuals, necessitating the use of intermittent self-catheterization, as well as urinary tract infections.

Although it is unknown which OAB patients are most suitable for SNM, important observations have been made. Scheepens et al. identified several predictive factors in a retrospective study evaluating 211 patients (29). They found that a history of intervertebral disc prolapse surgery and the duration of complaints are factors that may affect the chance of success. Everaert et al. reported that patients with a history of surgery for stress incontinence had significantly better long-term outcomes with SNM, whatever their symptoms were (30). In a group of 100 patients undergoing test stimulation, Koldewijn et al. did not show any predictors of success, although it appeared that patients with detrusor overactivity and urethral instability responded best to SNM (31). Groenendijk et al. studied the predictive value of urethral instability and other urodynamic parameters on the efficacy of sacral nerve stimulation in 19 patients (32). They found that 12 of the 13 successfully treated patients showed urethral instability at baseline, compared to 1 of the 6 patients with failure of SNM. Therefore, urethral instability appeared to be a valuable predictive factor for success. It has been postulated that increasing age has an adverse effect on neurologic integrity both within the central nervous system and to the bladder. Amundsen et al. demonstrated that age greater than 55 was associated with a poorer response to SNM (33). In predictive factor studies in the treatment of faecal incontinence, older age has also been identified as a negative predictor for PNE outcome (34, 35). Currently, a trial stimulation remains the only reliable factor in predicting success with permanent treatment.

Urinary retention

Voiding can be impaired by either bladder outlet obstruction or insufficient contractility of the detrusor. In turn, bladder outlet obstruction can be of anatomical or functional origin. Anatomical obstruction is often caused by an enlarged prostate, urinary tract tumours, bladder neck stenosis, or urethral strictures. Although poorly understood, functional aetiologies include detrusor external sphincter dyssynergia or detrusor bladder neck dyssynergia. In addition, pelvic floor dysfunction can cause inhibition of detrusor function, resulting in difficult voiding and varying degrees of urinary retention. Fowler et al. described over-activity of the urethral sphincter as a cause of urinary retention, especially in young women (Fowler's syndrome) (36, 37). Women with this disorder show abnormal activity of the external urethral sphincter on electromyography. As a result, the urethral sphincter is unable to relax, which causes inadequate bladder emptying.

Besides urological causes, neurological disorders (e.g. spinal cord disease, spinal disc herniation, multiple sclerosis, and small-fibre neuropathy) should be considered as a possible basis for non-obstructive urinary retention. Patients with 'idiopathic' urinary retention often have a history of a triggering event, such as pelvic surgery or even emotional stress. They also frequently have a history of dysfunctional disorders in their childhood, such as lifelong constipation or urinary tract infections. Multiple authors have demonstrated the association of childhood dysfunctional elimination symptoms and adult bladder symptoms (38).

Prior to SNM there was no effective treatment for functional urinary retention, apart from clean intermittent self-catheterization, as pharmacological agents, including α-blockers and muscle relaxants, often gave poor results. More invasive treatments, such as urethral dilatation and bladder neck incisions have been associated with inconsistent results, a high relapse rate, and complications. Sacral neuromodulation has been recognized as an effective treatment for patients with functional urinary retention. A large multicentre clinical trial in 1999 resulted in FDA approval of SNM for this indication (39). Later, the clinical efficacy was confirmed in several studies, and now SNM has become a well-established treatment modality for patients with non-obstructive urinary retention (1, 2, 5, 40). No predictors of success have currently been identified. It is important to note that an elevated cystometric capacity or absence of signs of detrusor contractility on urodynamic investigation do not predict failure of SNM. However, Bertapelle et al. demonstrated that patients who showed a lack of detrusor response to acute stimulation of the sacral nerve roots, might have a lower chance of treatment success (41). Patients with pelvic floor hypertonicity, such as in Fowler's syndrome, appear to have a higher success rate (42).

Neurogenic bladder dysfunction

Originally, SNM was not considered an option for neurogenic bladder dysfunction, because it has been assumed that the efficacy of SNM relies on the integrity of the spinal and supraspinal reflex arcs (43). Furthermore, SNM has been previously attempted without success in patients with complete spinal cord lesions (44). Nevertheless, several studies have demonstrated that SNM can be used successfully in patients with voiding symptoms due to neurological disorders (45–47). Chartier-Kastler showed that SNM was successful in nine patients with neurogenic urgency incontinence due to diseases that affect the spinal cord (48). After a mean follow-up of 44 months, all patients had clinically significant improvement of incontinence, and five were completely dry. Lombardi et al. evaluated the effect of SNM in 24 patients with lower urinary tract dysfunction due to spinal cord injury with a mean follow-up of 61 month (49). Of the 13 patients with urinary retention, 9 (69%) were successfully treated, with a significant decrease in the number of catheterizations and a significant increase in voided volume. Amongst the 11 patients with over-active bladder symptoms, an 80% reduction in daytime frequency was observed, with 3 out of 7 patients remaining completely dry during the study period.

Yet, Hohenfeller et al. found less promising results. They evaluated 27 patients with neurogenic bladder dysfunction after a follow-up of 89 months (50). The underlying neurologic disorders were lesions of the spinal cord in 16, pelvic surgery in 6, cerebral lesions in 3, and inflammatory disease of the central nervous system in 2 patients. In 8 patients (30%), symptoms of LUTD significantly improved for 54 months. After this time period, all implants became ineffective, except in one patient. This study illustrates that while SNM may be effective for neurogenic bladder dysfunction, the results may be temporary.

In a recent review and meta-analysis by Kessler et al., the efficacy of SNM for neurogenic voiding dysfunction was evaluated (51). The pooled success rate of 26 studies was 68% for the test phase and 92% for permanent SNM, with a mean follow-up of 26 months. This indicates that SNM may also be an effective treatment in neurogenic bladder dysfunction, although the number of investigated patients is low with high between-study heterogeneity and lack of randomized controlled trials.

Functional bowel disorders

In 1995, Matzel et al. adapted SNM for the treatment of functional disorders of the lower gastrointestinal tract. Patients who do not respond to maximal conservative treatments such as pelvic floor training, drugs, or retrograde colonic irrigation are eligible candidates for SNM. Several studies demonstrated treatment success in patients with faecal incontinence (52–54). A review of patients with faecal incontinence who received a permanent implant reported that complete continence for solids and liquid motions was reported in 41 to 75% of patients (55). More recently, SNM has also been successfully used in patients with constipation (56, 57). For patients with idiopathic slow transit constipation who received permanent implants, evacuations increased five-fold. The Cleveland Clinic Constipation score also improved, with less abdominal pain and bloating (55).

Some studies reported on the treatment of patients with mixed urinary and faecal incontinence. Ganio et al. evaluated 40 patients with faecal incontinence, of whom 12 had concomitant voiding symptoms, including retention and incontinence (58). During test stimulation, 6 of the 12 had complete resolution of symptoms and one reported improvement. Uludag et al. evaluated the effect of permanent SNM in 50 patients with faecal incontinence, of whom 18 had concomitant urinary incontinence (59). After a median follow-up of 12 months, 9 patients (50%) showed improvement in urinary leakage, although bladder symptoms were not recorded by using voiding diaries. In a recent study by El-Gazzaz et al., 24 patients who received implants for urinary incontinence associated with faecal incontinence were studied. Seven patients (31.8%) experienced improvement in both urinary and faecal incontinence symptoms. There was no improvement in urinary symptoms in 11 patients (50%) and faecal incontinence symptoms did not improve in 12 patients (54.5%) (60).

Still, the efficacy of SNM for the management of double incontinence depends on patient selection. For example, when the main indication for implantation is faecal incontinence, the results for urinary incontinence can be disappointing because patient selection has not been made according to these symptoms. As a result, the voiding symptoms may not necessarily have features suggesting improvement with SNM. Further prospective trials are needed to determine which patients with combined problems will most likely benefit.

Pelvic pain

Pelvic floor dysfunction is often associated with both voiding symptoms and pelvic pain symptoms. Hypertonia of the pelvic floor is a common source of pelvic pain and is also an important feature in the aetiology of LUTD (61). SNM has been postulated to inhibit inappropriate excitation of the pelvic floor muscles, therefore facilitating voiding by interrupting the outflow to the urethral sphincter (62). Although sacral neuromodulation is not an FDA-approved treatment, several authors have reported on the 'off label' treatment of patients with urological pain syndromes. Maher et al. prospectively evaluated the effect of test stimulation with PNE in 15 patients with interstitial cystitis who were unresponsive to standard oral or intravesical therapy (63). Besides an improvement in voiding symptoms, a significant reduction in mean bladder pain from 8.9 to 2.4 on a scale of 0 to 10 was reported. There was at least a 50% decrease in bladder pain in 87% of the cases and at least a 50% decrease in 24-hour urinary voiding in 47% after PNE. Everaert et al. performed a test stimulation in 26 patients after failure of conservative treatment for intractable chronic pelvic pain (including genital, urethral, inguinal, and perineal pain) (64). Significant pain relief was obtained in 16 patients (62%). After a follow-up of 37 months, 73% of the implanted patients were satisfied with the treatment. Although these initial results seem promising, larger prospective trials are needed to determine the efficacy of SNM in the treatment of pelvic pain.

Mechanism of action

Although the exact mechanism of SNM is not well understood, it seems to involve modulation of the spinal cord reflexes and brain networks by peripheral afferents, rather than direct stimulation of the motor response of the detrusor or urethral sphincter (36). In patients with over-active bladder, SNM is thought to inhibit detrusor activity without affecting urethral resistance or the strength of detrusor contractions during voiding (65). The observation that early, bilateral SNM initiated during spinal shock could prevent the development of detrusor over-activity in complete spinal cord injury, might indicate modulation at the level of the spinal cord itself (66). However, PET-studies indicated that at the level of the brain, the activity of centres involved in activation or inhibition of the micturition reflex, can be enhanced or reduced with SNM (67, 68). This results in the activation or inhibition of lower urinary tract activity. Blok et al. compared the effect of acute and chronic SNM on brain activity by evaluating the regional cerebral blood flow with PET (69). Their findings suggested that acute SNM predominantly modulates areas involved in sensorimotor learning, whereas chronic SNM influences areas related to the awareness of bladder filling, the urge to void, and the timing of micturition.

For urinary retention, different theories on the mechanism of action have been proposed. SNM has been postulated to suppress the guarding reflex, resulting in decreased urethral sphincter tone, and thereby facilitating voiding. Animal studies indicated that the guarding reflexes can be modulated by afferent nerve activation and inhibit bladder activity by spinal or supraspinal pathways (70, 71). In contrast, the results of a study of 30 women with Fowler's syndrome showed that the maximum urethral closure pressure did not change significantly. Instead, the return of voiding ability seemed to be attributable to a small increase in detrusor contractility (72). In a recent study, functional MRI was used to evaluate brain responses to bladder filling in patients with Fowler's syndrome (73). The data showed abnormal brain responses in these patients, which are most likely caused by abnormally strong inhibition of the bladder afferents by over-activity of the urethral sphincter. The authors suggested that SNM acts at a sacral level, by blocking the urethral inhibition of afferent information from the bladder. Because the transmission of afferent information to the brain is restored, bladder sensations return, as well as the ability to void.

A possible working mechanism for neuromodulation in the treatment of pain is based on the Gate Control Theory. This theory states that pain perception depends on a pattern of peripheral nervous input. It is assumed that a gate-control mechanism at the spinal segment level is present, which regulates the interaction between afferent nerve signals and pain sensation (74). Inter-neurones of the spinal cord dorsal horn create gating components, and inhibition or facilitation of afferent fibres modulates the input to the spinal transmission neurones. Furthermore, it is postulated that the impulses from the dorsal horn are controlled by a descending system containing fibres from the brainstem, thalamus, and limbic lobes (75). Neuromodulation is supposed to restore the control at the spinal segmental 'gate' as well as at supraspinal sites, such as the brainstem and the limbic system nuclei.

To summarize, the exact mechanism of action of SNM in the treatment of lower urinary tract dysfunction is complex, and still remains unclear. Most likely, it involves a combination of different modes of action, involving the neuroaxis at different levels.

Neuromodulation technique

In sacral neuromodulation, one of the sacral nerves (usually S3) is stimulated with a quadripolar lead, which is positioned in the sacral foramen. The lead is connected to an implantable, reprogrammable device. The device can be implanted by creating a sub-cutaneous pocket in the lower abdomen or buttock. Patients are selected for SNM treatment based on their response to test stimulation with a temporary electrode (Fig. 15.2) (1, 2, 76, 77). During the test procedure, a needle is inserted into the third sacral foramen. Next, it is connected to an external stimulator and current is applied. Correct placement is confirmed by evaluating the sensory and motor responses to stimulation. Typical responses are: paraesthesia in the anal, vaginal, or perineal area, contraction of the levator ani muscle, and flexion of the great toe on the ipsilateral side of stimulation (78). In addition, correct position of the needle can be confirmed by fluoroscopy. When adequate responses have been obtained, the electrode is inserted through the needle and the needle is removed. In turn,

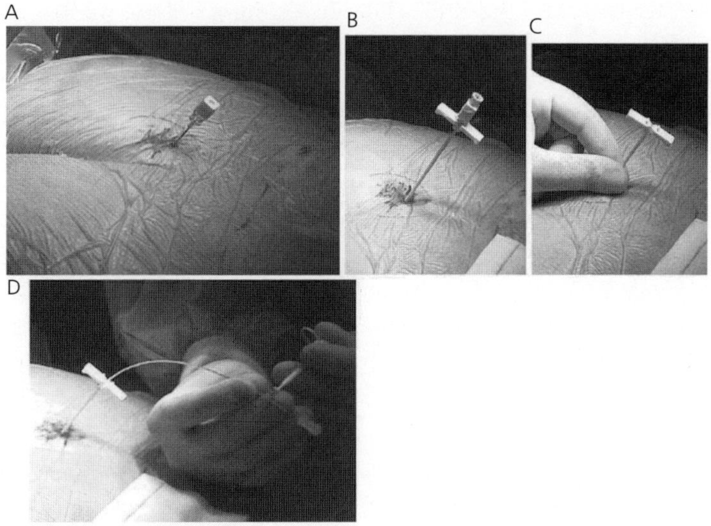

Fig. 15.2 Percutaneous technique of lead implantation. (**A**) After correct positioning of the patient, a test needle is used to probe and localise the third sacral foramen. (**B**) A lead introducer is inserted over a guide wire to provide access for the test lead into the sacral foramen. (**C**) The guide wire is removed. (**D**) The test lead is inserted through the introducer, and the contact points of the electrode are tested by applying electrical current.

the electrode is connected to an external stimulator. During the trial stimulation, which lasts for a minimum of 3 days, the response to sub-chronic stimulation can be evaluated.

Initially, test stimulation was performed with the 'percutaneous nerve evaluation' (PNE), in which a basic wire electrode (Medtronic™ number 041828–004) is connected to an external stimulator. However, due to the high risk of lead migration, the test duration is rather limited and the reported success rate is between 40 and 50% (2, 79). In 1997, the two-stage procedure was introduced, which aims at screening with the permanent electrode during a first stage (79, 80). If the patient is considered eligible for definitive SNM, the implantable neurostimulator (INS) is inserted in a second stage. This procedure enables prolonged screening for up to 1 month, resulting in a success rate of approximately 80%, which is significantly higher than with PNE testing (79, 80).

Originally, the permanent lead was implanted under direct vision and in turn secured to the sacral periosteum during an open surgical technique (81, 82). Spinelli et al. introduced a self-anchoring 'tined' lead in 2002, allowing percutaneous placement of the lead under radiological guidance (Fig. 15.3) (83, 84). Potential advantages of the tined lead include a shorter operation time, reduced risk of infection, less pain, and shorter post-operative recovery time. In addition, the lead can be inserted under local anaesthesia, enabling evaluation of the sensory responses to acute stimulation.

At the end of the test-stimulation period, the patient is evaluated for symptom improvement by using voiding diaries. In patients with urinary retention, a pressure-flow

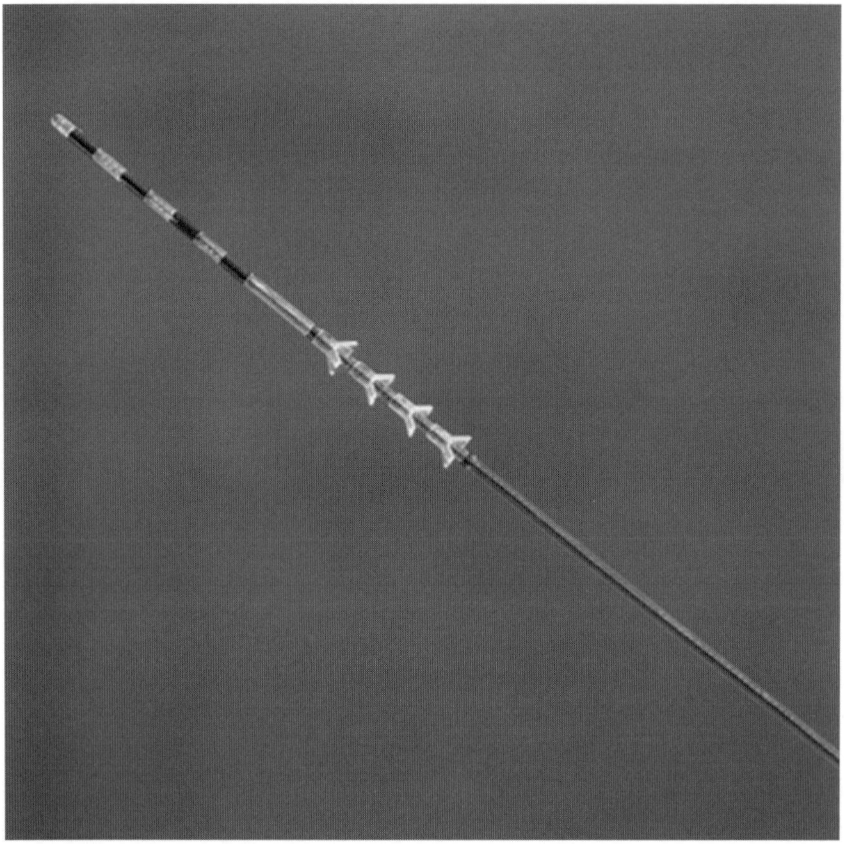

Fig. 15.3 Tined lead. Due to silicone barbs ('tines') the lead is self-anchored in the sub-cutaneous tissue. The tines deploy after removal of the introducer.

urodynamic investigation is additionally used to evaluate adequate voiding. If the voiding diaries and urodynamics show significant improvement, patients are considered eligible for definitive SNM treatment. A permanent stimulator and lead are implanted in the subcutaneous area of the buttock (85). The permanent lead has four electrodes at the tip that can be used as an anode or cathode during stimulation. After implantation, the electrode settings (polarity) and stimulation parameters (amplitude, pulse rate, and pulse width) are programmed and patients are taught how to use their personal programmer. Patients can turn their stimulator on and off, and are able to increase or decrease the amplitude within preset limits. The other stimulation parameters can only be altered by the physician.

Clinical results

If more than 50% improvement in voiding symptoms is observed during the test period, then patients are considered eligible candidates for SNM treatment. The voiding symptoms are measured by using voiding diaries, which are self-recorded by the patient. Preceding the test stimulation, patients keep a voiding diary to assess baseline symptoms. By comparing the results of the voiding diary that is kept during test stimulation, the degree of improvement can be evaluated. Depending on the type of complaint, different primary voiding parameters are used to evaluate the clinical effect. In patients with urgency incontinence, improvement of incontinence parameters is considered most important (number of leakages per day and the number of pads per day). In patients with urgency/frequency, the voiding frequency and voided volume per void are evaluated, and in patients with chronic urinary retention, reduction in the volume per catheterization and increase in voided volume is assessed.

Numerous reports on the clinical efficacy of SNM have been published. In early studies on SNM by Tanagho et al., stimulation of the S3 root resulted in restoration of continence in patients with detrusor over-activity due to suprasacral spinal cord injury (14). In 1995, Bosch et al. evaluated 18 implanted patients with urgency incontinence (86). The voiding diaries of these patients showed a highly significant drop in leakage episodes and frequency, with a significant increase in the average voided volume. The number of pads used per day dropped significantly as well. The effect was durable, as 13 patients who were followed for more than 2 years maintained the same initial improvement. Similar results were shown by Elabaddy et al. and Shaker et al. (87, 88). In addition, early studies reported on the use of SNM for the restoration of voiding in patients with non-obstructive urinary retention. Thon et al. reported long-lasting improvement in 70% of 33 implanted patients (89). Shaker et al. and Jonas et al. also reported a high success rate in these patients (2, 90).

Long-term outcome of SNM for lower urinary tract dysfunction has been assessed in several clinical trials. Table 15.1 presents an overview of a number of studies that evaluated the long-term efficacy. All studies showed that SNM treatment is safe and effective for patients with OAB, as well as patients with urinary retention, and most studies showed a higher success rate in the retention group. The largest prospective study, including 17 centres worldwide, reported a long-term success rate of approximately 70% (5).

Table 15.1 Long-term results of SNM treatment. Success of treatment was defined as the percentage of patients that had a successful outcome at last follow-up visit (more than 50% improvement in key voiding diary variables)

Study	Year	No. of patients	Success of treatment %	Follow-up (months)
Siegel et al. (1)	2000	112	62	26
Bosch et al. (76)	2000	45	60	47
Dasgupta et al. (91)	2004	26	77	37
Van Kerrebroeck et al. (5)	2007	105	70	49
Sutherland et al. (92)	2007	104	69	22

Follow-up and adverse events

Directly after implantation, the implantable neurostimulator (INS) is activated and optimal stimulation settings are chosen. These settings are determined by evaluating the sensory response to different combinations. The tip of the implanted lead contains four stimulation points and each one can be used as a cathode or anode. Also, the case of the stimulator can be used as an anode, which results in unipolar type of stimulation. When the lead itself is used for both the cathode and anode, bipolar stimulation is the result. The stimulation setting (uni- or bipolar) that gives the best sensory response (anal, vaginal, or perineal), at the lowest amplitude, is considered optimal. The amplitude of stimulation is initially set just above sensory threshold. Not much is known about the optimal pulse rate with chronic stimulation. Although it is generally advised to set the pulse rate between 10 and 16 Hz, the effect of different pulse rates on treatment efficacy has never been evaluated in clinical studies. This also applies for the pulse width, which is advised to set at 210 ms. Patients receive a 'patient programmer', which they can use to turn the INS on or off when necessary. Also, the programmer grants the ability to make small alterations in the stimulation amplitude. Patients are advised to keep the INS on both during the day and at night.

Patient follow-up after implantation of the neurostimulator is scheduled after 6 weeks, 6 months, and yearly thereafter. During each follow-up visit, the stimulation parameters are checked in order to evaluate patient compliance and correct use of the patient programmer. Next, the impedance is measured. If the impedance is less than 50 ohm or more than 4000 ohm, there may be a short cut or an open circuit, respectively. An abnormal impedance can be an indication for a broken wire, and a re-operation may be required to replace the damaged lead. In case of decreased efficacy, the impedances and battery lifespan are checked. When there are no signs of lead damage and the sensory response is preserved, parameter settings can be adjusted in attempt to restore efficacy. Different stimulation settings can be tried for 2 weeks. Also, an X-ray can be considered to rule out lead migration. If all these changes do not lead to any improvement, and all parameters and sensory responses are correct, it is often challenging to find a satisfactory solution. First of all, the patient's symptoms have to be re-evaluated to rule out other causes of therapy failure (e.g. stress incontinence or neurological disease), especially in patients who have been treated with SNM for several years. Subsequently, replacement of the lead or contralateral placement of a new lead can be considered. Before definitive placement of a new lead, a test stimulation can be conducted to assess the clinical response. Also, bilateral stimulation can be attempted. Although this has never been evaluated in clinical studies, data from animal studies suggest a stronger modulatory effect of bilateral stimulation (93, 94). If successful, a second device can be implanted and connected to the contralateral lead or a TWIN (Medtronic™) stimulator can be used.

Pain after implantation is not uncommon, occurring in 24–34% after long-term follow-up (1, 5, 30). Pain can be located at the site of the INS or at the site where the stimulation sensation is perceived. The cause of the pain can often be differentiated by turning the stimulator off. If pain symptoms persist, they are often a result of mechanical discomfort of the INS. If pain symptoms decrease, they are often stimulation-related. The physician can attempt to relieve pain symptoms by altering the stimulation settings. If no pain relief occurs, repositioning of the INS or lead can be necessary.

References

1 **Siegel SW, Catanzaro F, Dijkema HE et al.** Long-term results of a multicenter study on sacral nerve stimulation for treatment of urinary urge incontinence, urgency-frequency, and retention. Urology 2000;**56**:87–91.

2 **Jonas U, Fowler CJ, Chancellor MB et al.** Efficacy of sacral nerve stimulation for urinary retention: results 18 months after implantation. J Urol 2001;**165**:15–19.

3 **Schmidt RA, Jonas U, Oleson KA et al.** Sacral nerve stimulation for treatment of refractory urinary urge incontinence. Sacral Nerve Stimulation Study Group. J Urol 1999;**162**:352–57.

4 **Van Kerrebroeck PE.** A treatment algorithm for the overactive bladder. BJU Int 1999;**83**(Suppl. 2):29–30.

5 **van Kerrebroeck PE, van Voskuilen AC, Heesakkers JP et al.** Results of sacral neuromodulation therapy for urinary voiding dysfunction: outcomes of a prospective, worldwide clinical study. J Urol 2001;**178**:2029–34.

6 **Bullock TH.** The future of research on electroreception and electrocommunication. J Exp Biol 1999;**202**:1455–58.

7 **Saxtorph M.** Stricture urethrae-Fistula perineae-Retnetio urinae. Clinsk Chirurgi Gyldendalske Fortlag Copenhagen 1878;265–80.

8 **Katona F.** Stages of vegatative afferentation in reorganization of bladder control during intravesical electrotherapy. Urol Int 1975;**30**:192–203.

9 **van Balken MR, Vergunst H, Bemelmans BL.** The use of electrical devices for the treatment of bladder dysfunction: a review of methods. J Urol 2004;**172**:846–51.

10 **Ascoli R.** Treatment of neurogenic bladder. Acta Urol Belg 1965;**33**:76–83.

11 **Nashold BS, Jr.**, Friedman H, Boyarsky S. Electrical activation of micturition by spinal cord stimulation. J Surg Res 1971;**11**:144–47.

12 **Jonas U, Heine JP, Tanagho EA.** Studies on the feasibility of urinary bladder evacuation by direct spinal cord stimulation.I. Parameters of most effective stimulation. Invest Urol 1975;**13**:142–50.

13 **Schmidt RA, Bruschini H, Tanagho EA.** Sacral root stimulation in controlled micturition. Peripheral somatic neurotomy and stimulated voiding. Invest Urol 1979;**17**:130–34.

14 **Tanagho EA, Schmidt RA, Orvis BR.** Neural stimulation for control of voiding dysfunction: a preliminary report in 22 patients with serious neuropathic voiding disorders. J Urol 1989;**142**:340–45.

15 **Abrams P, Andersson KE, Birder L et al.** Fourth International Consultation on Incontinence Recommendations of the International Scientific Committee: Evaluation and treatment of urinary incontinence, pelvic organ prolapse, and fecal incontinence. Neurourol Urodyn 2010;**29**:213–40.

16 **Milsom I, Abrams P, Cardozo L, Roberts RG, Thuroff J, Wein AJ:** How widespread are the symptoms of an overactive bladder and how are they managed? A population-based prevalence study. BJU Int 2001;**87**:760–66.

17 **Stewart WF, Van Rooyen JB, Cundiff GW et al.** Prevalence and burden of overactive bladder in the United States. World J Urol 2003;**20**:327–36.

18 **Bump RC and Norton PA.** Epidemiology and natural history of pelvic floor dysfunction. Obstet Gynecol Clin North Am 1998;**25**:723–46.

19 **Grimby A, Milsom I, Molander U, Wiklund I, Ekelund P**. The influence of urinary incontinence on the quality of life of elderly women. Age Ageing 1993;**22**:82–9.

20 **Temml C, Haidinger G, Schmidbauer J, Schatzl G, Madersbacher S**. Urinary incontinence in both sexes: prevalence rates and impact on quality of life and sexual life. Neurourol Urodyn 2000;**19**:259–71.

21 **Elbadawi A, Yalla SV, Resnick NM**. Structural basis of geriatric voiding dysfunction. III. Detrusor overactivity. J Urol 1993;**150**:1668–80.

22 **Karram MM, Partoll L, Rahe J**. Efficacy of nonsurgical therapy for urinary incontinence. J Reprod Med 1996;**41**:215–19.

23 **Robert M, Ross S, Farrel SA et al**. Conservative management of urinary incontinence. J Obstet Gynaecol Can 2006;**28**:1113–25.

24 **Resnick NM**. Improving treatment of urinary incontinence. Jama 1998;**280**:2034–35.

25 **Sutherland SE, Goldman HB**. Treatment options for female urinary incontinence. Med Clin North Am 2004;**88**:345–66.

26 **Sahai A, Khan MS, Dasgupta P**. Efficacy of botulinum toxin-A for treating idiopathic detrusor overactivity: results from a single center, randomized, double-blind, placebo controlled trial. J Urol 2007;**177**:2231–36.

27 **Brubaker L, Richter HE, Visco A et al**. Refractory idiopathic urge urinary incontinence and botulinum A injection. J Urol 2008;**180**:217–22.

28 **Flynn MK, Amundsen CL, Perevich M, Liu F, Webster GD**. Outcome of a randomized, double-blind, placebo controlled trial of botulinum A toxin for refractory overactive bladder. J Urol 2009;**181**:2608–15.

29 **Scheepens WA, Jongen MMGJ, Nieman FHM, de Bie RA, Weil EHJ, van Kerrebroeck PEV**. Predictive factors for sacral neuromodulation in chronic lower urinary tract dysfunction. Urology 2002;**60**:598.

30 **Everaert K, De Ridder D, Baert L, Oosterlinck W, Wyndaele JJ**. Patient satisfaction and complications following sacral nerve stimulation for urinary retention, urge incontinence and perineal pain: a multicenter evaluation. Int Urogynecol J Pelvic Floor Dysfunct 2000;**11**:231–35; discussion 236.

31 **Koldewijn EL, Rosier PF, Meuleman EJ, Koster AM, Debruyne FM, Van Kerrebroeck PhE**. Predictors of success with neuromodulation in lower urinary tract dysfunction: results of trial stimulation in 100 patients. J Urology 1994;**152**:2071–75.

32 **Groenendijk PM, Heesakkers JP, Lycklama ANAA**. Urethral instability and sacral nerve stimulation-a better parameter to predict efficacy? J Urol 2007;**178**:568–72; discussion 572.

33 **Amundsen CL, Romero AA, Jamison MG, Webster GD**. Sacral neuromodulation for intractable urge incontinence: are there factors associated with cure? Urology 2005;**66**:746–50.

34 **Govaert B, Melenhorst J, Nieman FH, Bols EM, van Gemert WG, Baeten CG**. Factors associated with percutaneous nerve evaluation and permanent sacral nerve modulation outcome in patients with fecal incontinence. Dis Colon Rectum 2009;**52**:1688–94.

35 **Gourcerol G, Gallas S, Michot F, Denis P, Leroi AM**. Sacral nerve stimulation in fecal incontinence: are there factors associated with success? Dis Colon Rectum 2007;**50**:3–12.

36 **Kessler TM, Fowler CJ**. Sacral neuromodulation for urinary retention. Nat Clin Pract Urol 2008;**5**:657–66.

37 **Swinn MJ, Fowler CJ**. Isolated urinary retention in young women, or Fowler's syndrome. Clin Auton Res 2001;**11**:309–11.

38 **Minassian VA, Lovatsis D, Pascali D, Alarab M, Drutz HP**. Effect of childhood dysfunctional voiding on urinary incontinence in adult women. Obstet Gynecol 2006;**107**:1247–51.

39 **Tanagho EA, Schmidt RA**. Electrical stimulation in the clinical management of the neurogenic bladder. J Urol 1988;**140**:1331–39.

40 **Kessler TM, Buchser E, Meyer S et al**. Sacral neuromodulation for refractory lower urinary tract dysfunction: results of a nationwide registry in Switzerland. Eur Urol 2007;**51**:1357–63.

41 **Bertapelle P, Bodo G, Carone R**. Detrusor acontractility in urinary retention: detrusor contractility test as exclusion criteria for sacral neurostimulation. J Urol 2008;**180**:215–16.

42 **Swinn MJ, Kitchen ND, Goodwin RJ, Fowler CJ**. Sacral neuromodulation for women with Fowler's syndrome. Eur Urol 2000;**38**:439–43.

43 **Schmidt RA, Doggweiler R**. Neurostimulation and neuromodulation: a guide to selecting the right urologic patient. Eur Urol 1998;**34**(Suppl. 1):23–26.

44 **Schurch B, Reilly I, Reitz A, Curt A**. Electrophysiological recordings during the peripheral nerve evaluation (PNE) test in complete spinal cord injury patients. World J Urol 2003;**20**:319–22.

45 **Roth TM**. Sacral neuromodulation and lower urinary tract dysfunction in cerebral palsy. Int Urogynecol J Pelvic Floor Dysfunct 2007;**18**:567–69.

46 **Wallace PA, Lane FL, Noblett KL**. Sacral nerve neuromodulation in patients with underlying neurologic disease. Am J Obstet Gynecol 2007;**197**: 96 e1–5.

47 **Marinkovic SP, Gillen LM**. Sacral neuromodulation for multiple sclerosis patients with urinary retention and clean intermittent catheterization. Int Urogynecol J Pelvic Floor Dysfunct 2009;**21**:223–28.

48 **Chartier-Kastler EJ, Ruud Bosch JL, Perrigot M, Chancellor MB, Richard F, Denys P**. Long-term results of sacral nerve stimulation (S3) for the treatment of neurogenic refractory urge incontinence related to detrusor hyperreflexia. J Urol 2000;**164**:1476–80.

49 **Lombardi G, Del Popolo G**.Clinical outcome of sacral neuromodulation in incomplete spinal cord injured patients suffering from neurogenic lower urinary tract symptoms. Spinal Cord 2009;**47**:486–91.

50 **Hohenfellner M, Humke J, Hampel C et al**. Chronic sacral neuromodulation for treatment of neurogenic bladder dysfunction: long-term results with unilateral implants. Urology 2001;**58**:887–92.

51 **Kessler TM, La Framboise D, Trelle S et al**. Sacral neuromodulation for neurogenic lower urinary tract dysfunction: systematic review and meta-analysis. Eur Urol 2010;**58**(6):865–74.

52 **Melenhorst J, Koch SM, Uludag O, van Gemert WG, Baeten CG**. Sacral neuromodulation in patients with faecal incontinence: results of the first 100 permanent implantations. Colorectal Dis 2007;**9**:725–30.

53 **Kenefick NJ**. Sacral nerve neuromodulation for the treatment of lower bowel motility disorders. Ann R Coll Surg Engl 2006;**88**:617–23.

54 **Matzel KE, Kamm MA, Stosser M et al**. Sacral spinal nerve stimulation for faecal incontinence: multicentre study. Lancet 2004;**363**:1270–76.

55 **Jarrett ME, Mowatt G, Glazener CM et al**. Systematic review of sacral nerve stimulation for faecal incontinence and constipation. Br J Surg 2004;**91**:1559–69.

56 **Kenefick NJ, Nicholls RJ, Cohen RG, Kamm MA**. Permanent sacral nerve stimulation for treatment of idiopathic constipation. Br J Surg 2002;**89**:882–88.

57 **Malouf AJ, Wiesel PH, Nicholls T, Nicholls RJ, Kamm MA**. Short-term effects of sacral nerve stimulation for idiopathic slow transit constipation. World J Surg 2002;**26**:166–70.

58 **Ganio E, Masin A, Ratto C et al**. Short-term sacral nerve stimulation for functional anorectal and urinary disturbances: results in 40 patients: evaluation of a new option for anorectal functional disorders. Dis Colon Rectum 2001;**44**:1261–67.

59 **Uludag O, Koch SM, van Gemert WG, Dejong CH, Baeten CG**. Sacral neuromodulation in patients with fecal incontinence: a single-center study. Dis Colon Rectum 2004;**47**:1350–57.

60 **El-Gazzaz G, Zutshi M, Salcedo L, Hammel J, Rackley R, Hull T**. Sacral neuromodulation for the treatment of fecal incontinence and urinary incontinence in female patients: long-term follow-up. Int J Colorectal Dis 2009;**24**:1377–81.

61 **Butrick CW**. Pathophysiology of pelvic floor hypertonic disorders. Obstet Gynecol Clin North Am 2009;**36**:699–705.

62 **Leng WW, Chancellor MB**. How sacral nerve stimulation neuromodulation works. Urol Clin North Am 2005;**32**:11–18.

63 **Maher CF, Carey MP, Dwyer PL, Schluter PL**. Percutaneous sacral nerve root neuromodulation for intractable interstitial cystitis. J Urol 2001;**165**:884–86.

64 **Everaert K, Devulder J, De Muynck M et al**. The pain cycle: implications for the diagnosis and treatment of pelvic pain syndromes. Int Urogynecol J 2001;**12**:9–14.

65 **Groen J, Ruud Bosch JL, van Mastrigt R**. Sacral neuromodulation in women with idiopathic detrusor overactivity incontinence: decreased overactivity but unchanged bladder contraction strength and urethral resistance during voiding. J Urol 2006;**175**:1005–1009; discussion 1009.

66 **Sievert KD, Amend B, Gakis G et al**. Early sacral neuromodulation prevents urinary incontinence after complete spinal cord injury. Ann Neurol 2010;**67**:74–84.

67 **Blok BF**. Central pathways controlling micturition and urinary continence. Urology 2002;**59**:13–7.

68 **Dasgupta R, Critchley HD, Dolan RJ, Fowler CJ**. Changes in brain activity following sacral neuromodulation for urinary retention. J Urol 2005;**174**:2268–72.

69 **Blok BF, Groen J, Bosch JL, Veltman DJ, Lammertsma AA**. Different brain effects during chronic and acute sacral neuromodulation in urge incontinent patients with implanted neurostimulators. BJU Int 2006;**98**:1238–43.

70 **De Groat WC, Ryall RW**. Recurrent inhibition in sacral parasympathetic pathways to the bladder. J Physiol 1968;**196**:579–91.

71 **de Groat WC**. Mechanisms underlying recurrent inhibition in the sacral parasympathetic outflow to the urinary bladder. J Physiol 1976;**257**:503–13.

72 **DasGupta R, Fowler CJ**. Urodynamic study of women in urinary retention treated with sacral neuromodulation. J Urol 2004;**171**:1161–64.

73 **Kavia R, Dasgupta R, Critchley H, Fowler C, Griffiths D**. A functional magnetic resonance imaging study of the effect of sacral neuromodulation on brain responses in women with Fowler's syndrome. BJU Int 2010;**105**:366–72.

74 **Melzack R, Wall PD**. Pain mechanisms: a new theory. Science 1965;**150**:971–79.

75 **van der Pal F, Heesakkers JP, Bemelmans BL**. Current opinion on the working mechanisms of neuromodulation in the treatment of lower urinary tract dysfunction. Curr Opin Urol 2006;**16**:261–67.

76 **Bosch JL, Groen J**. Sacral nerve neuromodulation in the treatment of patients with refractory motor urge incontinence: long-term results of a prospective longitudinal study. J Urol 2000;**163**:1219–22.

77 **Hassouna MM, Siegel SW, Nyeholt AA et al**. Sacral neuromodulation in the treatment of urgency-frequency symptoms: a multicenter study on efficacy and safety. J Urol 2000;**163**:1849–54.

78 **Schmidt RA, Senn E, Tanagho EA**. Functional evaluation of sacral nerve root integrity. Report of a technique. Urology 1990;**35**:388–92.

79 **Janknegt RA, Weil EH, Eerdmans PH**. Improving neuromodulation technique for refractory voiding dysfunctions: two-stage implant. Urology 1997;**49**:358–62.

80 **Kessler TM, Madersbacher H, Kiss G**. Prolonged sacral neuromodulation testing using permanent leads: a more reliable patient selection method? Eur Urol 2005;**47**:660–65.

81 **Grunewald V, Hofner K, Thon WF, Kuczyk MA, Jonas U.** Sacral electrical neuromodulation as an alternative treatment option for lower urinary tract dysfunction. Restor Neurol Neurosci 1999;**14**:189–93.

82 **Schmidt RA.** Advances in genitourinary neurostimulation. Neurosurgery 1986;**19**:1041–44.

83 **Spinelli M, Giardiello G, Gerber M, Arduini A, van den Hombergh U, Malaguti S.** New sacral neuromodulation lead for percutaneous implantation using local anesthesia: description and first experience. J Urol 2003;**170**:1905–907.

84 **Spinelli M, Weil E, Ostardo E et al.** New tined lead electrode in sacral neuromodulation: experience from a multicentre European study. World J Urol 2005;**23**:225–29.

85 **Scheepens WA, Weil EH, van Koeveringe GA et al.** Buttock placement of the implantable pulse generator: a new implantation technique for sacral neuromodulation—a multicenter study. Eur Urol 2001;**40**:434–38.

86 **Bosch JL, Groen J.** Sacral (S3) segmental nerve stimulation as a treatment for urge incontinence in patients with detrusor instability: results of chronic electrical stimulation using an implantable neural prosthesis. J Urol 1995;**154**:504–507.

87 **Shaker HS, Hassouna M.** Sacral nerve root neuromodulation: an effective treatment for refractory urge incontinence. J Urol 1998;**159**:1516–19.

88 **Elabbady AA, Hassouna MM, Elhilali MM.** Neural stimulation for chronic voiding dysfunctions. J Urol 1994;**152**:2076–80.

89 **Thon WF, Baskin LS, Jonas U, Tanagho EA, Schmidt RA.** Neuromodulation of voiding dysfunction and pelvic pain. World J Urol 1991;**9**:138–41.

90 **Shaker HS, Hassouna M.** Sacral root neuromodulation in idiopathic nonobstructive chronic urinary retention. J Urol 1998;**159**:1476–78.

91 **Dasgupta R, Wiseman OJ, Kitchen N, Fowler CJ.** Long-term results of sacral neuromodulation for women with urinary retention. BJU Int 2004;**94**:335–37.

92 **Sutherland SE, Lavers A, Carlson A, Holtz C, Kesha J, Siegel SW.** Sacral nerve stimulation for voiding dysfunction: One institution's 11-year experience. Neurourol Urodyn 2007;**26**:19–28; discussion 36.

93 **Schultz-Lampel D.** Neurophysiologische Grundlagen und Klinische Anwendung der sakralen Neuromodulation zur Therapie der Blasenfunctionsstörungen: *Klinik für Urologie und Kinderurologie*. Wuppertal, Universität Witten/Herdecke 1997;1–280.

94 **Kaufmann S, Naumann CM, Hamann MF et al.** Unilateral vs bilateral sacral neuromodulation in pigs with formalin-induced detrusor hyperactivity. BJU Int 2009;**103**:260–63, 2009.

Chapter 16

Neuromodulation for faecal incontinence and constipation

Emma V. Carrington, Emma H. Horrocks, Charles Knowles, and Noel N. Thin

Key points

1 Sacral nerve stimulation (SNS) and percutaneous tibial nerve stimulation (PTNS) are effective treatments for faecal incontinence (FI).
2 SNS has some data on the treatment of chronic constipation (CC).
3 SNS may offer a >50% reduction of symptoms in 75–100% of patients with FI and an increase in stool frequency in 87% of patients with CC.
4 Clinical benefit of SNS in FI has been demonstrated in patients with varied disease aetiologies.
5 PTNS is an emerging minimally invasive form of neuromodulation with case series suggesting symptomatic improvement in up to 70% of patients with FI.

Introduction

Disease burden of faecal incontinence and chronic constipation

Faecal incontinence (FI) and chronic constipation (CC) have much in common: They are prevalent in Western populations, cause significant social and psychological disability, and consume considerable health resources. Further, they share a common broad pathophysiology, i.e. physiological disturbance of the normal process of defaecation. Until recently, it was under-appreciated that over 40% sufferers have co-existent symptoms of both FI and CC (1). For this reason, management strategies for these conditions have considerable overlap.

Varying degrees of FI are reported by 1–15% of UK adults outside nursing institutions (2, 3), that estimation allowing for a high degree of under-reporting as only 15–45% seek treatment (4, 5). Since prevalence and severity of FI increases with age (3, 4), it is likely that this condition will become a greater problem. Constipation is also common in both adults and children, and 20% of the population report this symptom at some point in their lives (2–28% adults; 0.7–30% children) (6, 7). Chronic constipation, usually defined as >6 months of persistent symptoms, is less common with a prevalence of 1–2% (8) and results in 0.5 million GP consultations per annum in the UK. Such patients, are usually female (9) and are referred to tertiary centres for specialist investigation. Nearly 80% of these patients feel that laxative therapy is unsatisfactory (10) and the effect of symptoms on quality of life (QoL) is significant (11).

Role of neuromodulation in the treatment algorithm of faecal incontinence and chronic constipation

Until the introduction of neuromodulation for bowel disorders, failure of conservative therapies (stool bulking ages, biofeedback, bowel retraining) invariably meant progression to invasive surgery. In the context of FI, this required repair of the sphincter complex (12–14), construction of a neosphincter (15), or formation of a permanent stoma (16). In the constipated patient, a colonic resection or permanent end stoma would be considered. The morbidity and failure rates associated with these strategies are significant (17, 18).

The advent of neuromodulation has offered a safer, more acceptable therapeutic option for these challenging patients. At present it is available in two forms, which will be considered separately: sacral nerve stimulation (SNS) and percutaneous tibial nerve stimulation (PTNS). Other neuromodulatory techniques such as pudendal nerve stimulation (PNS) are emerging and will be considered at the end of the chapter.

Sacral nerve stimulation

Direct electrical stimulation of the sacral nerve roots by SNS is a safe, effective, minimally invasive therapeutic option for FI patients failing non-interventional therapies, regardless of aetiology, e.g. sphincter injury, neurological impairment.

> Neuromodulation has offered a safer, more acceptable form of treatment for cases of severe faecal incontinence and chronic constipation unresponsive to conservative measures.

More recently, evidence has suggested effectiveness in patients with constipation (19). SNS is based on the concept that residual anorectal neuromuscular function pertinent to continence can be recruited by electrical stimulation of the contributing afferent and efferent nerve supplies. The first application of SNS to the management of functional bowel disorders was by Matzel in 1995 (20).

Patient selection and work-up

FI and CC occur secondary to a number of differing aetiologies (21) and patients present with a diverse constellation of symptoms. It is, therefore, recommended that patients should be assessed and managed in tertiary units with multidisciplinary teams available

(22). As no consensus has been reached regarding the degree of symptom severity necessary to warrant treatment with SNS, the decision to proceed should be based on clinical judgement of the effect of symptoms on the individual's quality of life and should be made together with the patient.

Specific absolute contraindications to treatment include: pregnancy or desire to become pregnant, and congenital malformations precluding placement of electrodes, e.g. sacral agenesis. Relative contraindications include: co-existent medical conditions requiring regular magnetic resonance scanning, participation in contact/high-impact sports, dermatological conditions affecting the implantation site, and psychological instability precluding permanent device implantation.

Pre-operative work up typically includes the performance of anorectal physiology and endoanal ultrasound, the findings of which may demonstrate pathologies better treated with an alternate approach (e.g. sphincter repair). In addition, antero-posterior and lateral view pelvic radiographs should be requested in patients who have previously undergone lumbar spinal fixation to exclude sacral neo-osteogenesis (23). Patients should then receive full pre-operative counselling outlining the implications of life with a permanent implant including the use of the hand held control.

Pre-operative work up for SNS should include anorectal physiology and endoanal ultrasound.

SNS has effectiveness in patients with both urge and passive predominant faecal incontinence. Although initial reports suggested that an intact external anal sphincter was a prerequisite for treatment, subsequent case series have suggested effectiveness in a number of underlying aetiologies, including: dysfunctional/disrupted anal sphincter (24), post-rectal resection syndrome (25), and partial spinal cord injury (26).

Case series' data suggest that SNS has effectiveness in FI secondary to several pathophysiologies.

With regard to the management of CC, case series' data suggest that SNS may be effective in treatment of slow transit constipation, normal transit constipation, and rectal evacuatory dysfunction (27).

Treatment technique

SNS typically follows a two-stage approach: a trial period of temporary stimulation with subsequent transfer to permanent stimulation, if an appropriate clinical response has been achieved (though it should be noted that there is no evidence for this).

Test stimulation

There are two methods of performing the test phase: the peripheral nerve evaluation (PNE) method and the staged approach. The PNE method uses a non-tined monopolar lead (3065USC; Medtronic, Minneapolis, Minnesota, USA) and can be performed under local anaesthetic (infiltration to the level of the sacral periosteum with care taken to avoid the sacral foramen preventing possible paralysis of the sacral nerve) with or without sedation (see Fig. 16.1).

The lead is inserted percutaneously through a needle introducer positioned in the appropriate sacral foramen (typically S3) using a Seldinger technique. During PNE, optimal electrode placement is ascertained by observation of pelvic floor contraction (lifting and tightening of the anus, known as the 'bellows' action) +/− flexion of the great toe. The external portion of the lead is connected to an extension wire and earth pad, both of which are secured with dressings. The extension wire is connected to an external pulse generator (3625; Medtronic). Stimulation is commenced the same day (stimulation parameters: 14 Hz frequency, pulse width 210 μs with amplitude controlled at a comfortable sub-sensory level by the patient, typically 1–3 mA).

Clinical response is assessed subjectively and with a 2-week bowel diary, with success typically defined as a ≥50% reduction in weekly FI episodes. Following cessation of the test period, the lead is removed in the outpatient setting.

The PNE method is widely practiced but poses the significant disadvantage that, should a second-stage implant be warranted, placement of a new lead is required and replication of the exact position may be difficult.

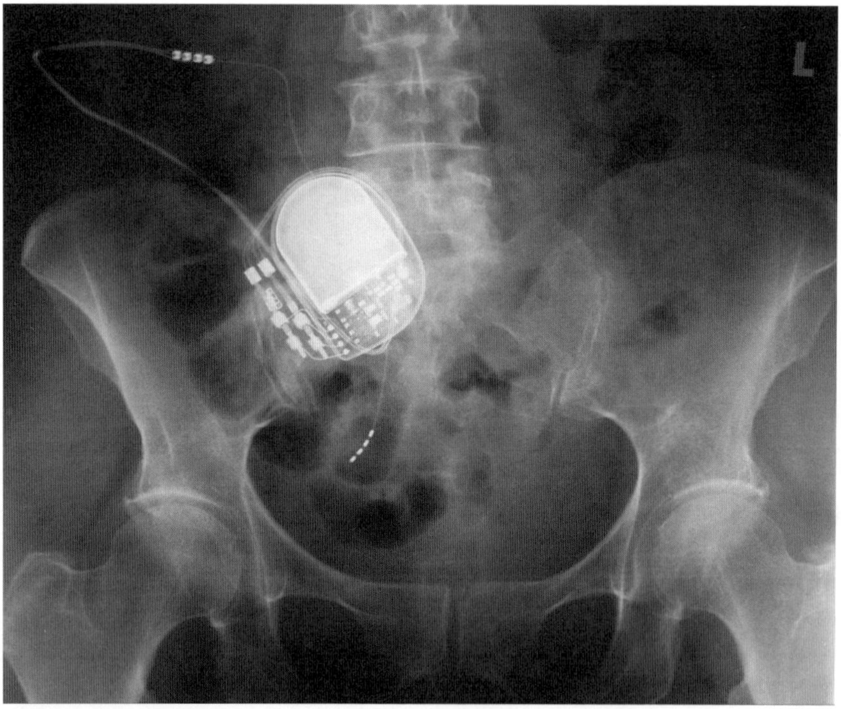

Fig. 16.1 Pelvic radiograph of sacral nerve stimulator *in situ*.
Reproduced courtesy of Medtronic.

An alternative test method uses the tined quadripolar lead (3093–28; Medtronic). This may be considered the first of a two-stage procedure. It requires more surgical skill than the PNE approach. The tined lead is barbed, thus allowing permanent implantation, as it anchors to the sacrum on passage through the sacral foramen. Before implantation the tined lead is soaked in an antibiotic solution to prevent bacterial colonization. Insertion of the tined lead is also performed under local anaesthetic with sedation.

First, an introducing needle is used to locate the optimum response from the sacral nerve. The guide wire is placed using a Seldinger technique. The depth of the introducer is assessed with fluoroscopy to ensure safe and accurate positioning of the lead. Following this, the lead is tunnelled sub-cutaneously to a small pocket created in the ipsilateral buttock. This pocket will house an interconnector to an exteriorized wire that connects to the external stimulator (3625; Medtronic). As the leads are sub-cutaneously tunnelled, infection risk is decreased, allowing the testing phase to be lengthened to 6 weeks.

The advantages of the tined lead are:

1 It allows the patient a more accurate representation of the improvement that could be expected from the permanent system.

2 The placement of the lead remains constant.

The disadvantages are:

1 A small surgical procedure is required to remove the tined lead if the test stimulation phase is not successful.

2 The tined lead is more expensive then the unipolar lead.

This approach requires careful planning to avoid unnecessary delays to the second stage of the procedure.

Permanent stimulation

If PNE has been carried out previously, the unilateral percutaneous insertion of a permanent tined lead (3093–28; Medtronic) and implantable pulse generator (IPG) (3023; Medtonic) is required. This may be performed under local anaesthesia with sedation or under a general anaesthetic. Where possible, the permanent lead should be inserted in the same sacral foramen as the temporary lead. The technique for the insertion of the tined lead is the same as already described. After correct insertion and positioning of the lead, a sub-cutaneous tunnel is created allowing the lead to be connected to the IPG. The IPG is then placed in a sub-cutaneous pocket in the ipsilateral buttock. There must be a concerted effort to get the size and depth of the sub-cutaneous pocket right. Too large and the IPG may rotate, too shallow and it will be uncomfortable for the patient, too deep and it will be difficult for the patient to use with their hand held controller (3037; Medtronic). It is also important to ensure the IPG is not located on the gluteal epimysium, and to ensure that the lead is tucked deep to the implant before closure, as this protects the lead in the event that an IPG replacement is necessary.

If the tined lead is already in position, then the second-stage procedure is simpler. The sub-cutaneous pocket already fashioned can be re-opened and the interconnector located.

The interconnector and externalized wire can be removed and the free end of the lead attached to the IPG. Once the implant has been inserted, stimulation can be commenced the same day using similar stimulation parameters as previously. Prophylactic intra-operative antibiotics may be given at induction with subsequent post-operative cover.

Complications include bleeding, wound or lead infection, sleep disturbance, perineal or leg pain, and lead displacement or damage (28). The implant should not be visible and does not restrict normal activities, although rigorous activities should be avoided for the first 6 weeks.

Clinical outcomes

Faecal incontinence

Five systematic reviews (29–33) and 26 review articles exist on SNS in the treatment of FI. There is also a single meta-analysis (34). Studies demonstrate that the majority of patients with successful PNE progress to successful permanent implantation in the medium term. Interpretation is limited by a paucity of high-quality trial evidence and the use of varied outcome measures. A predominance of case series and the possibility of selection bias mean a placebo effect still cannot be confidently excluded. In addition, treatment success has not been reported on an intention-to-treat basis (with most studies reporting successful progression from temporary to permanent, rather than baseline to permanent treatment) resulting in a possible over-estimation of effect.

There is now 15 years of experience with SNS, so long-term results are emerging (35, 36). Table 16.1 comprises the largest case series of SNS to date.

Quality of life after permanent SNS

The most commonly utilized QoL measures are the American Society of Colon and Rectal Surgeons (ASCRS) Faecal Incontinence Quality of Life (FIQL) (disease-specific), and the generic Social Function 36 (SF-36) questionnaires. A recent review (43) of larger case series (more than 10 patients), showed that 12 studies used the ASCRS FIQL score and 9 studies used the SF-36 scores to assess the medium- and long-term effects of SNS. These studies agreed that the frequency of involuntary stool loss and clinical scores were significantly improved in all patients after SNS therapy, resulting in overall improvements of QoL scores in both the medium and long term. The magnitude of improvement in QoL outcomes diminishes, however, in the longer term for both disease-specific and generic QoL measures, and this is particularly evident in the social and mental domains. Disease-specific QoL assessments mirrored improvements in clinical continence measures much more closely than the generic QoL measures (44). There is, however, still a paucity of evidence regarding long-term QoL assessments to determine the effectiveness of SNS in the treatment of FI. Furthermore, there is no consensus on the best QoL assessment tool in post-SNS patients, making meaningful comparisons between studies difficult, although the FIQL and SF-36 scores are by far the most widely reported.

Table 16.1 Summary treatment success as reported by the largest case series (>100 permanent SNS implants). Derived success rate calculated by the authors on an intention-to-treat basis

Primary author	Year	Number of recruited patients	Number of permanent implants	Follow-up (months)	Reported success rate (%)	Derived success rate (%)
Melenhorst (37)	2007	134	100	26[a]	79[d]	59[d]
Govaert (38)	2009	245	173	35[a]	77[d]	53[d]
Michelsen (35)	2010	167	126	36[b]	81[e]	52[e]
Maeda (39)	2011	245	176	33[c]	63[f]	44[f]
Mellgren (40)	2011	133	120	36[b]	86[d]	59[d]
Duelund-Jakobsen (41)	2011	n/s	158	46[c]	75[d]	n/s[d]
Gallas (42)	2011	n/s	200	6[b]	54[g]	n/s[g]
Summary: median (range)			**158 (100–200)**	**35 (6–46)**	**77 (54–86)**	**53 (44–59)**

KEY: [a]mean values (integer values), [b]values taken at time point, [c]median ITT: intention to treat, n/s not specified.

Success based on:

[d]>50% improvement in FI episodes / week.

[e]Decrease in Cleveland Clinic Incontinence Score.

[f]Good or acceptable outcome.

[g]>30% improvement in Cleveland Clinic Incontinence Score.

Chronic constipation

SNS is considered the first-line invasive procedure for patients failing conservative approaches for FI (45), but its roles in treating other lower GI and pelvic disorders, such as chronic pain (46) and chronic constipation (CC), are less established.

There is now a greater understanding that disordered defecation is often the sum of several disturbances to anorectal and colonic physiology. It is thought that SNS, therefore, is likely to affect changes in motor and/or sensory function of the colon, rectum, and anus common to the pathophysiologies of FI and CC, thus explaining the often cited 'paradox' of SNS effectiveness in both these conditions. SNS has clear advantages over more radical surgical alternatives for CC such as colectomy (47, 48); however, the high costs, while competitive in respect of utility analyses for FI (49), will be a source of obvious concern for health providers treating CC.

A recently published European study of SNS on 62 patients with CC (mixed pathophysiologies) (19) has shown a favourable 63% success rate on intent to treat. A recent study by Govaert et al. (50), with the largest series (117 patients) and longest follow-up (median 37 months) to date, also had a similar success rate of 52%; however, these data have not been replicated by others (51–53). Some data exist to support the use of SNS in patients with rectal evacuatory dysfunction (ED). A placebo-controlled cross-over trial of temporary SNS in the treatment of 13 patients with ED demonstrated improvement in clinical outcomes and Wexner constipation scores (27). Another study of SNS in CC included a cohort of patients (58% of 19) with rectal outlet obstruction. This study did not, however, present the results according to pre-operative pathophysiology (slow transit constipation (STC), ED, or both) other than to note that SNS had no symptomatic effect on either of the two patients with combined STC-ED (53). The study was also limited to the temporary phase of treatment.

PNE is in effect a screening stage of a two-stage treatment protocol and is considered (without statistical proof) to have reasonable utility in terms of predicting eventual outcome in patients with urinary problems or FI (45). Some studies suggest, however, that PNE is significantly less accurate as a screening tool in patients with CC, with less than 50% patients screened positive going on to successful permanent stimulation (51) (Table 16.2). Failure of test stimulation to accurately predict eventual outcome poses a major barrier to the viability of SNS as a treatment for CC from both patient benefit and economic perspectives. Whether this is due to the generally high placebo responses observed in trials of CC (54, 55), the greater influence of psychological comorbidities (56), or the need for more critical lead positioning is unknown.

Table 16.2 Summary of constipation treatment success as reported by the largest case series (>10 permanent SNS implants). Derived success rate calculated by the authors on an intention-to-treat bases

Primary author	Year	Number of recruited patients	N perm	Median Follow-up (months)	Reported success (%)	Derived success (%)
Kamm (19)	2010	62	45	28	87[a]	63[a]
Maeda (52)	2010	70	38	26	n/s	50[b]
Carriero (56)	2010	13	11	22	n/s	85[c]
Sharma (57)	2011	21	11	34	n/s	48[d]
Govaert (50)	2012	117	68	37	n/s	52[b]
van Wunnik (58)	2012	13	12	7	92[b]	92[b]
Knowles (27)	2012	13	11	19	82[b]	69[b]
Summary: medians (ranges)				26 (7–37)	87 (82–92)	63 (48–92)

KEY:

Success based on:

[a]Improvement in any one of: (1) bowel frequency changing from two or less to three or more evacuations per week; (2) a ≥50% reduction in the proportion of defecation episodes associated with straining; or (3) a ≥50% reduction in the proportion of defecation episodes associated with a sense of incomplete evacuation.

[b]Maintained clinical benefit and continuation of treatment.

[c]Improvement in the bowel movements per week of ≥50% and a decreased need of laxatives and received permanent implant.

[d]Patients with ≥50% improvement in bowel diaries.

Physiological outcomes

The question of how SNS works is a complex subject that can be approached by considering how a field of electrons influences conduction of action potentials within a mixed spinal nerve (59) or by a pragmatic approach that observes the effects on end-organ function.

Studies to date have predominantly focused on the end-organ effects of SNS. It is increasingly appreciated that SNS is likely to work not only by providing peripheral motor stimulation to the anal sphincter in patients with FI, but rather by affecting changes in motor and/or sensory function of the anus, rectum, and colon. SNS, therefore, is likely to be effective for both FI and constipation, not due to paradoxical actions in these conditions, but because it normalizes or improves pathophysiology or pathophysiologies that are common to both. The effects of SNS on rectal and anal physiological function have been studied mostly in case series. They are considered separately below.

Rectal motor effects

The role of the rectum as a responsive storage vessel in terms of its capacity, distensibility, and compliance is paramount for effective evacuatory function. Nevertheless, due to the relative complexity of techniques to study rectal wall dynamics and motor function, data are limited to three recent studies. Significant increases in rectal volume tolerability and rectal capacity were shown in two of these (60, 61). A further study demonstrated that SNS reduced postprandial changes in rectal tone but did not affect phasic rectal motility (62). More detailed studies utilizing prolonged ambulatory recording methods to measure diurnal and nocturnal motor activities are required.

Rectal sensory effects

The impact of abnormal rectal sensation on the development of defecatory symptoms is being increasingly appreciated and it is now accepted that rectal hypo- and hypersensitivity are associated with both FI and CC (63–67). Unfortunately, close examination of the literature reveals that inadequate reporting limits interpretation of the large number of case series examining sensory changes following treatment (68).

As both impaired and heightened sensitivity are important in FI, it is prudent to look for normalization of sensory thresholds within individuals or specific subgroups thus defined, rather than changes in average value. Unfortunately this has not been the case and the majority of studies analyse significantly hyper- and hyposensate patients together, i.e. physiologically significant changes may have occurred in subgroups but have been masked by an apparently constant mathematical mean.

Despite this, evidence for sensory modulation exists: first, in a double-blind, placebo-controlled, randomized trial of SNS in constipated patients with rectal hyposensitivity—during which a normalization of sensory thresholds was found concomitant with symptomatic improvement (27). Similar findings were demonstrated in a group of patients with post-anterior resection. In this study, neorectal sensation normalized during treatment with SNS, i.e. those with hyposensitivity showed a reduction in sensory thresholds and vice versa for those with hypersensitivity (69).

Experimental studies seem to support this afferent-predominant hypothesis. A study of electromyographic latencies following SNS electrode insertion in patients with urological dysfunction suggested longer latencies than would be expected if the actions of SNS were motor-mediated (70). Such changes may be mediated by alterations in neurotransmitter expression as previously shown in patients with FI (71).

Evidence suggests that modulation of rectal sensation may underlie the mechanism of action of SNS; however, poor data-reporting makes interpretation of case series' data difficult.

Other rectal effects

The effect of SNS on local efferent autonomic neuronal function has also been studied using laser Doppler mucosal blood flow. This demonstrated an increase in mucosal blood flow during periods of stimulation (72), which the authors suggested was likely to reflect increased net parasympathetic activity.

Anal motor effects

The fact that correct electrode placement is commonly confirmed via observation of the 'anal twitch', initially led to the widespread belief that the mechanism of SNS was one primarily of peripheral motor neurostimulation. This was supported by initial reports of augmentation of anal sphincter function (mainly squeeze) in patients undergoing temporary stimulation for FI (73–75). Although this has subsequently been questioned in the light of several studies attesting otherwise, some recent large studies from well-established investigators do appear to confirm these earlier findings (37, 76).

The effects of SNS on anal motor function have not been demonstrated conclusively.

Despite this, the majority of larger studies do not report significantly augmented sphincter function, with the exception of a single large case series (37) who demonstrated an increase in anal squeeze pressures maintained for 24 months. Again, however, this area is confounded by population heterogeneity and the need for confidence that measurements of anal sphincter pressures correlate reliably with symptomatology. In particular, several groups have reported significant changes in means and confidence intervals that would lie (before and after SNS) within most published normal parameters of anal pressures (77). Thus whether such changes are clinically significant must be questioned. Finally, when considering anal motor effects as the primary mechanism of action, it is vital to appreciate that SNS has been more recently shown to benefit patients with significant sphincter defects (24, 78, 79).

An interesting adjunct is the demonstration of a reduction in cortico-anal excitability after SNS (without change in anal pressures) through the use of transcranial magnetic stimulation (80). The authors postulated that this central inhibitory change may be secondary to reduced sphincter attention in response to an improvement in volitional control.

Anal sensory effects

Only one study has specifically sought changes in perianal (and perineal) sensation during treatment with SNS (74). In a cohort of patients predominantly with neurologically induced faecal incontinence, qualitative assessment suggested that the most consistent observation was one of improved anal sensation. Further, the finding that SNS can improve idiopathic anal pain perhaps supports an anal sensory effect (although the origin of pain in these patients is not necessarily the anus) (81). Certainly, it is tempting to postulate that normalization of anal sensation could contribute to improved discrimination during anal sampling and thus leading to improvements in continence.

Percutaneous tibial nerve stimulation

Percutaneous tibial nerve stimulation (PTNS) is increasingly recognized as a new treatment modality for FI. The concept is that via stimulation of the tibial nerve, similar changes in anorectal neuromuscular function can be achieved as with SNS without the need for a permanent surgically implanted device. It was first described in 1983 by McGuire in patients with urinary incontinence using a transcutaneous electrode over the common peroneal or posterior tibial nerve, producing data suggesting long-term effectiveness (82). The method was adjusted by Stoller in 1999, through the use of a percutaneous needle with a ground electrode on the ipsilateral extremity (83). In 2003, Shafik proposed using PTNS for FI and achieved a reported 78% functional success in 32 patients (84).

Patient selection and work-up

PTNS is a minimally invasive outpatient therapy. Adult patients with faecal incontinence from any aetiology, including those with a sphincter defect, may be considered for treatment. Prior assessment with anorectal physiology, endoanal ultrasound, or defecating proctography is helpful but not mandatory. Similar to the work up for SNS, patients should be selected by a suitable specialist with clinical experience of functional bowel disorders, and patients should have failed basic conservative measures, such as dietary advice and medications. There are few contraindications to the PTNS, however, these include: the presence of a pacemaker or implantable defibrillator, bleeding disorders, the presence of a painful or total peripheral neuropathy (which may result in over or under stimulation), and patients who are pregnant or intending to become pregnant whilst receiving the treatment. Prior to commencement of PTNS, patients should be counselled regarding expectations and should be willing and able to attend for 12 weekly sessions of therapy.

PTNS is a minimally invasive, outpatient form of neuromodulation for the treatment of faecal incontinence.

Treatment technique

PTNS is delivered using the Urgent ® PC neuromodulation system (Uroplasty Ltd. Manchester, UK) (85–87). The PTNS stimulator is a reusable external pulse generator that provides visual and auditory feedback. It has an adjustable current setting from 0–9 mA in pre-set 0.5-mA increments, a fixed-pulse frequency of 20 Hz and a pulse width of 200 μs. Therapy is given for a period of 12 weeks, in weekly 30-minute sessions, though there is some flexibility with regard to this. Following the 12 initial treatments, some patients may need occasional 'top-up' sessions to sustain symptom relief. Side-effects include occasional tenderness at the site of needle insertion (85, 86).

The site of needle insertion is identified at a location on the lower inner aspect of either leg, three finger-breaths (5 cm) cephalad to the medial malleolus and one finger-breadth (2 cm) posterior to the tibia. The area is cleaned with ethanol and the needle electrode-guide tube assembly placed over the identified insertion site at a 60-degree angle between electrode and ankle. The 34-gauge needle electrode is gently tapped to pierce the skin and thence advanced using a rotating motion approximately 2 cm. The lead wire is connected to the needle and the calcaneal reference electrode placed on the ipsilateral calcaneus. The lead wire is then connected to the Urgent PC stimulator box.

The setting for therapy is determined by increasing the current whilst observing the patient's response. An appropriate response is the perception of a stimulus down into the foot or toe, or a motor response of the foot or ankle. Once the appropriate level for therapy is found, the 30-minute treatment is given (see Fig. 16.2).

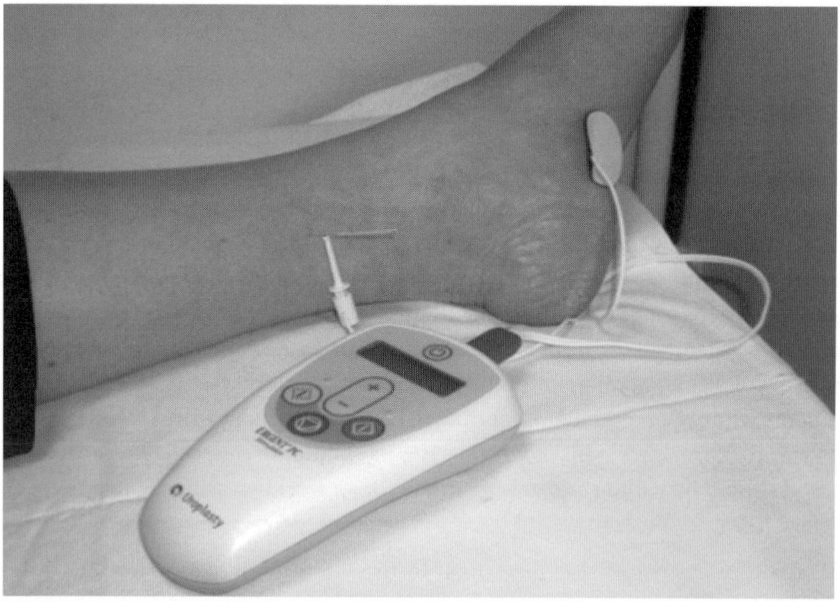

Fig. 16.2 Percutaneous tibial nerve stimulation.

Clinical outcomes

There are 12 studies examining the outcomes of tibial nerve stimulation for the treatment of FI published between 2003 and 2011, with series between 2 and 100 patients with FI from various aetiologies (total 309 patients). All studies are non-randomized case series, with one study including a control group for comparison (84). Of these studies, eight use PTNS, with either the Uroplasty Urgent PC or with the Stoller Afferent Nerve Stimulator (SANS; Urosurge, Coralville. Iowa), and four use transcutaneous tibial nerve stimulation, using TENS over the site of the tibial nerve (88–91). For the purposes of this chapter, we will consider only the studies that use PTNS.

Direct comparisons between the studies are difficult due to the heterogeneity of treatment protocols, outcome measures, and follow-up. Treatment regimens differ significantly between the different studies. Though all groups use 30-minute treatment sessions, session frequency ranges from alternate days to once weekly, and the duration from 1 month to 8 months, often with additional sessions for those who have had perceived success (92). Outcome measures also vary considerably and include: Wexner scores (a FI symptom severity score (93)); bowel diaries; analogue scales of perception of success; QoL measures; ability to defer defecation; and changes in end-organ function using techniques such as anorectal manometry. Follow-up duration of the patients ranges from 0 to 29 months following treatment cessation. Since Wexner scores and bowel diaries were the main determinants of treatment success, these have been discussed later.

The Wexner score was used as an outcome measure in seven of these studies, though reported in different ways, making comparison between these studies difficult. Two studies reported 65 and 81% of patients, respectively, had some improvement following treatment but the size of this improvement was not quantified (86, 92). A further four studies showed the mean Wexner score for the whole patient group improved (84, 94–96). One study reported that immediately after treatment, 38% of patients had a ≥50% reduction in Wexner Score (92). The reader should note in the studies that quote changes in the overall group mean, the individual patient experience may not be accurately represented. Further studies examining individual changes in symptom severity are required.

Two studies ($n = 22$ and $n = 31$) measured treatment success as the percentage of patients who achieved a ≥50% decrease in FI episodes per week (86, 96) and report 63.4 and 71% achievement, respectively. In one study, 12 of the 31 patients were reported fully continent following treatment (86). Interpretation of other studies using bowel diaries as a measure of treatment success is difficult as they have presented data as mean or improvements, rather than individual patient data (92, 94, 95).

Six studies collected data on QoL (86, 92, 95–98). This ranged from visual analogue scales to formal questionnaires. All showed improvement, but were mostly expressed as mean values over the whole group, with some domains reaching significance.

The long-term data relating to the effects of PTNS on symptoms are limited; however, there is the suggestion that treatment effect may be long-lasting, with one study demonstrating a >50% reduction in number of episodes of faecal incontinence in 31% of patients at 11 months (92).

Some studies have looked at different FI aetiologies in an attempt to classify success of PTNS. One study, of 88 females, reports no correlation between sphincter morphology and PTNS outcome, and no correlation between rectal sensation and PTNS outcome (94). Another study attempts to classify the effect of PTNS in patients with urge, passive, and mixed faecal incontinence (95). It seems that the median number of weekly FI episodes is significantly reduced in patients with urge and mixed FI, but not passive FI. Similarly, it seems the improvement in mean Wexner score is significant in patients with urge and mixed FI, but not passive FI. Again raw data and individual patient experiences are not alluded to, making these results difficult to interpret.

To date there are no data pertaining to the use of PTNS in chronic constipation.

Direct comparison between studies examining treatment effect of PTNS is difficult; however, case series suggest a symptomatic improvement in most patients.

Physiological outcomes

There are no studies in the literature regarding mechanism of action of PTNS in patients with faecal incontinence. The hypothesis of PTNS is based on its presumed similarity to SNS, since the tibial nerve contains afferent and efferent fibres and originates from the 4th, and 5th lumbar and 1st, 2nd, and 3rd sacral nerves, the same spinal nerves that innervate the bladder and rectum (99). Extrapolation from SNS would point to both sensory and motor neuromodulatory effects (68). Many of the publications on the clinical effectiveness of PTNS comment on the proposed mechanisms of action, but these too are mostly based on studies of SNS, citing examples such as altering sensation in the rectum, up-regulating the striated muscle function of the external sphincter, and reduction in detrimental spontaneous anal relaxations and rectal contractions (61, 74, 84, 92, 100–102). However, no studies have shown any convincing change in anorectal physiology tests (84, 92).

Experimental studies have mainly concentrated on the afferent mediated effects of PTNS. A study of the effect of electrical stimulation over the tibial nerve in the rat demonstrated an increase in the peak amplitude of primary cortical evoked potentials by 45.1% (103). This is supported in a clinical study for the treatment of over-active bladder. Treatment was associated with an increase in long latency somatosensory evoked potentials, whereas placebo was not (104). A further study suggested that PTNS inhibited bladder activity by depolarizing somatic sacral and lumbar afferent fibres (105).

Few data exist pertaining to the mechanism of action of PTNS; however, experimental studies suggest an afferent predominant modulation of neuronal function.

Pudendal nerve stimulation

Pudendal nerve stimulation (PNS) is a relatively well-documented treatment for voiding dysfunctions. The first evidence of its use in FI was reported by Matzel et al. in 2005 (106), with the first published paper by Bock et al. in 2010.

PNS offers an alternative neuromodulatory option in those who have failed SNS, or those who cannot undergo SNS, as they do not fulfil guidelines, e.g. anatomical anomalies or spinal lesions (32, 107–109). Results of a study on voiding dysfunction even suggest that PNS is superior to SNS in treating this disorder (110). It has also been suggested that the voltage amplitude required for PNS therapy may be less than that in SNS therapy for some patients, meaning battery life will be longer and avoiding such frequent generator exchange (111).

PNS may provide an alternative neuromodulatory option to SNS in FI.

Patient selection and work-up

There are no guidelines on the requirement for patient selection or work-up when using PNS in the treatment of FI, as publications are limited to feasibility studies and small case series. It seems appropriate though that since PNS uses the same equipment as in SNS (Medtronic, Minneapolis), similar cautions should be used. The authors suggest PNS should only be used by practitioners experienced in the treatment of FI and the technique of PNS, and in the setting of close monitoring, e.g. closely audited or research study, in order that efficacy and adverse events can be appropriately monitored. It seems prudent that patient selection should be based on those in whom FI is refractory to conservative measures, and those who fully understand and consent to this treatment, whose efficacy is not fully understood. Contraindications to treatment should be similar to those for SNS, including: pregnancy or desire to become pregnant, and congenital malformations precluding placement of electrodes. Relative contraindications should include: co-existent medical conditions requiring regular magnetic resonance scanning, participation in contact/high-impact sports, dermatological conditions affecting the implantation site, and psychological instability precluding permanent device implantation.

Treatment technique

The original technique described by Spinelli et al. in the treatment of neurogenic bladder has been modified by the two publications in FI (107). We will detail here the most recent modification by George et al. (109), where the procedure is carried out on patients in the prone position with 30-degree hip flexion and 30-degree knee flexion, and the buttocks taped apart, under general anaesthesia with no muscle relaxation. Insertion of the neurostimulator is a one- or two-stage procedure, in a similar way to SNS, depending on whether a 'test-stimulation period' is adopted. If being carried out as a one-stage procedure, the neurostimulator is inserted at this operation, and if a two-stage procedure is being adopted, the initial neurostimulator is an external preliminary one, which is replaced for an internal definitive one at the second operation.

First the surface marking of the ischial spine is identified by drawing a horizontal line through the level of the greater trochanters of the femur and a vertical line through the ischial tuberosity. Where these two lines bisect marks the anatomical location of the ischial spine. These landmarks can be confirmed using fluoroscopic guidance. A blunt lead introducer (Medtronic model 35550–18), consisting of a rigid metal obturator for peripheral nerve evaluation in a plastic sheath, can then be inserted through a small 5-mm incision over the landmark for the ischial spine, and using a gloved finger inside the anal canal, this can be directed towards the ischial spine. At this anatomical location, the pudendal nerve is running in the pudendal (Alcock's) canal and is a relatively isolated structure. Once satisfactory placement of the lead introducer is felt at the ischial spine, a stimulation wire (Medtronic, Inc.041831) can then be connected to the metal obturator and to the external neurostimulator (Medtronic model 3652). The neurostimulator is then set to a standard SNS pulse width of 210 μs and a frequency of 14 Hz and initially 5 V. The stimulator is then activated, whilst palpating with a gloved finger in the anal canal to feel for contraction of the anal sphincter, signifying correct electrode placement. If no contraction is felt, the needle tip can be repositioned until a response is obtained. The voltage of the neurostimulator can then gradually be reduced in 1-V increments until the minimum voltage required for adequate contraction is reached. A barbed quadripolar 'tined' lead (Medtronic 3093) can then be introduced via the sheath and connected to an extension lead (Medtronic 3093 extension kit) and pulse generator: external preliminary (Medtronic model 3625) or internal definitive (Medtronic model 3058). A final check of lead placement can then be made at the end of the procedure by assessing anal sphincter contraction as before. This technique was modified from that used by Bock et al. by the introduction of a blunt needle introducer in the place of the 20-gauge insulated needle (Medtronic model 141,829), which is sharp, in an attempt to reduce the risk of accidental damage to other structures. For permanent stimulation, the lead is tunnelled sub-cutaneously and the neurostimulator is buried, as with SNS.

Clinical outcomes

There are two publications regarding PNS in the treatment of FI. The first reports successful treatment of two patients who had failed SNS, both of whom remained completely continent at 4 months following permanent implantation (111). The second study reports results of 20 patients, of whom 7 had FI with failed SNS, and the remaining 13 had 'bowel dysfunction secondary to a complete cauda equina lesion' (109). Of these 20 patients, 14 had ≥50% reduction of symptoms during the temporary testing phase, and went on to have permanent implants, with one of these suffering loss of efficacy due to lead migration, thus resulting in a 65% success rate of treatment in this study. The authors note that there is currently a trial recruiting in Switzerland comparing SNS to PNS in patients with faecal incontinence, by means of a double-blind cross-over study. This may help add to the literature surrounding this treatment modality.

Very little literature exists to support the use of PNS in FI, and further studies are awaited prior to this comprising a viable treatment option.

Physiological outcomes

There are no published studies reporting the mechanism of action of PNS in FI or in urological disorders. The pudendal nerve is a mixed somatic and autonomic nerve, which is derived from the ventral rami of the S2, S3, and S4 nerve roots. It divides into the inferior rectal nerve, the perineal nerves, and the dorsal nerve of the penis or clitoris. It is the inferior rectal nerve that supplies the external anal sphincter. The mechanism by which pudendal nerve stimulation affects FI is not understood but it could be as a result of direct motor stimulation to the anal sphincter or a result of central effects on the somatic or autonomic nervous system (109, 111).

There are no publications in the literature pertaining to the use of PNS in constipation.

Conclusions

The advent of neuromodulation has revolutionized the treatment of faecal incontinence. SNS, PTNS, and PNS have provided the clinician with minimally invasive surgical options for the management of cases that previously would have proceeded to invasive, irreversible sphincter surgery or stoma formation. In particular, the introduction of PTNS has demonstrated clinical benefit in patients unfit for surgical intervention. As the prevalence of FI increases with age and infirmity, such outpatient modalities are likely to become increasingly sought after.

Case series exist detailing clinical effectiveness, in particular, for SNS are encouraging and suggest good outcomes. However, there remains a real need for adequately powered, robustly conducted randomized studies and a move towards reporting outcomes on an intention-to-treat basis.

The mechanistic effects of neuromodulation remain unclear, and interpretation of data is limited by differences in techniques employed, varied outcome of reporting, and lack of robust study design. The initial presumption of motor stimulation of the anal sphincter has now been superseded by the hypothesis of a mixed effect on anal motor and rectal sensory functioning. Experimental research on the effects of SNS on pelvic afferent signalling, spinal and cortical processing are required to gain an overall picture of the effects of these techniques.

The reported successes aside, there remain significant limitations in the current practice of neuromodulation and there is a continued on-going need to optimize therapy. It should be remembered that, in SNS, a significant number of patients fail temporary stimulation (approximately 25%) with a further 25% initially responding to temporary stimulation but having little lasting effect of a permanent implant. The latter group will almost certainly contain some placebo responders to temporary stimulation; however, failures in both groups may be due to poor electrode positioning and poor patient selection.

Ultimately, improvements in the understanding of the normal process of defecation and the actions of neuromodulation are required to provide the basis for improved patient selection. This will enable treatment tailored to pathophysiologically defined patient subgroups, allowing the optimization of this promising treatment modality.

References

1 **Burgell RE, Bhan C, Lunniss PJ.** Fecal incontinence in men: co-existent constipation and impact of rectal hyposensitivity. Gastroenterology 2010;**138**.

2 **Nelson RL.** Epidemiology of fecal incontinence. Gastroenterology 2004 Jan;**126**(1 Suppl. 1):S3–7.

3 **Perry S, Shaw C, McGrother C et al.** Prevalence of faecal incontinence in adults aged 40 years or more living in the community. Gut 2002 Apr;**50**(4):480–84.

4 **Edwards NI, Jones D.** The prevalence of faecal incontinence in older people living at home. Age Ageing 2001 Nov;**30**(6):503–07.

5 **Johanson JF, Lafferty J.** Epidemiology of fecal incontinence: the silent affliction. Am J Gastroenterol. 1996 Jan;**91**(1):33–36.

6 **Stewart WF, Liberman JN, Sandler RS et al.** Epidemiology of constipation (EPOC) study in the United States: relation of clinical subtypes to sociodemographic features. Am J Gastroenterol. 1999 Dec;**94**(12):3530–40.

7 **McCrea GL, Miaskowski C, Stotts NA, Macera L, Hart SA, Varma MG.** Review article: self-report measures to evaluate constipation. Aliment Pharmacol Ther 2008 Apr;**27**(8):638–48.

8 **Cook IJ, Talley NJ, Benninga MA, Rao SS, Scott SM.** Chronic constipation: overview and challenges. Neurogastroent Motil: the official journal of the European Gastrointestinal Motility Society. 2009 Dec;**21** Suppl 2:1–8. [Review]

9 **Knowles CH, Scott SM, Rayner C et al.** Idiopathic slow-transit constipation: an almost exclusively female disorder. Dis Colon Rectum 2003 Dec;**46**(12):1716–17.

10 **Wald A, Scarpignato C, Mueller-Lissner S et al.** A multinational survey of prevalence and patterns of laxative use among adults with self-defined constipation. Aliment Pharmacol Ther 2008 Oct 1;**28**(7):917–30.

11 **Irvine EJ, Ferrazzi S, Pare P, Thompson WG, Rance L.** Health-related quality of life in functional GI disorders: focus on constipation and resource utilization. Am J Gastroenterol 2002 Aug;**97**(8):1986–93.

12 **Malouf AJ, Norton CS, Engel AF, Nicholls RJ, Kamm MA.** Long-term results of overlapping anterior anal-sphincter repair for obstetric trauma. Lancet 2000 Jan 22;**355**(9200):260–65.

13 **Fang DT, Nivatvongs S, Vermeulen FD, Herman FN, Goldberg SM, Rothenberger DA.** Overlapping sphincteroplasty for acquired anal incontinence. Dis Colon Rectum 1984 Nov;**27**(11):720–22.

14 **Oliveira L, Pfeifer J, Wexner SD.** Physiological and clinical outcome of anterior sphincteroplasty. Br J Surg 1996 Apr;**83**(4):502–05.

15 **Williams NS, Ogunbiyi OA, Scott SM, Fajobi O, Lunniss PJ.** Rectal augmentation and stimulated gracilis anal neosphincter: a new approach in the management of fecal urgency and incontinence. Dis Colon Rectum 2001 Feb;**44**(2):192–98.

16 **Madoff RD, Williams JG, Caushaj PF.** Fecal incontinence. N Engl J Med 1992 Apr 9;**326**(15):1002–07.

17 **Yoshioka K, Keighley MR.** Sphincter repair for fecal incontinence. Dis Colon Rectum 1989 Jan;**32**(1):39–42.

18 **Nikiteas N, Korsgen S, Kumar D, Keighley MR.** Audit of sphincter repair. Factors associated with poor outcome. Dis Colon Rectum 1996 Oct;**39**(10):1164–70.

19 **Kamm MA, Dudding TC, Melenhorst J et al.** Sacral nerve stimulation for intractable constipation. Gut. 2010 Mar;**59**(3):333–40. [Clinical Trial Multicentre Study Research Support, Non-U.S. Gov't]

20 **Matzel KE, Stadelmaier U, Hohenfellner M, Gall FP.** Electrical stimulation of sacral spinal nerves for treatment of faecal incontinence. Lancet 1995 Oct 28;**346**(8983):1124–27.[Case Reports Research Support, Non-US Gov't]

21 **Rao SS, Ozturk R, Laine L.** Clinical utility of diagnostic tests for constipation in adults: a systematic review. Am J Gastroenterol 2005 Jul;**100**(7):1605–15. [Evaluation Studies Review]

22 **Vaizey CJ, Kamm MA, Nicholls RJ.** Recent advances in the surgical treatment of faecal incontinence. Brit J Surg 1998 May;**85**(5):596–603. [Review]

23 **Dudding TC, Hollingshead JR, Nicholls RJ, Vaizey CJ.** Sacral nerve stimulation for faecal incontinence: patient selection, service provision and operative technique. Colorectal Disease: the official journal of the Association of Coloproctology of Great Britain and Ireland Colorectal Dis. 2011 Aug;**13**(8):e187–95. [Review]

24 **Boyle DJ, Knowles CH, Lunniss PJ, Scott SM, Williams NS, Gill KA.** Efficacy of sacral nerve stimulation for fecal incontinence in patients with anal sphincter defects. Dis Colon Rectum 2009 Jul;**52**(7):1234–39. [Clinical Trial]

25 **de Miguel M, Oteiza F, Ciga MA, Armendariz P, Marzo J, Ortiz H.** Sacral nerve stimulation for the treatment of faecal incontinence following low anterior resection for rectal cancer. Colorectal Disease: the official journal of the Association of Coloproctology of Great Britain and Ireland Colorectal Dis. 2011 Jan;**13**(1):72–7.

26 **Jarrett ME, Matzel KE, Christiansen J et al.** Sacral nerve stimulation for faecal incontinence in patients with previous partial spinal injury including disc prolapse. Brit J Sury 2005 Jun;**92**(6):734–39. [Clinical Trial Controlled Clinical Trial Multicentre Study Research Support, Non-US Gov't]

27 **Knowles CH, Thin N, Gill K et al.** Prospective randomized double-blind study of temporary sacral nerve stimulation in patients with rectal evacuatory dysfunction and rectal hyposensitivity. Ann Surg 2012 Apr;**255**(4):643–49.

28 **Leroi AM, Lenne X, Dervaux B et al.** Outcome and cost analysis of sacral nerve modulation for treating urinary and/or fecal incontinence. Ann Surg 2011 Apr;**253**(4):720–32.

29 **Mowatt G, Glazener C, Jarrett M.** Sacral nerve stimulation for faecal incontinence and constipation in adults. Cochrane Database Syst Rev 2007(3):CD004464. [Review]

30 **Boyle DJ, Murphy J, Gooneratne ML et al.** Efficacy of sacral nerve stimulation for the treatment of fecal incontinence. Dis Colon Rectum 2011 Oct;**54**(10):1271–78. [Research Support, Non-US Gov't]

31 **Fraser C, Glazener C, Grant AM, Mowatt G.** Systematic review of the efficacy and safety of sacral nerve stimulation for faecal incontinence. In: Procedures RBfI (ed.) Aberdeen: National Institute for Clinical Excellence; 2004.

32 **Jarrett ME, Mowatt G, Glazener CM et al.** Systematic review of sacral nerve stimulation for faecal incontinence and constipation. Brit J Surg 2004 Dec;**91**(12):1559–69. [Research Support, Non-US Gov't Review]

33 **Maeda Y, Matzel K, Lundby L, Buntzen S, Laurberg S.** Postoperative issues of sacral nerve stimulation for fecal incontinence and constipation: a systematic literature review and treatment guideline. Dis Colon Rectum 2011 Nov;**54**(11):1443–60. [Review]

34 **Tan E, Ngo NT, Darzi A, Shenouda M, Tekkis PP.** Meta-analysis: sacral nerve stimulation versus conservative therapy in the treatment of faecal incontinence. Int J Colorectal Dis 2011 Mar;**26**(3):275–94.

35 **Michelsen HB, Thompson-Fawcett M, Lundby L, Krogh K, Laurberg S, Buntzen S.** Six years of experience with sacral nerve stimulation for fecal incontinence. Dis Colon Rectum 2010 Apr;**53**(4):414–21.

36 **Matzel KE, Lux P, Heuer S, Besendorfer M, Zhang W.** Sacral nerve stimulation for faecal incontinence: long-term outcome. Colorectal Dis 2009 Jul;**11**(6):636–41.

37 **Melenhorst J, Koch SM, Uludag O, van Gemert WG, Baeten CG.** Sacral neuromodulation in patients with faecal incontinence: results of the first 100 permanent implantations. Colorectal Dis 2007 Oct;**9**(8):725–30.

38 **Govaert B, Melenhorst J, Nieman FH, Bols EM, van Gemert WG, Baeten CG.** Factors associated with percutaneous nerve evaluation and permanent sacral nerve modulation outcome in patients with fecal incontinence. Dis Colon Rectum 2009 Oct;**52**(10):1688–94.

39 **Maeda Y, Lundby L, Buntzen S, Laurberg S.** Suboptimal outcome following sacral nerve stimulation for faecal incontinence. Br J Surg 2011 Jan;**98**(1):140–47.

40 **Mellgren A, Wexner SD, Coller JA et al.** Long-term efficacy and safety of sacral nerve stimulation for fecal incontinence. Dis Colon Rectum 2011 Sep;**54**(9):1065–75.

41 **Duelund-Jakobsen J, van Wunnik B, Buntzen S, Lundby L, Baeten C, Laurberg S.** Functional results and patient satisfaction with Sacral Nerve Stimulation for idiopathic faecal incontinence. Colorectal Disease 2012;**14**(6):753–9.

42 **Gallas S, Michot F, Faucheron JL et al.** Predictive factors for successful sacral nerve stimulation in the treatment of faecal incontinence: results of trial stimulation in 200 patients. Colorectal Disease: the official journal of the Association of Coloproctology of Great Britain and Ireland. Colorectal Dis. 2011 Jun;**13**(6):689–96. [Clinical Trial Multicentre Study]

43 **Thin NN, Knowles CH, Allison ME.** Sacral nerve stimulation for faecal incontinence. Gastrointest Nursing 2012 Feb 2012;**10**(1):36–44. [Review]

44 **Matzel K.** Sacral nerve stimulation. In: Ratto C, Doglietto GB (eds) Fecal Incontinence: Diagnosis and Treatment. Milan: Springer; 2007:244.

45 **Wexner SD, Coller JA, Devroede G et al.** Sacral nerve stimulation for fecal incontinence: results of a 120-patient prospective multicenter study. Ann Surg 2010 Mar;**251**(3):441–49.

46 **Feler CA, Whitworth LA, Fernandez J.** Sacral neuromodulation for chronic pain conditions. Anesthesiol Clin North America 2003 Dec;**21**(4):785–95.

47 **Knowles CH, Dinning PG, Pescatori M, Rintala R, Rosen H.** Surgical management of constipation. Neurogastroenterol Motil 2009 Dec;**21** Suppl 2:62–71.

48 **Knowles CH, Scott M, Lunniss PJ.** Outcome of colectomy for slow transit constipation. Ann Surg 1999 Nov;**230**(5):627–38.

49 **Dudding TC, Meng Lee E, Faiz O et al.** Economic evaluation of sacral nerve stimulation for faecal incontinence. Brit J Surg 2008 Sep;**95**(9):1155–63. [Research Support, Non-US Gov't]

50 **Govaert B, Maeda Y, Alberga J, Buntzen S, Laurberg S, Baeten CG.** Medium-term outcome of sacral nerve modulation for constipation. Dis Colon Rectum 2012 Jan;**55**(1):26–31.

51 **Vitton V, Roman S, Damon H, Barth X, Mion F.** Sacral nerve stimulation and constipation: still a long way to go. Dis Colon Rectum 2009 Apr;**52**(4):752–53; author reply 3–4.

52 **Maeda Y, Lundby L, Buntzen S, Laurberg S.** Sacral nerve stimulation for constipation: suboptimal outcome and adverse events. Dis Colon Rectum 2010 Jul;**53**(7):995–99.

53 **Holzer B, Rosen HR, Novi G et al.** Sacral nerve stimulation in patients with severe constipation. Dis Colon Rectum 2008 May;**51**(5):524–29; discussion 9–30.

54 **Camilleri M, Kerstens R, Rykx A, Vandeplassche L.** A placebo-controlled trial of prucalopride for severe chronic constipation. N Engl J Med 2008 May 29;**358**(22):2344–54.

55 **Enck P, Vinson B, Malfertheiner P, Zipfel S, Klosterhalfen S.** The placebo response in functional dyspepsia—reanalysis of trial data. Neurogastroenterol Motil 2009 Apr;**21**(4):370–77.

56 **Carriero A, Martellucci J, Talento P, Ferrari CA.** Sacral nerve stimulation for constipation: do we still miss something? Role of psychological evaluation. Int J Colorectal Dis 2010 Aug;**25**(8):1005–10.

57 **Sharma A, Liu B, Waudby P, Duthie GS.** Sacral neuromodulation for the management of severe constipation: development of a constipation treatment protocol. Int J Colorectal Dis 2011 Dec;**26**(12):1583–87.

58 **van Wunnik BP, Peeters B, Govaert B, Nieman FH, Benninga MA, Baeten CG.** Sacral neuromodulation therapy: a promising treatment for adolescents with refractory functional constipation. Dis Colon Rectum 2012 Mar;**55**(3):278–85.

59 **Krames ES, Hunter Peckham P, Rezai AR.** Fundamentals of electrical stimulation. In: Krames E.S.HPP, Rezai A.R. (eds) Neuromodulation, 1st edn. London: Elsevier; 2009:109–21.

60 **Uludag O, Morren GL, Dejong CH, Baeten CG.** Effect of sacral neuromodulation on the rectum. Br J Surg 2005 Aug;**92**(8):1017–23.

61 **Michelsen HB, Buntzen S, Krogh K, Laurberg S.** Rectal volume tolerability and anal pressures in patients with fecal incontinence treated with sacral nerve stimulation. Dis Colon Rectum 2006 Jul;**49**(7):1039–44. [Comparative Study]

62 **Michelsen HB, Worsoe J, Krogh K et al.** Rectal motility after sacral nerve stimulation for faecal incontinence. Neurogastroenterol Motil 2010 Jan;**22**(1):36–41, e6.

63 **Gladman MA, Lunniss PJ, Scott SM, Swash M.** Rectal hyposensitivity. Am J Gastroenterol 2006 May;**101**(5):1140–51.

64 **Lunniss PJ, Gladman MA, Benninga MA, Rao SS.** Pathophysiology of evacuation disorders. Neurogastroenterol Motil 2009 Dec;**21**(Suppl. 2):31–40.

65 **Chan CL, Scott SM, Williams NS, Lunniss PJ.** Rectal hypersensitivity worsens stool frequency, urgency, and lifestyle in patients with urge fecal incontinence. Dis Colon Rectum 2005 Jan;**48**(1):134–40.

66 **Gladman MA, Dvorkin LS, Lunniss PJ, Williams NS, Scott SM.** Rectal hyposensitivity: a disorder of the rectal wall or the afferent pathway? An assessment using the barostat. Am J Gastroenterol 2005 Jan;**100**(1):106–14.

67 **Gladman MA, Scott SM, Chan CL, Williams NS, Lunniss PJ.** Rectal hyposensitivity: prevalence and clinical impact in patients with intractable constipation and fecal incontinence. Dis Colon Rectum 2003 Feb;**46**(2):238–46.

68 **Carrington EV, Knowles CH.** The influence of sacral nerve stimulation on anorectal dysfunction. Colorectal Disease: the official journal of the Association of Coloproctology of Great Britain and Ireland Colorectal Dis. 2011 Mar;**13** Suppl 2:5–9. [Research Support, Non-US Gov't Review]

69 **Ratto C, Grillo E, Parello A, Petrolino M, Costamagna G, Doglietto GB.** Sacral neuromodulation in treatment of fecal incontinence following anterior resection and chemoradiation for rectal cancer. Dis Colon Rectum 2005 May;**48**(5):1027–36.

70 **Fowler CJ, Swinn MJ, Goodwin RJ, Oliver S, Craggs M.** Studies of the latency of pelvic floor contraction during peripheral nerve evaluation show that the muscle response is reflexly mediated. J Urol 2000 Mar;**163**(3):881–83.

71 **Gooneratne ML, Facer P, Knowles CH et al.** Normalization of substance P levels in rectal mucosa of patients with faecal incontinence treated successfully by sacral nerve stimulation. Br J Surg 2008 Apr;**95**(4):477–83.

72 **Kenefick NJ, Emmanuel A, Nicholls RJ, Kamm MA.** Effect of sacral nerve stimulation on autonomic nerve function. Br J Surg 2003 Oct;**90**(10):1256–60.

73 **Ganio E, Masin A, Ratto C et al.** Short-term sacral nerve stimulation for functional anorectal and urinary disturbances: results in 40 patients: evaluation of a new option for anorectal functional disorders. Dis Colon Rectum 2001 Sep;**44**(9):1261–67.

74 **Rosen HR, Urbarz C, Holzer B, Novi G, Schiessel R.** Sacral nerve stimulation as a treatment for fecal incontinence. Gastroenterology 2001 Sep;**121**(3):536–41. [Clinical Trial]

75 **Ripetti V, Caputo D, Ausania F, Esposito E, Bruni R, Arullani A.** Sacral nerve neuromodulation improves physical, psychological and social quality of life in patients with fecal incontinence. Tech Coloproctol 2002 Dec;**6**(3):147–52.

76 **Holzer B, Rosen HR, Novi G, Ausch C, Holbling N, Schiessel R.** Sacral nerve stimulation for neurogenic faecal incontinence. Br J Surg 2007 Jun;**94**(6):749–53.

77 **Scott SM, Gladman MA.** Manometric, sensorimotor, and neurophysiologic evaluation of anorectal function. Gastroenterol Clin North Am 2008 Sep;**37**(3):511–38, vii.

78 **Melenhorst J, Koch SM, Uludag O, van Gemert WG, Baeten CG.** Is a morphologically intact anal sphincter necessary for success with sacral nerve modulation in patients with faecal incontinence? Colorectal Dis 2008 Mar;**10**(3):257–62.

79 **Dudding TC, Pares D, Vaizey CJ, Kamm MA.** Sacral nerve stimulation for the treatment of faecal incontinence related to dysfunction of the internal anal sphincter. Int J Colorectal Dis 2010 May;**25**(5):625–30. [Clinical Trial]

80 **Sheldon R, Kiff ES, Clarke A, Harris ML, Hamdy S.** Sacral nerve stimulation reduces corticoanal excitability in patients with faecal incontinence. Br J Surg 2005 Nov;**92**(11): 1423–31.

81 **Falletto E, Masin A, Lolli P et al.** Is sacral nerve stimulation an effective treatment for chronic idiopathic anal pain? Dis Colon Rectum 2009 Mar;**52**(3):456–62.

82 **McGuire EJ, Zhang SC, Horwinski ER, Lytton B.** Treatment of motor and sensory detrusor instability by electrical stimulation. J Urol 1983 Jan;**129**(1):78–79. [Case Reports]

83 **Stoller ML.** Afferent nerve stimulation for pelvic floor dysfunction. Eur Urol 1999;**35**:16.

84 **Shafik A, Ahmed I, El-Sibai O, Mostafa RM.** Percutaneous peripheral neuromodulation in the treatment of fecal incontinence. Eur Surg Res. 2003;**35**:103–07.

85 **Allison M.** Percutaneous tibial nerve stimulation for patients with faecal incontinence. Nurs Stand 2011 Feb 16–22;**25**(24): 44–8.

86 **Boyle DJ, Prosser K, Allison ME, Williams NS, Chan CL.** Percutaneous tibial nerve stimulation for the treatment of urge fecal incontinence. Dis Colon Rectum 2010 Apr;**53**(4):432–37. [Research Support, Non-US Gov't]

87 **Peters KM, Carrico DJ, Perez-Marrero RA et al.** Randomized trial of percutaneous tibial nerve stimulation versus Sham efficacy in the treatment of overactive bladder syndrome: results from the SUmiT trial. J Urol 2010 Apr;**183**(4):1438–43. [Comparative Study Multicentre Study Randomized Controlled Trial Research Support, Non-US Gov't]

88 **Queralto M, Portier G, Cabarrot PH, et al.** Preliminary results of peripheral transcutaneous neuromodulation in the treatment of idiopathic fecal incontinence. Int J Colorectal Dis 2006 Oct;**21**(7):670–72.

89 **Vitton V, Damon H, Roman S, Nancey S, Flourie B, Mion F.** Transcutaneous posterior tibial nerve stimulation for fecal incontinence in inflammatory bowel disease patients: a therapeutic option? Inflamm Bowel Dis 2009 Mar;**15**(3):402–405. [Comparative Study]

90 **Vitton V, Damon H, Roman S, Mion F.** Transcutaneous electrical posterior tibial nerve stimulation for faecal incontinence: effects on symptoms and quality of life. Int J Colorectal Dis 2010 Aug;**25**(8):1017–20. [Clinical Trial]

91 **Eleouet M, Siproudhis L, Guillou N, Le Couedic J, Bouguen G, Bretagne JF.** Chronic posterior tibial nerve transcutaneous electrical nerve stimulation (TENS) to treat fecal incontinence (FI). Int J Colorectal Dis 2010 Sep;**25**(9):1127–32. [Clinical Trial]

92 **de la Portilla F, Rada R, Vega J, Gonzalez CA, Cisneros N, Maldonado VH.** Evaluation of the use of posterior tibial nerve stimulation for the treatment of fecal incontinence: preliminary results of a prospective study. Dis Colon Rectum 2009 Aug;**52**(8):1427–33. [Comparative Study Evaluation Studies]

93 **Rockwood TH, Church JM, Fleshman JW et al.** Patient and surgeon ranking of the severity of symptoms associated with fecal incontinence: the fecal incontinence severity index. Dis Colon Rectum 1999 Dec;**42**(12):1525–32. [Research Support, Non-US Gov't]

94 **Hotouras A, Thaha MA, Boyle D et al.** Short-term outcome following percutaneous tibial nerve stimulation (PTNS) for faecal incontinence: a single-centre prospective study. Colorectal Disease: the official journal of the Association of Coloproctology of Great Britain and Ireland 2011 Dec 6. Colorectal Dis. 2012 Sep;**14**(9):1101–5.

95 **Hotouras A, Thaha MA, Allison ME, Currie A, Scott SM, Chan CL.** Percutaneous tibial nerve stimulation (PTNS) in females with faecal incontinence: the impact of sphincter morphology and rectal sensation on the clinical outcome. Int J Colorectal Dis. 2012 Jul;**27**(7):927–30.

96 **Govaert B, Pares D, Delgado-Aros S, La Torre F, Van Gemert WG, Baeten CG.** A prospective multicentre study to investigate percutaneous tibial nerve stimulation for the treatment of faecal incontinence. Colorectal Disease: the official journal of the Association of Coloproctology of Great Britain and Ireland Colorectal Dis. 2010 Dec;**12**(12):1236–41. [Clinical Trial Multicentre Study Research Support, Non-US Gov't]

97 **Mentes BB, Yuksel O, Aydin A, Tezcaner T, Leventoglu A, Aytac B.** Posterior tibial nerve stimulation for faecal incontinence after partial spinal injury: preliminary report. Tech Coloproctol 2007 Jun;**11**(2):115–19. [Case Reports]

98 **Findlay JM, Yeung JM, Robinson R, Greaves H, Maxwell-Armstrong C.** Peripheral neuromodulation via posterior tibial nerve stimulation—a potential treatment for faecal incontinence? Ann Roy Coll Surg 2010 Jul;**92**(5):385–90. [Evaluation Studies]

99 **Agur AMR, Dalley AF.** Grant's Atlas of Anatomy, 12th edn. Philadelphia: Wolters Kluwer Health/ Lippincott Williams & Wilkins; 2009.

100 **Vaizey CJ, Kamm MA, Turner IC, Nicholls RJ, Woloszko J.** Effects of short term sacral nerve stimulation on anal and rectal function in patients with anal incontinence. Gut 1999 Mar;**44**(3):407–12.

101 **Jarrett ME, Varma JS, Duthie GS, Nicholls RJ, Kamm MA.** Sacral nerve stimulation for faecal incontinence in the UK. Brit J Surg 2004 Jun;**91**(6):755–61.

102 **Leroi AM, Parc Y, Lehur PA et al.** Efficacy of sacral nerve stimulation for fecal incontinence: results of a multicenter double-blind crossover study. Ann Surg 2005 Nov;**242**(5):662–69. [Comparative Study Multicentre Study Randomized Controlled Trial Research Support, Non-US Gov't]

103 **Griffin KM, Pickering M, O'Herlihy C, O'Connell PR, Jones JF.** Sacral nerve stimulation increases activation of the primary somatosensory cortex by anal canal stimulation in an experimental model. Brit J Surg 2011 Aug;**98**(8):1160–69. [Research Support, Non-US Gov't]

104 **Finazzi-Agro E, Rocchi C, Pachatz C et al.** Percutaneous tibial nerve stimulation produces effects on brain activity: study on the modifications of the long latency somatosensory evoked potentials. Neurourol Urodynam 2009;**28**(4):320–24.

105 **Vodusek DB, Light JK, Libby JM.** Detrusor inhibition induced by stimulation of pudendal nerve afferents. Neurourol Urodynam 1986;**5**(4):381–89.

106 **Matzel KS, U. Besendorfer, M. Hohenberger, W.** Pudendal stimulation for anorectal dysfunction—the first application of a fully implantable microstimulator. Colorectal Disease: the official journal of the Association of Coloproctology of Great Britain and Ireland Colorectal Dis. 2005;**7**(Suppl. 1):103.

107 **Spinelli M, Malaguti S, Giardiello G, Lazzeri M, Tarantola J, Van Den Hombergh U.** A new minimally invasive procedure for pudendal nerve stimulation to treat neurogenic bladder: description of the method and preliminary data. Neurourol Urodynam 2005;**24**(4):305–09. [Clinical Trial]

108 **Spinelli M, Sievert KD**. Latest technologic and surgical developments in using InterStim Therapy for sacral neuromodulation: impact on treatment success and safety. Eur Urol 2008 Dec;**54**(6):1287–96. [Research Support, Non-US Gov't Review]

109 **George AT, Dudding TC, Nicholls RJ, Vaizey CJ**. A new minimally invasive technique for pudendal nerve stimulation. Colorectal Disease: the official journal of the Association of Coloproctology of Great Britain and Ireland Colorectal Dis. 2012 Jan;**14**(1):98–103.

110 **Peters KM, Feber KM, Bennett RC**. Sacral versus pudendal nerve stimulation for voiding dysfunction: a prospective, single-blinded, randomized, crossover trial. Neurourol Urodynam 2005;**24**(7):643–47. [Comparative Study Randomized Controlled Trial Research Support, Non-US Gov't]

111 **Bock S, Folie P, Wolff K, Marti L, Engeler DS, Hetzer FH**. First experiences with pudendal nerve stimulation in fecal incontinence: a technical report. Tech Coloproctol 2010 Mar;**14**(1):41–4. [Case Reports]

Chapter 17

Gastric stimulation for obesity and gastroparesis

Edy E. Soffer

Key points

Gut electrical stimulation (GES) is an evolving therapeutic modality for a number of clinical conditions.

1 Gastric electrical stimulation for gastroparesis has been in clinical use for almost two decades. It can improve symptoms in carefully selected patients (in particular those with diabetic gastroparesis).

2 Lower oesophageal sphincter (LOS) stimulation is used to treat gastro-oesophageal reflux disease (GORD). Limited experience over the last few years have shown good efficacy and safety of this intervention.

3 Vagal electrical stimulation has been recently introduced as a treatment for obesity. Clinical trials showed that this therapy can safely reduce weight in obese patients.

4 In spite of the expanding clinical application of electrical stimulation, our understanding of its mechanisms of action remains limited. Data from larger number of patients, obtained over longer duration of follow-up, are needed to establish the role of electrical stimulation in clinical practice.

Introduction

Interest in electrical stimulation of the gut stems from the fact that organs along the gastrointestinal tract, like the heart, have natural pacemakers, and the myoelectric activity they generate may be controlled and manipulated by the application of electrical stimuli. Electrical stimulation of the gut was reported as early as five decades ago, in an attempt to resolve post-operative ileus (1). In the decade that followed, experimental works, primarily in the canine model, began to elucidate the nature of gastrointestinal myoelectric activity and its relation to contractile activity (2, 3–5). These studies showed that the natural gastric pacesetter potential arose in the body of the stomach, and that rectangular electric pulses given in that region, at a frequency slightly higher than the intrinsic gastric slow wave frequency, can control (entrain) gastric electrical activity. Subsequent research in animals and humans addressed the effect of different pulse parameters on gastric motor physiology (6–13).

The era of clinical use of GES was prompted by studies in animals and humans that showed that GES with higher frequency and shorter pulse duration (in microseconds) can improve nausea and vomiting and enhance gastric emptying (14, 15). The low-power consumption of this type of pulse, unlike long-duration pulses used for pacing, allowed for incorporation of such pulses in devices using current battery technology. A number of clinical studies then followed and, based on their results, the FDA granted the Enterra system under the restriction of a Humanitarian Use Device (HUD) status, which provides treatment for uncommon conditions (less than 4000 implantations/year) for which no effective therapy is available. A Humanitarian Device Exemption (HDE) allows for marketing of the system under restricted conditions, as described earlier, and also requires approval by Institutional Review Boards. It is important to note that such restrictions do not imply that treatment with the Enterra system is experimental.

This chapter reviews three application of gut electrical stimulation: GES for gatroparesis, GES for obesity and stimulation of the LOS for GERD.

Gut electrical stimulation for gastroparesis

The gastric phase is an important step in the process of digestion. Its repertoire of motor functions ensures proper accommodation of meals, mixing and trituration of ingested food to small particles that can be delivered to the small bowel at an appropriate rate that allows for optimal intestinal absorption of nutrients. Central to these functions are smooth muscle cells, which perform mechanical work in the form of phasic and tonic contractions under the integrated control of autonomic and enteric neurones, which convey sensory information, exert efferent control, and generate reflex patterns; and interstitial cells of Cajal, which serve as rhythm generators and as an interface between nerves and smooth muscle (16–19). Abnormalities of these elements were documented in patients with gastroparesis (20), resulting in impaired myoelectrical activity, abnormal contractile activity and impaired gastric emptying of food (21).

Two types of electrical stimulation have been used for gastroparesis. One type delivers pulses with duration in milliseconds (usually few hundreds), at a frequency of a few cycles per minute. Hence, it is also commonly referred to as low-frequency or high-energy stimulation, since the amount of energy delivered to the tissue depends, among others, on the product of pulse duration and its frequency. Previous experimental works, primarily in the canine model, showed that the natural gastric pacesetter potential arose in the body of the stomach, and that rectangular electric pulses given in that region can control (entrain) gastric electrical activity. Subsequent studies in animals and humans showed that stimulation at a frequency that is slightly higher than the intrinsic gastric slow wave frequency (approximately three cycles per minute in humans), and with pulse duration in the range of milliseconds, achieves the best pacing results, and can also improve gastric emptying in health and disease (6–8, 12, 13).

The high-power consumption of this type of stimulation has limited its clinical use. The second type of stimulus delivers pulses with duration in microseconds, at a Hertz frequency (cycles per seconds), hence also referred to as high-frequency or low-energy stimulation. Studies in animals and early reports in humans showed that GES with these parameters can improve nausea and vomiting and enhance gastric emptying (14, 15). The low-power consumption of this type of pulse, unlike long-duration pulses used for pacing, allowed for incorporation of such pulses in devices using current battery technology. GES with trains of high-frequency, short-duration pulses is currently the only type in clinical use for gastroparesis (Fig. 17.1).

Equipment and implantation procedure

The Enterra gastric stimulation system consists of three main elements: a pair of leads, a pulse generator, and a programming system. Two leads are surgically placed in the gastric wall, on the greater curvature, 10 cm proximal to the pylorus. The leads are connected to a pulse generator, placed in a sub-cutaneous pocket in the abdominal wall, in the left or right upper quadrants. The pulse generator was adapted from existing devices in clinical use that can sustain the long-term requirements of a low-energy type of stimulation. The permanent implantable pulse generator is controlled by an external programmer, which allows for interrogation and programming of stimulation parameters via a radio-telemetry link. The pulse generator is programmed to specific parameters, shown in Fig. 17.1, that derive from earlier canine and human studies (14, 15).

The Enterra system is implanted surgically, by laparotomy or, increasingly, by laparoscopy. Hospital stay following laparoscopic insertion is short, approximately 2 days (22), and is shorter when compared to placement via laparotomy (23). The battery life extends to 5–10 years, depending on the pulse parameters used (24). When the battery is depleted, the pulse generator is replaced by local intervention. In the US, the system is approved for patients with idiopathic or diabetic gastroparesis who are markedly symptomatic in spite of maximal medical therapy.

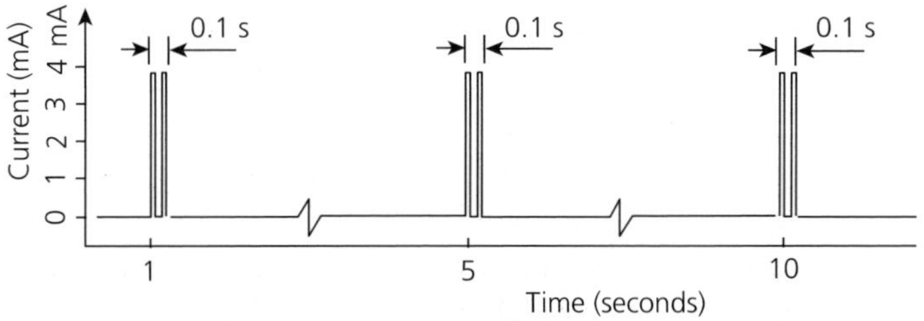

Fig. 17.1 An illustration of the type of electrical stimulation delivered by the Enterra system. Short bursts of short-duration rectangular pulses (330 μs each) are given at a frequency of 14 Hz in each burst. Bursts in turn last 0.1 s and are delivered every 5 s. This type of stimulus is referred to as short-pulse duration/high frequency, and also as low energy.

Clinical experience with gut electrical stimulation

Published data on GES for gastroparesis derive almost entirely from open-label studies, performed mostly in a select number of centres with large experience in this therapy (22, 25–33). Published studies consistently demonstrate that GES has a beneficial effect in patients with gastroparesis. The few studies that had a double-blind phase reported comparable outcome (26, 33), but their results were questioned because of study design issues. Besides improvement in symptoms, GES was found to improve nutritional status (25, 34) and quality of life (26, 35). GES was also found to reduce healthcare utilization, thus reducing healthcare costs associated with gastroparesis (36). Lately, the use of GES was expanded to aetiologies beyond diabetic and idiopathic gastroparesis. GES was tried in patients with post-surgical gastroparesis (37–39), with intestinal pseudo-obstruction (40), and patients who underwent organ transplant (41), with encouraging results. Data, however, are too few, and more studies are needed to determine the efficacy of GES in these groups of patients.

Different concepts of stimulation are also being investigated in order to maximize efficacy. A variation on the single-channel gastric stimulation is the use of a number of electrodes, positioned at intervals along the long axis of the stomach, with application of sequential stimulation. Multichannel pacing requires a fraction of the energy used in single-channel pacing (42), and it improves gastric emptying and symptoms in experimental models of gastroparesis (43), and in diabetic patients with gastroparesis (44). A different approach delivers high-frequency stimulation, applied to circumferential electrodes. Sequential stimulation induces sequential contractions that facilitate gastric empting (45). The technical feasibility and clinical efficacy of such systems remain to be explored in clinical trials.

Long-term studies report a complication rate of 7–10%, the main one being infection of the sub-cutaneous pocket (46, 47). Less common complications include erosion of the abdominal wall by the device, penetration of the leads through the gastric wall, or tangling of wires in the generator pocket and formation of adhesions. These complications are generally managed surgically. In case of infection of the pocket, the pulse generator needs to be removed; however, it can be reinserted once infection is fully controlled (46).

Given the invasive nature of this intervention, efforts were made to identify factors that can predict good response to therapy. A few clinical features were found to be associated with less than optimal response, such as the use of opiates (48) and idiopathic, rather than diabetic, aetiology (26, 49). Also, pain and bloating do not improve as well as nausea and vomiting (48). Thus, diabetic patients with gastroparesis, with nausea and vomiting as their predominant symptoms, appear to be the best candidates for GES. Unfortunately, individual response to GES remains unpredictable. The need to predict response generated an interest in the use of temporary gastric electrical stimulation. Gastric stimulation using trans-nasal mucosal electrodes is delivered for a few days, and the response to therapy is assessed to predict response to long-term therapy with the Enterra system (50). However, there are no data thus far from double-blind, control studies to support this concept. Also, once implantation is performed, there is no clear strategy for addressing patients who do not respond to GES. Various manipulations of the Enterra pulse parameters have been suggested (51) but data are not yet sufficient to demonstrate the efficacy of different pulse variables.

Mechanisms of gastric electrical stimulation

In general, electrical stimulation of gut tissue can modulate the neuromuscular function of the organs involved, affect afferent neural activity emanating from the organs, or both. This concept has been tested in both animal models and humans; however, the mechanisms of action of GES in gastroparesis remain poorly understood. Studies in animals (2) and later in humans (6) have clearly shown that entrainment (pacing) of gastric slow waves can be achieved with GES using low-frequency/long-duration pulse parameters, and that these parameters can enhance gastric emptying (7, 8). Initial reports from animal and human studies suggested that similar effects can be achieved with GES when using short-duration pulses (14, 15). However, subsequent studies, using the pulse parameters of the implantable Enterra system, did not support these initial observations. Enterra parameters did not control vasopressin-induced gastric dysrhythmia in an animal model, though it improved vomiting (52); while in humans, GES did not affect gastric electrical activity in patients with gastroparesis, as measured by electrogastrography (53). The effect of GES on gastric emptying is inconsistent, with some studies showing enhancement of gastric emptying (22, 28), observed only in diabetics (26), or no improvement (47, 54). Given the variable correlation between gastric emptying and symptoms of gastroparesis (55), and keeping in mind the possibility of spontaneous resolution of idiopathic gastroparesis over time (56), the system should not be used to achieve a prokinetic effect, such as to treat patients who suffer from gastric bezoars or severe gastro-oesophageal reflux disease.

A more plausible mechanism is perhaps the effect of GES on gastric biomechanical activity. Both low-frequency/long-duration and high-frequency/short-duration pulses were shown to reduce gastric tone in animal models (57, 58) and reduced symptoms induced by gastric distension (58). Impairment of gastric accommodation has been documented in patients with functional dyspepsia and diabetic gastropathy (59, 60), and such impairment in turn is associated with gastrointestinal symptoms, primarily early satiety and weight loss (59), suggesting a possible mechanism for GES in relief of symptoms. The case for afferent modulation/central mechanism of GES remains unclear. In dogs, the anti-emetic effect is vagally mediated, since it is abolished by vagal disruption (52), but GES was also shown to improve symptoms in post-surgical gastroparesis, some with vagal disruption (37–39). GES was found to increase activity in the thalamus of patients with gastroparesis, as detected by positron emission tomography (61). These data are difficult to interpret, particularly since perturbation of the gut is likely to have a central representation, and hence its mere presence may not necessarily indicate a neural mechanism.

Areas of uncertainty

In spite of the encouraging data provided by the studies published thus far, there remains an element of scepticism with regard to this intervention (62), driven by the lack of a convincing double-blind, placebo (sham-stimulation) controlled study, sufficiently powered to provide conclusive data regarding efficacy. However, clinical experience and, most importantly, the lack of effective therapy for gastroparesis, support the use of GES in refractory patients with debilitating symptoms who have exhausted all available medical regimens. The lack of a reliable measure to predict response to therapy in individual patients, particularly given the invasive nature of this intervention, continues to limit the application of this intervention.

What the future holds

Considerable clinical evidence supports the use of GES for the treatment of drug refractory gastroparesis. The Enterra system is the only one approved for such purpose. Improvement of pulse parameters, the potential use of temporary stimulation, and the incorporation of variables that can predict better response to stimulation may improve the efficacy of the current system. New systems under investigation may prove more efficacious and provide control of symptoms coupled with a prokinetic effect.

Electrical stimulation of the lower oesophageal sphincter for GERD

Gastro-oesophageal reflux disease is one of the most common gastrointestinal disorders, affecting up to 30% of the population in developed countries, with increasing prevalence worldwide (63, 64). Its negative impact on the quality of life and economic burden are substantial (65, 66). The mainstay of therapy is acid suppression, primarily in the form of proton pump inhibitors (PPI). These drugs have revolutionized the treatment of GERD, however, up to 40% of GERD patients complain of continued symptoms while receiving adequate acid suppression (67, 68), in part because acid suppression agents reduce the acid content of the refluxed material, but not reflux itself (69). Incomplete control of symptoms by acid suppression therapy, as well as concern about side effects of PPIs, are among the main reasons cited by patients who choose to undergo alternative therapy, primarily anti-reflux surgery (70–72). Fundoplication has been the standard anti-reflux surgery and the primary alternative to pharmacotherapy, however, it is associated with adverse effects (73,) and its numbers are in decline (74). The unmet need of patients who are not satisfied with medical therapy and the traditional surgical approach has been driving a search for alternative treatment modalities, both endoscopic and surgical. One such alternative is application of electrical stimulation to the lower oesophageal sphincter.

Human studies of LOS electrical stimulation

Studies in animal models were the impetus for LOS stimulation in humans. While such studies, performed mostly in a canine model, used different techniques, pulse parameters and protocols, they all demonstrated a consistent enhancement of LOS pressure with LOS electrical stimulation (75–77). The results led to two acute studies in humans, conducted as a proof of concept, in order to evaluate the effect of electrical stimulation on LOS pressure in humans. The first study consisted of stimulation with temporary electrodes, implanted laparoscopically in GERD patients undergoing elective cholecystectomy (78). In the second study, patients with GERD symptoms were fitted with a temporary pacemaker lead, placed endoscopically at the level of the LOS (79). Both groups were stimulated with high frequency pulses of short duration, with significant increase in LOS pressure. The results of these studies prompted further assessment of this technology in GERD patients, by applying chronic stimulation using a permanently implanted system.

Chronic Human Studies

The safety and efficacy of LOS stimulation in patients with GORD have been evaluated by a single-center and a multi-center open label studies, as well as a registry of commercially implanted patients. The system consists of two electrodes, implanted in the muscular layer of the gastroesophageal junction, connected to a pulse generator located in a subcutaneous pocket in the left upper quadrant of the abdomen. The system delivers pulses with a width of 215 μs, nominal amplitude of 5 mA (range 3–8 mA) at a frequency of 20 Hz, up to twelve sessions a day, for 30 min a session. All implanted patients had documented abnormal oesophageal acid exposure, and the majority suffered from GORD symptoms with only partial response to PPI. Most patients were considering a surgical antireflux surgery for control of symptoms. After three years of stimulation, patients in the single -center study showed a sustained and significant improvement in Health Related Quality of Life (HRQL) metric (Fig. 17.2), and in oesophageal acid exposure (Fig. 17.3) (80).

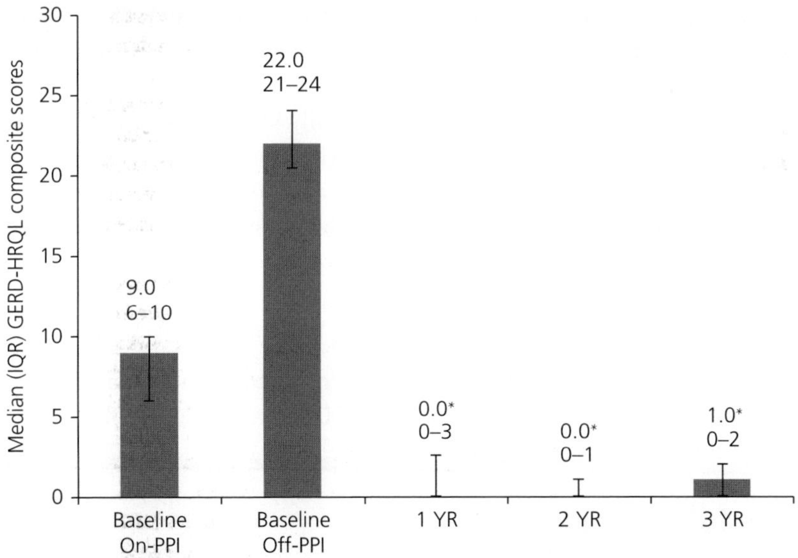

Fig. 17.2 Sustained and significant improvement in GERD symptoms as measured by the composite GERDHRQL scores at 3-year follow-up. Data: Median, IQR. *p<0.001 vs. baseline off-PPI at all time points, p<0.01 vs. baseline on-PPI at all time points (from reference 80)

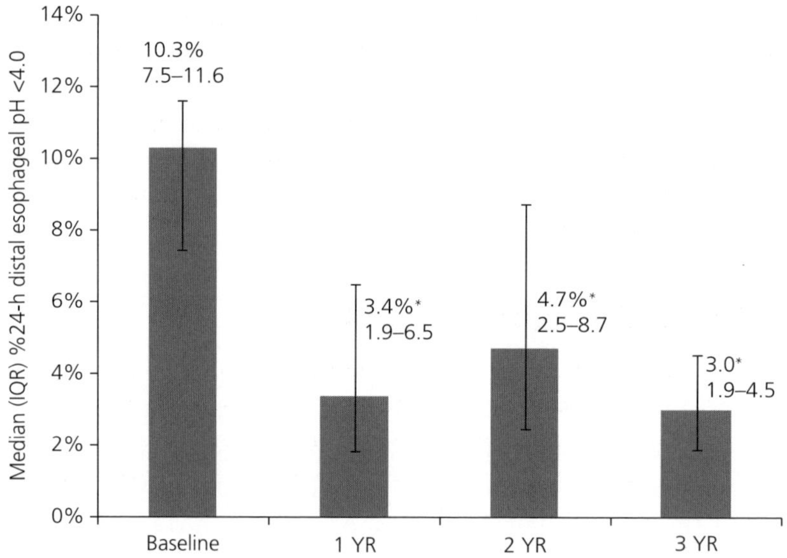

Fig. 17.3 Sustained and significant improvement in the distal oesophageal acid exposure on LOS stimulation at 3-year follow-up. Data: Median, IQR. 73% reported normalization (<4.0% of 24h) in their distal oesophageal acid exposure at their 3 year follow-up. *p<0.001 vs. baseline (from reference 80)

Comparable results were observed in the multi-center study at 6 months follow up (81). Safety profile has been good, and most adverse effects have been surgical or perioperative in nature. There was one episode of electrode migration requiring removal. There were no new episodes of dysphagia.

The mechanisms of action of LES-EST are not fully known, and stimulation-induced increase in LES pressure that was observed primarily in acute and short-term studies in both animals and humans may be only one factor accounting for the beneficial effect of this intervention. Other mechanisms affecting such pathophysiological aspects of GERD such as transient LES relaxation or the acid pocket remain to be elucidated.

Areas of uncertainty

Experience with LOS electrical was obtained from open label studies and data from control trial with a sham stimulation arm are lacking. Data from Longer follow up, obtained from a larger number of patients are needed.

What the future holds

Experience with LOS electrical stimulation showed that the therapy significantly improves symptoms of GORD and oesophageal acid exposure, with a very satisfactory safety profile thus far. The intervention is technically simple, is non-disruptive and pulse parameters and stimulation sessions can be adjusted. The studies conducted thus far applied restrictive enrolment criteria (such as limiting hiatal hernia size, degree of erosive esophagitis etc.) hence, the applicability of electrical stimulation therapy to the wider population of GERD patients remains to be determined by future studies and further experience. The technology is promising, and further experience and longer follow up of implanted patients will determine the place of LES electrical stimulation in the armamentarium of anti-reflux interventions in patients with GERD.

Gastric Electrical Stimulation for Obesity

Obesity is a leading cause of morbidity and mortality with an increasing prevalence worldwide (82). The financial cost to society of obesity-related medical conditions (such as the metabolic syndrome, cardiovascular disease and cancer) is very high (83). Treatment consists of non-invasive measures, such as diet, behaviour modifications and pharmacotherapy, or invasive, primarily traditional bariatric surgery procedures. Non-invasive modalities have been shown consistently to have limited efficacy and sustainability (84). Traditional bariatric surgery, including Roux-en-Y gastric bypass, sleeve gastrectomy, and restrictive gastric band (though numbers of the latter have been greatly reduced with the advent of sleeve gastrectomy), are comparatively successful, but they are associated with morbidity and mortality (85), and the number of traditional bariatric procedures remains a fraction of the number of people suffering from obesity (86). These factors have led over the years to a quest for less invasive interventions for control of body weight, among them the application of electrical stimulation to the gut, primarily the stomach. It is an attractive concept because the intervention is minimally invasive, reversible, does not alter gastrointestinal anatomy, and as a result has a better safety profile.

The ingestion of food triggers various integrated physiological responses involving gut motor and secretory function (87). Among these responses, gastric distension and the release of certain regulatory peptides such as CCK and GLP1 induce a sensation of satiety, with resulting inhibition of food intake (88). The vagus nerve serves an important role in these processes. Satiety signals from gastric distension, as well as from regulatory peptides are conveyed to the central nervous system by way of vagal afferents that project to the nucleus of the solitary tract (NTS) in the caudal hindbrain (88). Electrical stimulation of the stomach is thought to affect food intake by modulating some of the above mechanisms. Impairment of motor function was attempted by application of stimulation that disrupts the normal pacemaker activity or reverses its direction. Application of a pacing stimulus at the distal antrum in a canine model resulted in reverse pacing, reversing the direction of antral slow waves and contractions, thus disrupting gastric electromechanical activity and delaying gastric emptying (89). The same effect was achieved by sequential stimulation in retrograde direction of sets of electrodes, implanted along the stomach, using high-frequency trains of pulses (90). The utility of such methods in humans remains unclear. A different concept applies non-disruptive stimuli to the stomach or the vagus, intended to modulate satiety and vagal signalling. Three variations of this concept were tested in humans, with mixed results.

Clinical experience with Electrical Stimulation for Obesity

Transcend Implantable gastric electrical stimulation device

The system consists of two leads, each lead contain a bipolar electrode, implanted in the anterior medial wall of the stomach about 8 cm above the pylorus, connected to an implantable subcutaneous pulse generator. Pulse parameters consisted of a width of 450 μs and pulse frequency of 40 Hz, delivered at a cycle of 2 sec on and 3 sec off. A decade of studies with this technology, culminated in a large prospective, randomized, sham-controlled, double- blinded, multicentre study involving 190 obese subjects. All subjects were implanted with gastric stimulators and were randomized to either a control group (stimulation off) or treatment group (stimulation on) and were followed for one year (91). At the conclusion of the 12- month study, there was no statistically significant difference between the two groups in excess weight loss.

The Tantalus™ Implantable gastric electrical stimulation Device

This system uses electrical stimuli that are synchronized with the gastric slow waves, resulting in augmentation of the force of gastric contractions without disruption of the natural gastric electrical rhythm. This augmentation, in turn, increases afferent vagal activity thought to induce satiety (92). The system consists of two pairs of electrodes implanted in the anterior and posterior wall of the antrum that can detect gastric slow waves and deliver a pulse. Animal experiments were followed by a small prospective, non-randomized, open-label, single-center trial that assessed the effect of stimulation on body weight and eating behaviour in obese subjects. At 1 year effect on weight loss was promising and safety profile was good (93), but results were inconclusive given the small number of enrolled subjects.

Vagal Nerve Blockade Therapy System

The rationale behind this technology is the observation that bilateral truncal vagotomy (used in the past for the treatment of peptic ulcer disease) resulted in decreased appetite and weight loss in some patients (94). Initial human studies showed that the technique can induce a significant weight loss in obese subjects (95) and the electrical stimulation was further refined (96), leading to a prospective, multicentre, randomized, double-blind, sham-controlled clinical trial in obese patients (97). During laparoscopy, electrodes were placed around the anterior and posterior vagus nerves at the gastro-oesophageal junction. The treatment group received biphasic pulses, at a frequency of 5000 Hz and amplitude of 6–8 mA, in an alternating mode, for at least 12 hours a day. At the end on one year, weight loss in the vagal block group was statistically greater than in the sham device group, though the study results did not meet the prespecified coprimary efficacy objectives. The treatment was well tolerated, having met the primary safety objective.

What the future holds

Reported data on electrical stimulation have confirmed the good safety profile of this intervention, compared to traditional bariatric surgery. Two new systems of gastric electrical stimulation for obesity are currently undergoing trials. Long-term follow-up and data on sustainability of weight loss, in well-designed sham-controlled trials, should help determine the value of electrical stimulation as a therapeutic modality for obesity.

References

1 **Bigutay AM, Win grove R, Griffin WO et al**. Gastro-intestinal pacing: a new concept in the treatment of ileus. Ann Surg 1963;**158**(3):338–48.

2 **Kelly KA, La Force RC**. Pacing the canine stomach with electrical stimulation. Am J Physiol 1972;**222**:588–94.

3 **Sarna SK and Daniel EE**. Gastrointestinal electrical activity: terminology. Gastroenterology 1975;**68**:1631–35.

4 **Hinder RA, Kelly KA**. Human gastric pacemaker potential: Site of origin, spread, and response to gastric transaction and proximal gastric vagotomy. Am J Surg 1977;**133**:29–33.

5 **Bellahsène B-E, Schirmer BD, Updike OL et al**. Effect of electrical stimulation on gastric emptying. Dig Dis Sci 1987;**32**:902.

6 **Lin ZY, McCallum RW, Schirmer BD et al**. Effects of pacing parameters in the entrainment of gastric slow waves in patients with gastroparesis. Am J Physiol 1998;**274**:G186–91.

7 **Eagon JC, Kelly KA**. Effects of gastric pacing on canine gastric motility and emptying. Am J Physiol 1993;**265**:G767–74.

8 **McCallum RW,Chen JDZ, Lin ZY et al**. Gastric pacing improves gastric emptying and symptoms in patients with gastroparesis. Gastroenterology 1998; **114**:456–61.

9 **Hocking MP, Vogel SB, Sninsky CA**. Human gastric myoelectrical activity and gastric emptying following gastric surgery and with pacing. Gastroenterology 1992;**103**:1811–16.

10 **Miedema BW, Sarr MG, Kelly KA**. Pacing the human stomach. Surgery 1992;**111**:143–50.

11 **Lin ZY, McCallum RW, Schirmer BD et al**. Effects of pacing parameters in the entrainment of gastric slow waves in patients with gastroparesis. Am J Physiol 1998;**274**:G186–91.

12 **Bellahsène B-E, Schirmer BD, Updike OL et al**. Effect of electrical stimulation on gastric emptying. Dig Dis Sci 1987;**32**:902.

13 **Bellahsène B-E, Lind CD, Schirmer BD et al**. Acceleration of gastric emptying with electrical stimulation in a canine model of gastroparesis. Am J Physiol 1992;**262**:G826–34.

14 **Familoni BO, Abell TL, Nemoto D et al**. Efficacy of electrical stimulation at frequencies higher than basal rate in canine stomach. Dig Dis Sci 1997;**42**:892–97.

15 **Familoni BO, Abell TL, Voeller G et al**. Electrical stimulation at a frequency higher than basal rate in human stomach. Dig Dis Sci 1997;**42**:885.

16 **Huizinga JD**. Gastrointestinal peristalsis: joint action of enteric nerves, smooth muscle, and interstitial cells of Cajal. Microsc Res Tech 1999;**47**:239–47.

17 **Sanders KM**. Regulation of smooth muscle excitation and contraction. Neurogastroenterol Motil 2008;**20**(Suppl. 1):39–53.

18 **Furness JB**. The enteric nervous system: normal functions and enteric neuropathies. Neurogastroenterol Motil 2008;**20**(Suppl. 1):32–38.

19 **Farrugia G**. Interstitial cells of Cajal in health and disease. Neurogastroenterol Motil 2008; **20**(Suppl. 1):54–63.

20 **Grover M. Farrugia G. Lurken MS et al.** Cellular changes in diabetic and idiopathic gastroparesis. Gastroenterology 2011;**140**:1575–85.

21 **Tack J, Piessevaux H, Coulie B, Caenepeel P, Janssens J.** Role of impaired gastric accommodation to a meal in functional dyspepsia. Gastroenterology 1998;**115**(6):1346.

22 **Brody F, Vaziri K, Saddler A et al.** Gastric electrical stimulation for gastroparesis. J Am Coll Surg 2008;**207**:533–38.

23 **Al-Jubury A, Granger S, Barnes J et al.** Laparoscopy shortens the length of stay in patients with gastric electrical stimulation. J Soc Laparoendo Surg 2005;**9**:305–10.

24 **Curuchi AP, Al-Juburi A, Familoni B et al.** Gastric electrical stimulation-a ten year experience. Gastroenterology 2004;**126**:A1284.

25 **Abell T, Lou J, Tabbaa M et al.** Gastric electrical stimulation for gastroparesis improves nutritional parameters at short, intermediate, and long-term follow-up. JPEN 2003;**27**(4):277–81.

26 **Abell T, McCallum R, Hocking M et al.** Gastric electrical stimulation for medically refractory gastroparesis. Gastroenterology 2003;**125**:421–28.

27 **Cutts T, Luo J, Starkebaum W et al.** Is gastric electrical stimulation is superior to standard pharmacologic therapy in improving gi symptoms, healthcare resources, and long-term health care costs? Neurogastroenterol Motil 2005;**17**:35–43.

28 **Abell T, Custem EV, Abrahamsson H et al.** Gastric electrical stimulation in intractable symptomatic gastroparesis. Digestion 2002;**66**:204–21.

29 **Gourcerol G, Leblanc I, Leroi AM et al.** Gastric electrical stimulation in medically refractory nausea and vomiting. Eur J Gastroenterol Hepatol 2007;**19**:29–35.

30 **Islam S, Vick LR, Runnels MJ et al.** Gastric electrical stimulation for children with intractable nausea and gastroparesis. J Pediatr Surg 2008;**43**(3):437–42.

31 **Mason RJ, Lipham J, Eckerling G et al.** Gastric Electrical Stimulation: an alternative surgical therapy for patients with gastroparesis. Arch Surg 2005;**140**: 841–48.

32 **McKenna D, Beverstein G, Reichelderfer M et al.** Gastric electrical stimulation is an effective and safe treatment for medically refractory gastroparesis. Surgery 2008;**144**:566–74.

33 **McCallum RW, Snape W, Brody F et al.** Gastric electrical stimulation with Enterra therapy improves symptoms from diabetic gastroparesis in a prospective study. Clin Gastroenterol Hepatol 2010;**8**:947–54.

34 **Lin Z, Sarosiek I, Forster J et al.** Symptom responses, long-term outcomes and adverse events beyond 3 years of high-frequency gastric electrical stimulation for gastroparesis. Neurogastornterol Motil 2006;**18**:18–27.

35 **Forester J, Sarosiek I, Lin Z et al.** Further experience with gastric stimulation to treat drug refractory gastroparesis. Am J Gastro 2003;**186**:690–95.

36 **Lin Z, McElhinney C, Sarosiek I et al.** Chronic gastric electrical stimulation for gastroparesis reduces the use of prokinetic and/or antiemetic medications and the need for hospitalizations. Dig Dis Sci 2005 Jul;**50**:1328–34.

37 **McCallum RW, Lin Z, Wetzl P et al.** Clinical response to gastric electrical stimulation in patients with postsurgical gastroparesis. Clin Gastroenterol Hepatol 2005;**3**:49–54.

38 **Oubre B, Luo J, Al-Juburi A et al.** Pilot study on gastric electrical stimulation on surgery-associated gastroparesis: long-term outcome. South Med J 2005 Jul;**98**:693–97.

39 **Salameh J, Schmieg RE, Runnels JM et al.** Refractory gastroparesis after roux-en-y gastric bypass: surgical treatment with implantable pacemaker. J Gastrointest Surg 2007**11**:1669–72.

40 **Andersson S, lonroth H, Simren M et al.** Gastric electrical stimulation for intractable vomiting in patients with chronic intestinal pseudiobstruction. Neurogastroenterol Motil 2006;**18**:823–30.

41 **Filichia LA, Cendan JC.** Small case series of gastric electrical stimulation for the management of transplant-induced gastroparesis. J Surg Res 2008;**148**:90–3.

42 **Chen JD, Xu X, Zhang J et al.** Efficiency and efficacy of multi-channel gastric electrical stimulation. Neuogastroenterol Motil 2005;**17**:878–82.

43 **Song G, Hou X, Yang B et al.** Two-channel gastric electrical stimulation accelerates delayed gastric emptying induced by vasopressin. Dig Dis Sci 2005;**50**:662–68.

44 **Sarosiek I, Forester J, Roeser k et al.** Effect of multi-point gastric electrical pacing (MGP. on symptoms, gastric emptying and electrical activity in diabetic gastroparesis. Gastroenterology 2008;**134**:A847.

45 **Mintchev MP, Sanmiguel CP, Amaris M et al.** Microprocessor-controlled movement of solid gastric content using sequential neural electrical stimulation. Gastroenterology 2000;**118**:258–63.

46 **Anand C, Al-Juburi A, Familoni B et al.** Gastric electrical stimulation is safe and effective: a long-term study in patients with drug-refractory gastroparesis in three regional centers. Digestion 2007 Feb 5;464. Online < www.karger.com/dig >

47 **McCallum RW, Zhiyue L, Forester J et al.** Gastric electrical stimulation improves outcomes of patients with gastroparesis for up to 10 years. Clin Gastroenterol Hepatol 2011;**9**:314–19.

48 **Forster J, Damjanov I, Lin Z et al.** Absence of the interstitial cells of Cajal in patients with gastroparesis and correlation with clinical findings. J Gastrointest Surg 2005 Jan;**9**:102–08.

49 **Maranki JL, Lytes V, Meilahn JE et al.** Predictive factors for clinical improvement with Enterra gastric electric stimulation treatment for refractory gastroparesis. Dig Dis Sci 2008;**53**:2072–78.

50 **Ayinala S, Bastita O, Al-Juburi A et al.** Temporary gastric electrical stimulation can be safely performed with oral or PEG placed electrodes in patients with drug refractory gastroparesis. Gastrointest Endosc 2005;**61**(3):455–61.

51 **Abidi N, Starkebaum WL, Abell TL.** An energy algorithm improves symptoms in some patients with gastroparesis and treated with gastric electrical stimulation. Neurogastroenterol Motil 2006;**18**:334–38.

52 **Chen JDZ, Qian L, Ouyang H et al.** Gastric electrical stimulation with short pulses reduces vomiting but not dysrhythmia in dogs. Gastroenterolgy 2003;**124**:401–09.

53 **Lin Z, Forster J, Sarosiek I et al.** Effect of high-frequency gastric electrical stimulation on gastric myoelectrical activity in gastroparetic patients. Neurogastroenterol Motil 2004;**16**:205–12.

54 **Lin Z, Forster J, Sarosiek I et al.** Treatment of gastroparesis by high-frequency gastric electrical stimulation. Diabetes Care 2004;**27**:1071–76.

55 **Horowitz M, Harding PE, Maddox AF et al.** Gastric and esophageal emptying in patients with type 2 (non insulin-dependent. diabetes mellitus. Diabetologia 1989;**32**:151–9.

56 **Bityutskiy LP, Soykan I, McCallum RW.** Viral astroparesis; a subgroup of idiopathic gastroparesis-clinical characteristics and long-term outcomes. Am J Gastroenterol 1997;**92**:1501–04.

57 **Xing JH, Brody F, Brodsky J et al.** Gastric electrical stimulation at proximal stomach induces gastric relaxation in dogs. Neurogastroenterol Motil 2003;**15**:15–23.

58 **Xing JH, Chen JDZ.** Gastric electrical stimulation with parameters of gastroparesis enhances gastric accommodation and alleviates distension-induced symptoms in dogs. Dig Dis Sci 2006;**51**:2160–64.

59 **Tack J, Piessevaux H, Coulie B et al J.** Role of impaired gastric accommodation to a meal in functional dyspepsia. Gastroenterology 1998;**115**:1346–52.

60 **Samson M, Roelfus JM, Akkermans LM et al.** Proximal gastric motor activity in response to a liquid meal in type 1 diabetes mellitus with autonomic neuropathy. Dig Dis Sci 1998;**43**:491–6.

61 **McCallum RW, Dusing RW, Sarosiek I et al.** Mechanisms of high-frequency electrical stimulation in the stomach in gastroparetic patients. Conf Proc and Intern conf IEEE Engin Med Biol Soc 2006;**1**:5400–540. PMID: 17945898 [PubMed - indexed for MEDLINE]

62 **Stanghellini V**. Unfulfilled wishes by gastric electrical stimulation. Clin Gastroentero & Hepatol 2011;**9**:447–8.

63 **Sandler RS, Everhart JE, Donowitz M, et al**. The burden of selected digestive diseases in the United States. Gastroenterology 2002;**122**:1500–11.

64 **El-Serag HB, Sweet S, Winchester CC, et al**. Update on the epidemiology of gastro-oesophageal reflux disease: a systematic review. Gut 2014;**63**:871–80.

65 **Becher A, Al-Serag H**. Systematic review: the association between symptomatic response to proton pump inhibitors and health-related quality of life in patients with gastro-oesophageal reflux disease. Aliment Pharmacol Ther 2011;**34**:618–27.

66 **Joish VN, Donaldson G, Stockdale W, et al**. The economic impact of GERD and PUD: examination of direct and indirect costs using a large integrated employer claims database. Curr Med Res Opin 2005;**21**:535–44.

67 **Kaltenback T, Crockett S, Gerson LB**. Are lifestyle measures effective in patients with gastroesophageal reflux disease? An evidence-based approach. Archives of Internal Medicine 2006;**166**:965–71.

68 **El-Serag H, Becher A, Jones R**. Systematic review: persistent reflux symptoms on proton pump inhibitor therapy in primary care and community studies. Aliment Pharmacol Ther 2010;**32**:720–37.

69 **Sifrim D, Zerbib F**. Diagnosis and management of patients with reflux symptoms refractory to proton pump inhibitors. Gut 2012;**61**:1340–54.

70 **Vakil N, Shaw M, Kirby R**. Clinical effectiveness of laparoscopic fundoplication in a US community. Am J Med 2003;**114**:1–5.

71 **Fass R, Sifrim D**. Management of heartburn not responding to proton pump inhibitors. Gut 2009;**58**:295–309.

72 **Johnson DA, Oldfield EC**. Reported side effects and complications of long-term proton pump inhibitor use: dissecting the evidence. Clin Gastro Hepatol 2013;**11**:458–64.

73 **Richter JE**. Gastroesophageal reflux disease treatment: side effects and complications of fundoplication. Clin Gastro Hepatol 2013;**11**:465–71.

74 **Wang YR, Dempsey DT, Richter JE**. Trends and perioperative outcomes of inpatient antireflux surgery in the United States. Dis Esophagus 2011;**24**:215–23.

75 **Ellis F, Berne TV and Settevig K**. The Prevention of Experimentally Induced Reflux by Electrical Stimulation of the Distal Esophagus. Am J Surg 1968;**111**:482–7.

76 **Clarke JO et al**. An endoscopically implantable device stimulates the lower esophageal sphincter on demand by remote control: a study using a canine model. Endoscopy 2007;**39**:72–6.

77 **Sanmiguel CP, et al**. Effect of electrical stimulation of the LES on LES pressure in a canine model. Am J Physiol Gastrointest Liver Physiol 2008;**295**:389–94.

78 **Rodriguez L, Rodriguez P, Neto MG, et al**. Short-term electrical stimulation of the lower esophageal sphincter increases sphincter pressure in patients with gastroesophageal reflux disease. Neurogastroenterol Motil 2012;**24**:446–50.

79 **Banerjee R, Pratap N, Kalpala R, Reddy DN**. Effect of electrical stimulation of the lower esophageal sphincter using endoscopically implanted temporary stimulation leads in patients with reflux disease. Surg Endosc 2014;**28**:1003–9.

80 **Rodriguez L, Rodriguez P, Gomez B, Ayala J, Oxenberg D, Perez-Castilla A, Netto M, Soffer E, Crowell M**. Electrical Stimulation Therapy (EST) of the Lower Esophageal Sphincter (LES) Is Successful in Treating GERD—Long-Term 3 Year Results. Surg Endosc (in press).

81 **Kappelle WF, Bredenoord AJ, Conchillo JM, et al**. Electrical stimulation therapy of the lower esophageal sphincter for refractory gastroesophageal reflux disease—interim results of an international multicenter trial. Aliment Pharmacol Ther 2015 Sep;**42**(5):614–25.

82 WHO Fact sheet N311, May 2014.

83 **Dee A, Kearns K, O'Neill C, Sharp L, Staines A, O'Dwyer V, et al.** The direct and indirect costs of both overweight and obesity: a systematic review. BMC Res Notes 2014;**7**:242.

84 **Jensen MD, Ryan DH, Apovian CM, Ard JD, Comuzzie AG, Donato KA, et al.** 2013 AHA/ACC/TOS guideline for the management of overweight and obesity in adults: a report of the American College of Cardiology/American Heart Association Task Force on Practice Guidelines and The Obesity Society. Circulation 2014;**129**(25 Suppl):S102–38.

85 **Chang SH, Stoll CRT, Song J, Varela JE, Eagon CJ, Colditz GA.** The effectiveness and risks of bariatric surgery an updated systematic review and meta-analysis. 2003–2012. JAMA Surg 2014;**149**(3):275–87.

86 **Finkelstein EA, Trogdon JG, Cohen JW, Dietz W.** Annual medical spending attributable to obesity payer-and-service-specific estimates. Health Aff (Millwood) 2009;**28**:w822–31.

87 **Camilleri M.** Integrated upper gastrointestinal response to food intake. Gastroenterology 2006;**131**:640–58.

88 **Morton GJ, Meek TH, Schwartz MW.** Neurobiology of food intake in health and disease. Nat Rev Neurosci 2014;**15**:367–78.

89 **Eagon JC, Kelly KA.** Effects of gastric pacing on canine gastric motility and emptying. Am J Physiol 1993;**265**:G767–74.

90 **Onen D, Jalilian D, Neshev E, Mintchev MP.** Parametric study of neural gastric electrical stimulation in acute canine models. Trans Biomed Eng 2007;**54**(3):429–35.

91 **Shikora SA, Bergenstal R, Bessler M, Brody F, Foster G, Frank A, et al.** Implantable gastric stimulation for the treatment of clinically severe obesity: results of the SHAPE trial. Surg Obes Relat Dis 2009;**5**(1):31–7.

92 **Peles S, Petersen J, Aviv R, Policker S, Abu-Hatoum O, Ben- Haimm SA, et al.** Enhancement of antral contractions and vagal afferent signaling with synchronized electrical stimulation. Am J Physiol Gastrointest Liver Physiol 2003;**285**:G577–85.

93 **Bohdjalian A, Prager G, Ricardo A, Policker S, Schindler K, Kretschmer S, et al.** One-year experience with Tantalus™: a new surgical approach to treat morbid obesity. Obes Surg 2006;**16**:627–34.

94 **Kral JG.** Vagotomy for treatment of severe obesity. Lancet 1978;**1**:307–8.

95 **Camilleri M, Toouli J, Herrera MF, Kulseng B, Kow L, Pantoja JP, et al.** Intra-abdominal vagal blocking (VBLOC therapy): clinical results with a new implantable medical device. Surgery 2008;**143**(6):723–31.

96 **Camilleri M, Toouli J, Herrera MF, Kow L, Pantoja JP, Bilington CJ, et al.** Selection of electrical algorithms to treat obesity with intermittent vagal block using an implantable medical device. Surg Obes Relat Dis 2009;**5**(2):224–9.

97 **Ikramuddin S, Blackstone RP, Brancatisano A et al.** Effect of reversible intermittent intra-abdominal vagal nerve blockade on morbid obesity. ReCharge Randomized Clin Trial. JAMA 2014;**312**(9):915–22.

Chapter 18

Hyperhidrosis: pathophysiology and available therapies

Brian Perri, Shoshanna Vaynman, Samer Ghostine, Srinath Samudrala, J. Patrick Johnson, and Khawar Siddique

Key points

1 Hyperhidrosis is characterized by excessive sweating.
2 Standard medical therapies include anticholinergics or aluminium salts.
3 Minimally invasive (thoracoscopic) sympathectomy was introduced in 1951.
4 Selective ganglionectomy is now the treatment of choice.
5 Sympathectomy is effective and safe.

Introduction

Primary hyperhidrosis is an idiopathic condition characterized by excessive sweating beyond the physiological amount required to maintain thermal homeostasis, which can manifest with or without the presence of an offensive odour (bromhidrosis) (1). Hyperhidrosis can be a functionally morbid and even disabling disease, causing physical discomfort and social embarrassment, and negatively impacting occupational and daily activities. The onset of symptoms is usually during childhood or adolescence, and as such it can greatly impact psychosocial and educational development. Although studies have reported a spontaneous resolution of symptoms in patients after their mid-20s (2), for many, hyperhydrosis persists into adulthood and causes life-long social, and in some cases, debilitating functional morbidities.

Numerous treatments have been utilized for primary hyperhidrosis, such as the application of aluminium salts or oral anticholinergics. However, when conservative treatment options fail to control excessive sweating, a surgical approach may be considered. Surgical technology has advanced over the past few years in the treatment for primary hyperhidrosis.

Especially with the advent of minimally invasive surgical and imaging modalities, surgical treatment of hyperhydrosis, such as endoscopic transthoracic sympathectomy (ETS), is becoming a viable option. We discuss the history, clinical findings, pathophysiology, and treatment options for primary hyperhidrosis, including new developments in ETS.

Epidemiology

Although epidemiologic data is limited, hyperhidrosis is a relatively common condition with a reported incidence of 0.15–0.25% in young Israelis (3). Hyperhidrosis occurs in as high as 1% of the Western population, which is 20 times more frequent than in the Japanese or other Asian ethnic populations (4, 5). This condition is believed to have an autosomal recessive inheritance pattern with incomplete penetration (6).

Pathophysiology

Primary hyperhidrosis comprises one of two main categories of the general disease (7). Any part of the body may be affected, but the condition is usually focal with the palms, axillae, and soles of the feet, representing the most common areas of complaint (3).

Secondary hyperhidrosis can be generalized or focal but results from a myriad of medical conditions, such as chronic infections, dermatological ailments, neurological problems, cancer, the use of certain drugs, endocrine disorders, and conditions associated with excess catecholamine (7), as well as gustatory sweating auxiliary to diabetes or parotid gland surgery (8, 9). In contrast, primary hyperhidrosis is mediated by an abnormally hyperactive sympathetic nervous system. Complex regional pain syndrome (causalgia or reflex sympathetic dystrophy) and Raynaud's syndrome are conditions similarly caused by abnormal sympathetic nervous system regulation.

The sympathetic system is controlled by the hypothalamus, which sends fibres to the thoracic and upper lumbar intermediolateral zone of the spinal cord where the sympathetic cell bodies reside. From there, the sympathetic fibres travel to the sympathetic chain found lateral to the spinal column. It can be thought of as a parallel nerve circuit to the spinal cord with bilateral intervertebral segment relays from the spinal cord to the sympathetic chain. Surgical correction of primary hyperhidrosis aims to interrupt the sympathetic signalling to palmar and axillary cholinergic sweat glands by cutting and removing the T3 (and sometimes T4) ganglia and intervening sympathetic chain bilaterally. Because the sympathetic chain is, in effect, a parallel nerve circuit, the distal aspect of the sympathetic nervous system innervation is not disrupted.

Medical therapy

Anticholinergics

Primary hyperhidrosis is treated medically, first with systemic anticholinergic drugs, which may have variable effectiveness. Unfortunately, these drugs commonly cause undesirable side-effects that include blurry vision, dilated pupils, constipation, hastened micturation, heart palpitations, and mydriasis. As such, systemic anticholinergics have been unpopular with hyperhidrosis patients. Alternatively, topical anticholenergics, such as Drysol, have been used to avoid the adverse effects of systemic anticholinergics. These agents have variable success but can cause skin irritation requiring further specialized care (10).

Iontophoresis

Iontophoresis is another treatment option first introduced by Bouman et al. in the 1950s (11). This procedure entails directly applying a low-level electric current, about 15–20 mA, to the skin under an electrolyte solution for 30 minutes. The current creates a 'shock' that is perceived by many to be uncomfortable. Skin irritation and even burns are other side-effects that are not uncommon. Given the accompanying pain and discomfort, the major drawback to this form of therapy is that the procedure must be performed frequently, initially a few times per week and eventually once every couple weeks, in order to be effective. Results with iontophoresis are variable but typically produce the most successful results in patients with mild symptoms.

Botulinum toxin injections

More recently, injection of botulinum toxin (Botox) directly into the palmar subepidermal tissue has been implemented as an available treatment option for hyperhidrosis. Reports by Shelley et al. (12) and Schnider et al. (13) give a general outline of the treatment, which typically consists of 6–50 injections into each palm. Shelley et al. (12) found that each injection of 2 mouse units of botulinum toxin can effectively produce a 1.2-cm diameter of anhydrosis. The use of botulinum toxin injection to treat hyperhidrosis has been tested against the use of sodium chloride solution (13). Overall results using Botox showed a 26% reduction in sweating 3–8 weeks post-injection and 31% reduction after 13 weeks. Injection of botulinum toxin had a common side-effect of mild transient muscle weakness that resolved within 2–5 weeks (12, 13). The associated thumb weakness typically resolved in 3 weeks. Botox injections have to be repeated at various intervals (usually between 1 and 6 months) to treat recurrences (13). One report published a case of severe atrophy of the intrinsic muscles of the hand in a patient treated with intra-palmar Botox (14). Although the immediate short-term efficacy of Botox use for hyperhidrosis appears good, data on long-term use is not fully available.

Surgical treatments

It is important to reserve surgical intervention of primary hyperhidrosis for cases that are refractory to medical management. In many patients, the non-surgical treatments have limited efficacy, require a life-long use of the medications, or repeated treatment modalities in the case of electric current application or Botox injection. Furthermore, these treatments are often time-consuming, expensive, and entail significant side-effects. As such, the quest for a more definitive treatment for this condition has led to developing options through surgical intervention.

Pre-operative work-up

A pre-operative work-up is necessary to rule out secondary hyperhidrosis that can potentially be treated medically. Some of the most important causes of secondary hyperhidrosis are paraneoplastic/neurologic syndrome, thyroxicosis, diabetes mellitus, gout, menopause, pheochromocytoma, chronic alcoholism, and spinal cord injury, and medications such as tricyclic antidepressants and propranolol. Nocturnal hyperhidrosis can be associated with tuberculosis and Hodgkin disease. Psychological stimuli, in addition to thermoregulatory signals from the cerebral cortex, have also been shown to cause regional palmar sweating (10). Thyroid function panel, serum glucose levels, uric acid, and urine catecholamine level should be considered. Imaging should include at least a chest radiograph to rule out pulmonary lesions.

History and evolution of surgical sympathectomy

Thoracic sympathectomy was first introduced by Kotzareff in 1920 (15). Resection of the upper thoracic sympathetic ganglia has been shown to be an effective and definitive treatment for primary hyperhidrosis. However, the early approaches to the high thoracic sympathetic chain were highly invasive. They were achieved through a posterior paraspinal, supraclavicular, or an open thoracotomy. Historically, these surgeries were performed predominantly by cardiothoracic surgeons. The surgical incision required to gain adequate surgical exposure was commonly greater than 10 cm long. The approach was associated with significant morbidity and proved to be more traumatizing and time-consuming than the actual sympathectomy itself.

Minimally invasive sympathectomy

In 1951, Kux first described the thoracic endoscopic procedure for the treatment of tuberculosis (16). The urologic endoscope was adapted for use in these early surgeries. The technology was subsequently enhanced by integrating it with endoscopic monitoring technology to produce the minimally invasive video-assisted thoracoscopic surgery (VATS). Video-assisted monitoring enabled surgeons to obtain magnified and detailed images of the sympathetic ganglia through percutaneous portals, thereby eliminating the need to perform an open thoracotomy. Thoracoscopic sympathectomy surgery decreased the morbidity associated with early open procedures. VATS has been shown to accelerate patient recovery and improve patient satisfaction. In one series, 65 hyperhidrosis patients, 112 sympathectomies were performed by VATS endoscopic sympathectomy and ganglionectomy. Overall, VATS endoscopic sympathectomies were as successful as the open surgical techniques for treating hyperhidrosis but had the added benefit of substantially decreasing morbidity, length of hospital stay, and the time it took to return to normal activity. Complications and recurrence of symptoms were comparable with those demonstrated in previous reports. Furthermore, patient satisfaction and willingness to undergo a repeat operative procedure ranged from 66 to 99%. VATS sympathectomy has proven to be a successful treatment modality with high patient satisfaction in treating patients with palmar and axillary hyperhidrosis. Upper thoracic sympathectomy with ganglionectomies at T3 and T4 levels has been performed by multiple centres for the treatment of these conditions.

Technological advancements have continued to pave the way for improving endoscopic sympathectomy surgery. Today, for example, the instruments are smaller in diameter and they have a higher resolution quality. Thus, fewer and smaller access ports are used to perform the surgery. At our institution, we have been using a two small port technique to introduce the endoscope and a working endoscopic instrument. Different instruments can be inserted through the working port at the same time the endoscope is inserted, including scissors, electrocautery, and a suction/irrigator. In addition to making the incision more cosmetically desirable, this approach provides safe, easy access to the thoracic cavity. The modern high-quality endoscopes provide excellent resolution imaging to perform the sympathectomy surgery.

Nuances of surgical sympathectomy

The authors are now performing only T3 ganglionectomies and sympathetic chain resection, by dividing and removing the sympathetic chain above and below the T3 ganglion, for patients with symptoms of isolated bilateral palmar hyperhidrosis. If an accessory nerve of Kuntz is identified (often branching off the T2 ganglion), it is divided and resected. It is necessary to identify these common accessory nerve branches to completely eliminate the patient's excessive sweating. Additionally, the authors are performing bilateral T3 ganglionectomy and intervening sympathectomy in patients who experience symptoms of both palmar and axillary hyperhidrosis. It is worthwhile to note that patients with unilateral symptoms of hyperhidrosis must be thoroughly evaluated pre-operatively for possible causes of secondary hyperhidrosis.

The authors do not employ the *previous* technique of carbon dioxide insufflation for surgical exposure. This avoids the small but potential risk of decreasing cardiac stroke volume secondary to increased intra-thoracic pressure. Instead, a double-lumen endotracheal intubation is used for single-lung ventilation. This technique allows the ipsilateral lung to partially deflate and expose the upper thoracic sympathetic chain. Additionally, even though the authors are using smaller ports (2–5 mm versus 10-mm) for access to the thoracic cavity, they can intentionally allow atmospheric pressure to equilibrate with the intra-pleural cavity to cause a controlled pneumothorax. This provides enough exposure to successfully perform the sympathectomy. The partial lung collapse may be reversed after the sympathectomy by having the anaesthetist hold the patient's breath and provide positive pressure briefly while the surgeon aspirates intra-pleural air with the endoscopic suction. Once the lung is endoscopically visualized for full expansion, the endoscopic instruments can be withdrawn from the chest cavity.

Description of thoracoscopic sympathectomy

The first port is introduced above the fourth rib in the axilla. The endoscope is introduced through this port and the thoracic cavity is visually explored. The partially deflated lung

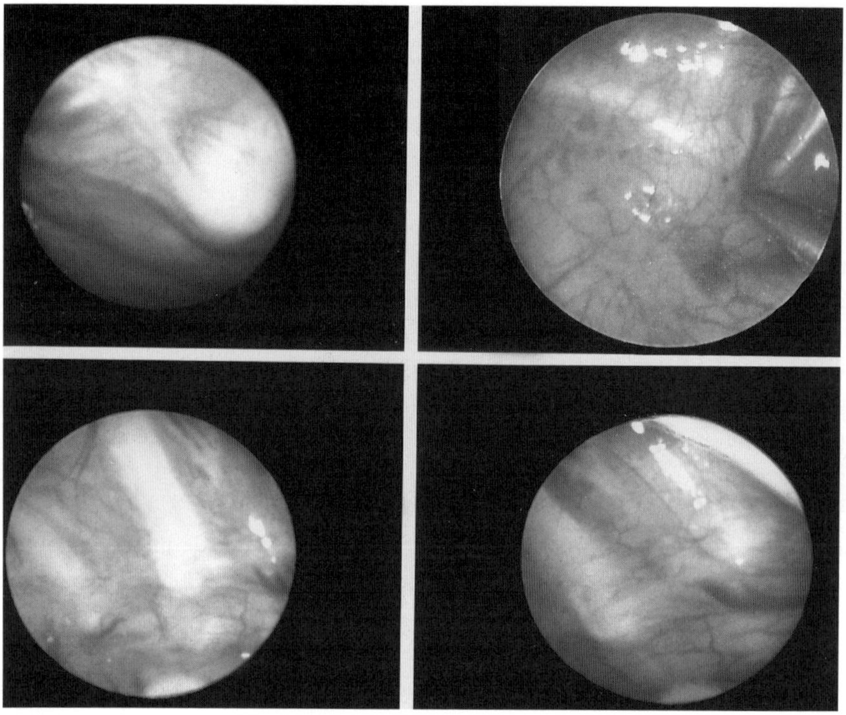

Fig. 18.1 Endoscopic view of the left thoracic cavity. The image shows the sympathetic chain coursing over the second and third rib heads and deep to the semi-transparent parietal pleura. (See Plate 5.)

is identified and gently swept away, if necessary. The first rib is most often not visible. The rib heads from T2 to T4 are easily identifiable through the parietal pleura and are important landmarks during the thoracoscopic sympathectomy surgery. The sympathetic chain courses superficial to the segmental and intercostal vessels. The stellate ganglion lies within the first intercostal space cephalad to the second rib head (Fig. 18.1).

The sympathetic chain is easily seen as it is a slightly raised, longitudinal structure running parallel to the spine and coursing over the rib heads. The parietal pleura from the second to third rib head are divided. Each sympathetic ganglion is located over or just caudal to the corresponding numbered rib (Fig. 18.2). The exposed sympathetic chain and associated T3 (and T4) ganglion is isolated, divided, then removed from the thoracic cavity. Haemostasis is achieved when necessary using bipolar cautery. The T2 ganglion is inspected to identify the accessory nerve of Kuntz. If this is identified, it is divided to ensure complete resolution of the hyperhidrosis.

The optimal ganglion selected for resection in the treatment of palmar hyperhidrosis remains a topic open to debate. Studies have investigated the effectiveness of T2 versus T3 ganglion resection (17) and T2 versus T4 ganglion resection (18). It appears that resecting any combination of the T2, T3, or T4 ganglion set is equally effective in providing

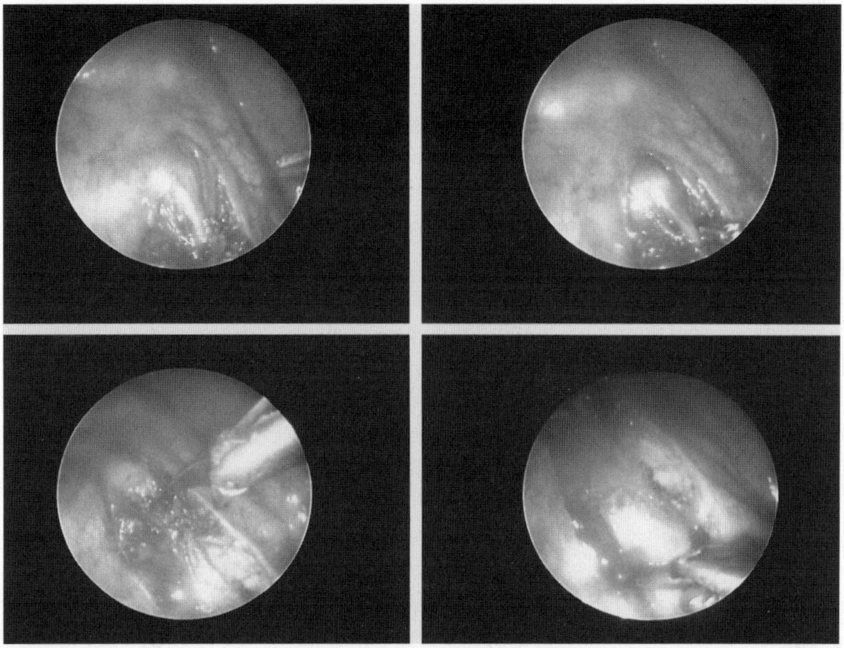

Fig. 18.2 The sympathetic chain and T3 ganglion are visible through the parietal pleura that has been divided. The endoscopic grasper lies adjacent to the sympathetic chain below the third rib and T3 ganglion. (See Plate 6.)

greater than 98% symptomatic improvement in palmar hyperhidrosis (17, 18). Current literature also suggests that there is less severe compensatory truncal hyperhidrosis when the T3 versus T2 ganglion is resected (17, 19) and infrequent compensatory hyperhidrosis when the T4 ganglion versus the T2 ganglion is resected (18). Yoon et al. (19) chose to perform T3 ganglionectomy in patients with palmar hyperhidrosis and both T3 and T4 ganglion resection in patients who exhibited axillary hyperhidrosis. In their study of 27 patients (24 with palmar hyperhidrosis, 3 with both palmar and axillary hyperhidrosis), all reported high satisfaction at a mean follow-up of 19 months. All patients had complete resolution of hyperhidrosis with the exception of one patient who continued to have axillary symptoms and required revision T4 ganglion resection. One patient experienced mild truncal compensatory hyperhidrosis for 1 month following surgery. Thus, T3 selective ganglion resection for palmar hyperhidrosis symptoms and T3 and T4 ganglion resection for symptomatic palmar and axillary hyperhidrosis provides a high success rate with a low incidence of compensatory truncal hyperhidrosis. In an additional study, Riet et al. (20) looked at selectively resecting T3 ganglion for palmar hyperhidrosis. They found 100% of patients had resolved hyperhidrosis, no recurrence of hyperhidrosis symptoms, and no incidence of compensatory hyperhidrosis at 3.5 years post-operative (20).

The accessory nerve of Kuntz is typically a rami communicantes of T2, but can arise from T3 or T4. This accessory nerve (more than one may be present) can be identified prior to incising the parietal pleura, as it courses parallel to the sympathetic chain. This small nerve branch may continue to carry neural signals past the transected segment of the sympathetic nerve trunk and should be divided when identified to increase the probability for successfully decreasing palmar hyperhidrosis.

Several monitoring systems are available to assess the success of an intra-operative sympathectomy at the level of the palms. Palmar cutaneous temperature transducers are the simplest means to detect a 1 to 2 degree increase in hand temperature, and laser Doppler flowmetry or arterial Doppler of the hands can measure for blood flow increase to the hands (21, 22, 23).

Risks associated with surgical sympathectomy

Compensatory hyperhidrosis

The physiologic response of the body following sympathectomy can result in compensatory sweating in previously unaffected areas (24). Compensatory hyperhidrosis is usually experienced on the trunk, face, posterior knees, or inner thighs. This effect is usually transient, lasting less than 6 months. Nevertheless, current technologies and a better understanding of the anatomical causes of compensatory hyperhidrosis have reduced its incidence.

Other surgical risks

Horner's syndrome is another complication, which is associated with a T1, stellate ganglion injury (25). Recalcitrant hyperhidrosis can also occur. These problems are typically avoided by simply dividing the accessory nerve(s) of Kuntz, avoiding stapling of the sympathetic chain (staples have been reported to dislodge), and removing the short segment of the sympathetic chain and ganglion (the nerve can otherwise grow back and re-anastomose). Interocostal neurovascular injury and post-operative intercostal neuralgia used to be more common with use of the larger ports and instruments. These have been largely absent since the introduction of the smaller diameter instruments and ports of 3 to 5 mm, and with the careful insertion of the port over the superior border of the rib. Pneumothoraces, which naturally result after opening the pleural cavity, are desirable during the surgical procedure but are subsequently easily reversed by having the anaesthetist return ventilation to the lung and provide a Valsalva manoeuvre, while one intra-thoracic instrument is placed on suction and the endoscope is used to visualize complete re-inflation of the lung at the apex. Our current understanding of the neural anatomy, advances in surgical instrumentation, and technical experience make complications associated with VATS sympathectomy extremely rare.

Conclusions

Primary hyperhidrosis is a disabling disease. A work-up must be performed to rule out secondary hyperhidrosis, which may be treated medically. Medications, topical therapies, and treatments such as ionophoresis and Botox injections should be attempted before resorting to a surgical intervention. Sympathectomy surgery for primary hyperhidrosis is an effective and safe treatment, which provides permanent improvement of palmar and axillary symptoms. Recent advances in endoscopic technology have enabled this procedure to be performed in a minimally invasive manner that produces minimal and discrete scarring in the patient's axilla and have advanced its status as an effective and safe treatment option.

References

1 **Atkins JL, Butler PE**. Hyperhidrosis: a review of current management. Plast Reconstr Surg 2002;**110**:222–28.

2 **Coulson IH**. Disorders of sweat glands. In: Burns T, Breathnach S, Cox N, Griffiths C (eds) Rook's Textbook of Dermatology, 7th edn, **vol. 3**. Blackwell Science Ltd; 2004:1–23.

3 **Adar R, Kurchin A, Zweig A, Mozes M**. Palmar hyperhidrosis and its surgical treatment: a report of 100 cases. Ann Surg 1977;**186**(1):34–41.

4 **Cloward RB**. Treatment of hyperhidrosis palmaris (sweaty hands); a familial disease in Japanese. Hawaii Med J 1957;**16**(4):381–87.

5 **Cloward RB**. Hyperhidrosis. J Neurosurg 1969;**30**(5):545–51.

6 **Ro KM**. 'Palmar Hyperhydrosis: evidence of genetic transmission.' J Vasc Surg 2002;**35**(2);382–86.

7 **Boni R**. Generalized hyperhidrosis and its systemic treatment. Curr Probl Dermatol 2002;**30**:44–47.

8 **Laskawi R, Ellies M, Rodel R, Schoenebeck C**. Gustatory sweating: clinical implications and etiologic aspects. J Oral Maxillofac Surg 1999;**57**:642–48.

9 **Restivo DA, Lanza S, Patti F et al**. Improvement of diabetic autonomic gustatory sweating by botulinum toxin type A. Neurology 2002;**59**:1971–73.

10 **Sato K, Kang WH, Saga K, Sato KT**. Biology of sweat glands and their disorders. II. Disorders of sweat gland function. J Am Acad Dermatol 1989;**20**(5 Pt 1):713–26.

11 **Bouman HD, Lentzer EM**. The treatment of hyperhidrosis of hands and feet with constant current. Am J Phys Med 1952;**31**(3):158–69.

12 **Shelley WB, Talanin NY, Shelley ED**. Botulinum toxin therapy for palmar hyperhidrosis. J Am Acad Dermatol 1998;**38**(2 Pt 1):227–29.

13 **Schnider P, Binder M, Auff E, ittler H, Berger T, Wolff K**. Double-blind trial of botulinum A toxin for the treatment of focal hyperhidrosis of the palms. Br J Dermatol 1997;**136**(4):548–52.

14 **Glass GE, Hussain M, Fleming AN, Powell BW**. Atrophy of the intrinsic musculature of the hands associated with the use of Botulinum toxin-A injections for hyperhidrosis: a case report and review of literature. J Plast Reconstr Anesthet Surg, 2009; **62**(8):e274–76.

15 **Kotzareff A**. Resection partielle de trone sympathetique cervical droit pour hyperhidrose unilaterale. Rev Med Suisse Romande 1920;**40**:111–13.

16 **Kux EF**. Endoscopic resection of the autonomic nervous system of the thoracic cavity. Rev Esp Tuberc 1951;**20**(190):19–24.

17 **Yazbek G, Wolosker N, de Campos JR, Kauffman P, Ishy A, Puech-Leao P**. Palmar hyperhidrosis-which is the best level of denervation using video-assisted thoracoscopic sympathectomy: T2 or T3 ganglion? J Vasc Surg 2005;**42**(2):281–85.

18 **Chou SH, Kao EL, Li HP, Lin CC, Huang MF**. T4 sympathectomy for palmar hyperhidrosis: an effective approach that simultaneously minimizes compensatory hyperhidrosis. Kaohsiung J Med Sci 2005 Jul:**21**(7):310–13.

19 **Yoon do H, Ha Y, Park YG, Chang JW**. Thoracoscopic limited T3 sympathicotomy for primary hyperhidrosis: prevention for compensatory hyperhidrosis. J Neurosurg 2003;**99**(Suppl. 1):39–43.

20 **Riet M, Smet AA, Kuiken H, Kazemier G, Bonjer HJ**. Prevention of compensatory hyperhidrosis after thoracoscopic sympathectomy for hyperhidrosis. Surg Endosc 2001;**15**(10):1159–62 (ISSN: 1432–2218).

21 **Crandall CG, Meyer DM, Davis SL, Dellaria SM**. Palmar skin blood flow and temperature responses throughout endoscopic sympathectomy. Anesth Analg 2005;**100**(1)277–83.

22 **Dickman, CA**. Thorascopic sympathectomy. In: Regan JJ and Lieberman IH (eds) Atlas of Minimal Access Spine Surgery, 2nd edn. Quality Medical Publishing, Inc: St. Louis, Missouri; 2004;321–40.

23 **Klodell CT, Lobato EB, Willert JL, Gravenstein N**. Oximetry-derived perfusion index for Intraoperative indentification of successful thoracic sympathectomy. Ann Thorac Surg 2005;**80**(2):467–70.

24 **Drott C, Gothberg G, Claes G**. Endoscopic transthoracic sympathectomy: an efficient and safe method for the treatment of hyperhidrosis. J Am Acad Dermatol 1995; **33**(1):78–81.

25 **Johnson JP, Patel NP**. Uniportal and biportal endoscopic thoracic sympathectomy. Neurosurgery 2002; **51**(Suppl. 2):79–83.

Chapter 19

Vagus nerve stimulation in the treatment of epilepsy I: history, vagus nerve physiology, and putative mechanisms

Benjamin I. Rapoport and Joseph R. Madsen

Key points

1 Vagus nerve stimulation is a safe therapeutic alternative for the treatment of patients suffering from medically refractory epilepsy.

2 The technology was first approved in 1997 by the United States Food and Drug Administration (FDA) 'for use as an adjunctive therapy in reducing the frequency of seizures in adults and adolescents over 12 years of age with partial onset seizures, which are refractory to anti-epileptic medication'. Approval was based on data from a series of randomized, sham-controlled trials demonstrating a small reduction in patient- and caregiver-reported seizure frequency among patients receiving therapeutic stimulation of the vagus nerve.

3 While the safety of vagus nerve stimulation has been adequately established over the last quarter-century, a careful, comprehensive review of human and animal studies raises questions as to the true efficacy of vagus nerve stimulation in the treatment of epilepsy. The efficacy of vagus nerve stimulation is certainly limited, and an unambiguous benefit relative to the natural history of refractory epilepsy remains to be clearly demonstrated.

4 There are neither known predictors of therapeutic efficacy in specific patients, nor validated techniques for tuning stimulation parameters to improve efficacy after implantation.

5 While the afferent autonomic pathways activated by stimulation of the vagus nerve have known targets within the central nervous system, no mechanism of action has been demonstrated by which stimulation of the vagus nerve should act to suppress epileptiform activity in the cerebral cortex, even after a quarter-century of experience with vagus nerve stimulation in human patients.

Introduction

Epilepsy and the autonomic nervous system

It might at first seem surprising to find a discussion of neuromodulation for the treatment of medically refractory epilepsy in a volume dedicated to surgery on the autonomic nervous system. Perhaps even more surprising, however, is that peripheral stimulation of the autonomic nervous system, through electrical stimulation of the vagus nerve, is thought to have an effect on seizures originating in the cerebral cortex. Yet seizures do frequently present with autonomic signatures, and some of the most dangerous seizures, including those associated with a high risk of sudden death, have the greatest autonomic impact (1). It is with these ideas in mind that we begin our discussion of vagus nerve stimulation for the treatment of epilepsy.

The need for alternatives to medical therapy in the treatment of epilepsy

Epilepsy is a common manifestation of central nervous system disease, and while seizures have a variety of aetiologies, epilepsy as a whole has been estimated to affect approximately 5–10 per 1000 people in the general population worldwide (2). In approximately two-thirds of those with epilepsy, pharmacotherapy affords good control of the disorder; in the remaining approximately one-third, epilepsy is refractory to medical therapy (3, 4). Surgical approaches to the treatment of some forms of epilepsy are available (4, 5), involving the resection or lesioning of brain regions responsible for generating or propagating seizures, but not all medically refractory patients are appropriate surgical candidates. There is consequently a clinical need for further alternatives to the pharmacologic treatment of epilepsy: electrical stimulation of the vagus nerve, a reversible form of neuromodulation, is an appealing technique, and is presently used as one such therapeutic option.

Electrical stimulation of the vagus nerve for medically intractable epilepsy

In its contemporary form, electrical stimulation of the vagus nerve has been systematically investigated and used as an approach to treating medically intractable epilepsy in human patients since the 1980s. An implantable device designed for vagus nerve stimulation (VNS) was first approved in 1997 by the United States Food and Drug Administration (FDA) 'for use as an adjunctive therapy in reducing the frequency of seizures in adults and adolescents over 12 years of age with partial onset seizures, which are refractory to antiepileptic medication' (6). Although a body of clinical literature has developed over the past three decades in support of VNS for use in the palliative management of some forms of epilepsy, the approach remains subject to important scientific and clinical criticisms concerning its efficacy and mechanism of action. The central scientific criticism of VNS is that its mode of action has not been elucidated, even after a quarter-century of experience with the technique. Clinically, the principal objections to VNS are, first, that its efficacy has not been demonstrated in randomized, double-blind, placebo-controlled trials; and, second, that the outcome measures used to quantify and justify its efficacy are partially subjective, and therefore subject to substantial reporting bias, especially in studies involving incomplete blinding of patients and investigators.

In Chapters 19 and 20, we present a critical review of VNS for intractable epilepsy from a practical, neurosurgical perspective. In this chapter, we begin by reviewing the evidence base for VNS in epilepsy. We then discuss the conceptual and technical development of VNS from a historical perspective, and review proposed mechanisms of action together with areas of controversy and continuing uncertainty concerning both efficacy and proposed mechanisms of action. In Chapter 20, we focus on the technical aspects of VNS as currently employed in clinical practice. We begin with discussions of indications and patient selection, and of the devices used for VNS. We then discuss in detail the operative techniques used in placing the vagus nerve electrode leads and implanting the generator, and address heuristics for programming the stimulator. Finally, we discuss post-operative management, including anticipation, avoidance, and management of complications. We hope that this multifaceted presentation will enable surgeons and scientists to appreciate in detail the best current practices associated with VNS for epilepsy, together with the important scientific questions and clinical limitations facing this therapeutic technique, and the implications of those limitations for candidate patients.

Evidence supporting use of vagus nerve stimulation in managing intractable epilepsy

The primary body of evidence used to justify VNS in the management of medically refractory epilepsy consists of the set of five clinical trials conducted for the initial review process by the United States Food and Drug Administration (FDA). These trials were funded by Cyberonics, manufacturer of the 'NeuroCybernetic Prosthesis' vagus nerve stimulator that ultimately received FDA approval in 1997. The trials are referred to in the literature as E01, E02, E03, E04, and E05, respectively, and many of the patients enrolled were followed through open extension periods of varying duration (6). In addition, the manufacturer compiled a registry of effectiveness data submitted by physicians on a voluntary basis, for 4743 patients (7). In this section we briefly review each of the initial trials and the evidence it generated.

The original justification for moving forward with human clinical trials was derived from a small set of animal studies, which we review and discuss in the section entitled 'Areas of controversy and uncertainty'. Results obtained in further clinical studies conducted by various groups since 1997 have in general been consistent with those of the initial trials, and have been reviewed systematically by several authors (8). Some readers may wish to skim the following technical description of the initial human clinical trials, which we provide both for completeness and as background for reference in later discussions of 'Areas of controversy and uncertainty' concerning the evidence provided by these clinical trials.

The E01 and E02 pilot trials

The first implantation of a vagal nerve stimulation device in a human patient was performed in 1988, and the associated four-patient case series described 'complete seizure control in two, a 40% reduction of seizure frequency in one, and no change in seizure frequency in the other' but qualified the results by disclaiming that: 'The results, however, are inconclusive because of the brief duration (6–12 months) of follow-up' (9). This series has subsequently been referred to in the literature as the 'E02 study' and will presently be discussed further.

The E01 study was a pilot longitudinal study that treated 10 patients with partial seizures (simple and complex) at three centres (6, 10, 11). The patient age range was 20–58 years, the interval between diagnosis of epilepsy and study enrolment was 13–22 years, and enrolled patients experienced mean and median numbers of 3.0 and 0.7 seizures per day, respectively, at baseline. All of the patients were concurrently treated with one or two anti-epileptic medications, but serum levels were required to remain in a steady state. Patients were given a 2-week recovery period after stimulator implantation, after which they were monitored through a 'placebo stimulation control period' of 3–4 weeks without stimulation. The subsequent treatment period consisted of 16 weeks of VNS. Each patient served as his or her own control, and analysis was based on differences in seizure rates between the treatment and post-operative control periods. Seizure frequency was determined using seizure diaries maintained by patients, often with the assistance of caregivers. Following the end of the initial stimulation period, patients were permitted to continue receiving VNS, and were followed for varying lengths of time. During the initial treatment phase of the trial, 30% (3 of 10) patients were considered 'responders', where a responder was defined as a patient experiencing greater than 50% reduction in seizure frequency. Mean and median reductions in seizure frequency were 24% and 32%, respectively. During the extension phase of the trial, all 10 patients were followed to 18 months, during which time median per cent seizure reduction remained between 42% and 46%, though the responder rates were 20%, 30%, and 50% (2, 3, and 5 of 10) at 6, 12, and 18 months, respectively. Eight patients were followed to 24 months, at which point the responder rate was 63% (5 of 8), with a mean per cent seizure reduction of 59%. Four patients were followed to 36 months, at which point the responder rate was 50% (2 of 4), with a mean per cent seizure reduction of 65%.

The E02 study, like E01, was a pilot longitudinal study. It treated four patients with partial seizures (simple and complex) at two centres (6, 10, 11). The patient age range was 18–42 years, the interval between diagnosis of epilepsy and study enrolment was 5–36 years, and enrolled patients experienced mean and median numbers of 0.4 seizures per day at baseline. All of the patients were concurrently treated with one or two anti-epileptic medications, and serum levels were required to have been in steady state for 1 month prior to the start of the study. The study design and analysis were identical to those of E01, although the electrical stimulation parameters differed between the two studies. During the initial treatment phase of the trial, 50% (two of four) patients were 'responders'; these two patients were historically the first two human patients to receive the therapy, and the initial, apparent success in these two cases generated enthusiasm for further human trials. Mean and median reductions in seizure frequency were 40% and 48%, respectively. During the extension phase, all four patients were followed to 12 months. Median per cent seizure reduction was 3% at 6 months (at which time only one of four patients was a responder), and 30% at 12 months (again with one of four patients responding). Three patients were followed to 18 months, at which point median per cent seizure reduction was 68% (with two of three patients responding). Two patients were followed to 36 months: at 24 months, median per cent seizure reduction was 60% (with two of two patients responding); and at 36 months, median per cent seizure reduction was 32% (with neither patient 'responding,' as defined by the 50% reduction criterion).

The E03 randomized controlled trial

The E03 study was a randomized, prospective study of the long-term effects of VNS. It has been described in a number of papers (6, 12), of which two by the First International Vagus Nerve Stimulation Study Group are most notable (13, 14). The study was designed as an 'active control' study, in which half of patients were initially randomized to receive low-frequency stimulation with stimulator parameters thought to be non-therapeutic. Because patients in previous trials had been able to sense stimulator activity, this design was considered by the investigators to offer a better control condition than absence of stimulation, in that all patients would sense some stimulator activity, and patients would nominally be blinded as to whether they were receiving high-frequency ('therapeutic') or low-frequency ('placebo') stimulation.

The study included 114 patients with partial seizures (simple and complex) at 17 centres, with 57 randomized to each arm; 126 patients were initially enrolled, and intention-to-treat analysis was used to minimize exclusion bias. The patient age range was 13–57 years (similar across arms), the interval between diagnosis of epilepsy and study enrolment was 4–47 years (similar across arms), and overall the enrolled patients experienced mean and median numbers of 1.6 and 0.8 seizures per day at baseline, respectively (similar across arms). Patients were concurrently treated with zero to three anti-epileptic medications, and were permitted steady-state serum level variation of 20% over 3 months. Patients were monitored for 12 weeks prior to simulator implantation, in order to establish baseline seizure frequency.

During the initial 12-week treatment phase, patients were randomized to receive stimulation with either presumed-therapeutic ('HIGH') or 'active control' ('LOW') stimulation parameters; both sets of parameters differed from those used in the E01 and E02 studies. Following this initial phase, all patients who elected to continue treatment were followed through an indefinite extension phase during which all patients received stimulation according to the presumed therapeutic parameters used for the 'HIGH' group. Seizure frequency calculations were again based on seizure diaries kept by patients and caregivers throughout the trial. The primary outcome measure was the change in reported seizure frequency between the stimulation and baseline periods for the two groups, as recorded in the seizure diaries. During the initial treatment phase of the trial, 30% of patients in the 'HIGH' arm and 14% of those in the 'LOW' arm were responders; mean and median seizure frequencies were reduced by 23% in the 'HIGH' arm and 6% in the 'LOW' arm, respectively. The difference in seizure reduction rates was considered statistically significant, with $p<0.02$ between the groups. During the extension phase, patients were followed, with considerable attrition, to 36 months and beyond. At 6 months, responder rate was 24% (28 of 108 patients), with median seizure frequency reduction of 27%. At 12 months, responder rate was 30% (31 of 102 patients), with median seizure frequency reduction of 33%. At 18 months, responder rate was 45% (32 of 71 patients), with median seizure frequency reduction of 46%. At 24 months, responder rate was 39% (20 of 51 patients), with median seizure frequency reduction of 41%. At 36 months, responder rate was 39% (19 of 49 patients), with median seizure frequency reduction of 40%.

The E04 open-label compassionate use trial

The E04 study was an uncontrolled, unblinded, open-label, compassionate use trial. Only a subset of the results, corresponding to the 24 of 116 treated patients with generalized seizures, have been published in the primary scientific literature (12, 15); the full results were described by Cyberonics in documentation submitted to the FDA (6). Overall, the E04 study treated 116 patients with medically refractory epilepsy, without regard for seizure type, at 24 centres. The patient age range was 4–63 years, the interval between diagnosis of epilepsy and study enrolment was 1–48 years, and enrolled patients experienced mean and median numbers of 25 and 0.7 seizures per day, respectively, at baseline. Concurrent use of anti-epileptic medications was permitted (the average number of anti-epileptic medications used by trial participants was 2.2), and no attempt was made to control for medication level changes during the trial. Vagus nerve stimulator implantation was performed after establishing seizure frequency during a 1-month-long baseline period; the stimulation parameters used were similar to those used for the 'HIGH' (presumed therapeutic) arm of the E03 study. As in the E01 and E02 studies, each patient served as his or her own control, and seizure frequency was monitored throughout the trial by seizure diaries maintained by patients and their caregivers. Outcome analysis was based on differences in seizure rates between the 'Pre-Implant Baseline Period' and a 12-week 'Acute Phase Stimulation' period; patients could subsequently elect to continue to receive VNS, and were followed on a voluntary basis, with considerable attrition, through an indefinite extension phase.

During the initial treatment phase of the trial, 29% of patients were considered 'responders,' experiencing greater than 50% reduction in seizure frequency. Mean and median reductions in seizure frequency were 7% and 22%, respectively. During the extension phase of the trial, 107 of the initial 116 patients were followed to 6 months, at which time the responder rate was 37% (40 of 107 patients), and the median per cent seizure reduction was 32%. At 12 months, responder rate was 31% (27 of 86 patients), with median seizure frequency reduction of 27%. At 18 months, responder rate was 39% (28 of 72 patients), with median seizure frequency reduction of 41%. At 24 months, responder rate was 35% (12 of 34 patients), with median seizure frequency reduction of 32%.

The E05 randomized controlled trial

The E05 study was similar in structure to E03, and like E03 it was a randomized, prospective study of the long-term effects of VNS. It has been described in a number of papers (16–18). Study design and analysis were identical to those used in E03; the primary difference between E03 and E05 was the larger study size of E05, which included 196 patients with partial seizures (simple and complex) at 20 centres. Ninety-four and 102 patients were prospectively randomized to the 'HIGH' (presumed therapeutic) and 'LOW' (active control) arms, respectively; 262 patients were initially enrolled, and intention-to-treat analysis was used to minimize exclusion bias. The overall patient age range was 13–60 years (similar across arms), and the overall interval between diagnosis of epilepsy and study enrolment was 2–52 years (similar across arms). Patients in the 'HIGH' arm experienced mean and median numbers of 1.6 and 0.6 seizures per day at baseline, respectively, while those in the 'LOW' arm respectively experienced mean and median numbers of 1.0 and 0.5 seizures per day at baseline. Patients were concurrently treated with an average of two anti-epileptic medications, and as in E03 were permitted steady-state serum level variation of 20% over 3 months. Stimulation parameters were similar to those used in E03. Following the initial treatment phase, all patients who elected to continue treatment were followed through an indefinite extension phase, referred to as XE5, during which all patients received stimulation according to the presumed therapeutic parameters used for the 'HIGH' group. Seizure frequency calculations were again based on seizure diaries kept by patients and caregivers throughout the trial.

During the initial treatment phase of the trial, 23% of patients in the 'HIGH' arm and 16% of those in the 'LOW' arm were responders; this difference in responder rates was not considered statistically significant, with $p = 0.17$ between the groups. Mean and median seizure frequencies were reduced by 28% and 23%, respectively, in the 'HIGH' arm; and 15% and 21%, respectively, in the 'LOW' arm. The difference in seizure reduction rates was considered statistically significant, with $p<0.05$ between the groups by Analysis of Variance ($p = 0.032$) and Cochran–Mantel–Haenszel Aligned Ranks ($p = 0.040$). The interquartile ranges (25th and 75th percentiles) for the per cent difference in seizure frequency between baseline and stimulation periods were (–9%, –49%) for the 'HIGH' arm and (+4%, –43%) for the 'LOW' arm (negative signs here denote reductions in seizure frequency, while the positive sign indicates increased seizure frequency during the stimulation period). During the early extension phase, 89 of the original 196 patients were followed to 6 months, at which point the responder rate was 40%, with median seizure frequency reduction of 33%. At 9 months, responder rate was 40% (16 of 40 patients), with median seizure frequency reduction of 34%.

History of vagus nerve stimulation for the treatment of epilepsy

In retrospect, the history of VNS as a treatment for epilepsy can be traced back at least as far as the late nineteenth century, with some of the seminal work on the physiology of the vagus nerve having been performed in the first half of the twentieth century. Nevertheless, the degree to which early investigations informed later ones is not always evident. For example, although Corning studied VNS for epilepsy as early as the 1880s, and developed a variety of devices that he used in treating epileptic patients, his work seems to have been all but forgotten during the twentieth century (19); certainly it is not referenced in the work of Zabara and the modern developers of the NeuroCybernetic Prosthesis system. Several authors also reference the work of Soma Weiss as anticipating later interest in stimulation of the vagus nerve, as Weiss proposed in 1934 that the carotid sinus reflex response to compression was mediated through a direct cerebral pathway, and that the associated syncopal response in humans was separate from the effects of carotid sinus compression on blood pressure, heart rate, and carotid artery blood flow (20).

Systematic investigations into the physiology of the vagus nerve began in the late nineteenth and early twentieth century. A series of experiments by Veach and colleagues beginning in 1924 investigated the frequency-dependent effects of electrical stimulation of the vagus nerve (21–24). In 1938, Bailey and Bremmer proposed that the vagus nerve had a representation within the sensory cortex, on the basis of experimental observations in a cat 'isolated encephalon' model (25), though later experiments by Sachs and colleagues were unable to confirm those findings (26). Nevertheless, a decade-and-a-half later, Zanchetti and colleagues observed variation in the electroencephalogram as a function of vagal afferent stimulation, using the same experimental preparation as Bailey and Bremmer (27). Several investigators maintained interest in the question of whether and to what degree vagus afferents have cortical projections, and a small amount of work in this area was conducted over the ensuing three decades, as reflected by references cited in the initial patent applications related to VNS (28–30). Yet as late as the 1980s, a series of detailed studies by Radna and MacLean in awake squirrel monkeys revealed variable responses of forebrain structures to vagal stimulation, with no clear pattern of single-unit excitation or inhibition (31, 32).

The present era of clinical interest in VNS began in the early 1980s with the work of Jacob Zabara. Zabara had evidently first considered VNS as a therapeutic intervention in 1971, while watching his wife manage her labour pains by consciously regulating her breathing during the birth of their first child. Aware that central nervous system control of respiration was mediated in part by vagal efferents, he wondered whether the ability to modulate labour pains and their associated autonomic symptoms through conscious control of respiration might imply the existence of vagal afferents capable of modulating central nervous system activity. In 1983, Zabara filed a United States Patent Application entitled 'NeuroCybernetic Prosthesis', which describes an implantable device:

> For controlling or preventing epileptic seizures and other motor disorders include[ing] a pulse generator . . . enclosed in an epoxy-titanium shell and . . . implanted in the body, preferably in the

> axilla. Electrode leads pass from the generator through a subcutaneous tunnel and terminate in an electrode patch on the vagus nerve. Provisions are made for varying the electrical signal from the generator after it has been implanted to 'tune' the same to the patient (28).

No patient had yet been treated, and the application presented no experimental evidence to support its claims, yet a first patent for the 'NeuroCybernetic Prosthesis' was granted in 1987, with subsequent patents granted to Zabara in 1989 and 1991 (28–30).

The first publications in the scientific literature pertaining to the device are a pair of conference abstracts written by Zabara, one of which was for the American Epilepsy Society and published in its 1985 Society Proceedings (33, 34):

> Long lasting control of seizures was observed during application of brief, repetitive stimulus trains to afferent, inhibitory neurons. Stimulation was initiated prior to, or during a seizure episode in dogs. . . . Nerve bundles were stimulated via cuff electrodes by spectral discrimination to activate neurons inhibitory to hypersynchronous discharge. . . . This research is the basis for the design of an antiepileptic, microprocessor-based, pulse generator which is being tested for clinical trials.

Zabara cofounded Cyberonics in 1987, in partnership with Reese Terry, an electrical engineer; the first implantation of a vagus nerve stimulator in a human patient soon followed, in November 1988, and was performed by neurosurgeon William Bell and neurologist J. Kiffen Penry at Wake Forest Medical School in North Carolina (35). In what proved to be striking yet atypical successes, the first two patients treated experienced complete cessation of seizure activity during 12 and 9 months of follow-up, respectively, including complex and simple partial seizures, as well as secondarily generalized seizures. The first patient had developed epilepsy 15 years earlier as a result of childhood encephalitis, whereas the second patient had a 20-year history of epilepsy associated with a partially resected arteriovenous malformation; both received concurrent therapy with anti-epileptic drugs during the trial of VNS. Of note, 'Patient 1 was the only patient with an aura and therefore was given a magnet to activate the stimulator at will to prevent seizures' (9). Results in the nine patients subsequently enrolled in this initial clinical trial were considerably less favourable. Of the two other patients treated at Wake Forest University, one experienced a 40% reduction in seizure frequency (a reduction of greater than 50% was required to qualify as 'treatment success'), while the other experienced no reduction in seizure frequency. The remaining seven patients in the trial included two at the University of Miami, neither of whom experienced a reduction in seizure frequency with VNS; and five at the University of Florida, of whom two experienced reductions in seizure frequency in the 7 to 9 months after implantation.

The initial pilot studies demonstrated that VNS for epilepsy appeared safe, even if its efficacy was still in doubt, and so Phase II clinical trials were begun. The entire series of human clinical trials of VNS for the treatment of epilepsy has been discussed in detail in another section.

In January 1997, Cyberonics submitted its completed application to the Food and Drug Administration for approval of the NeuroCybernetic Prosthesis System, its vagal nerve stimulator, including the results of all clinical trials (6). In July of that year, the FDA issued premarket approval of the NeuroCybernetic Prosthesis System: 'A vagus nerve stimulator . . . indicated for use as an adjunctive therapy in reducing the frequency of seizures in adults and adolescents over 12 years of age with partial onset seizures, which are refractory to anti-epileptic medications' (6).

United States patents filed by Zabara and colleagues since 1983, and others assigned to Cyberonics, reflect an interest in using VNS (as well as stimulation of other cranial nerves) to treat a wide variety of conditions, including psychiatric disorders, pain, eating disorders, obesity, thyroid and other endocrine disorders, hypertension, dementia, and coma (36–44). Clinical evidence supporting the claims made in these patents is limited. In 1998, however, following the approval of VNS for epilepsy, a pilot study began at the University of Texas Southwestern Medical Center to investigate the use of VNS in the treatment of severe depression in 30 patients. After 9 months, more than half of the patients experienced significant improvement in their symptoms, as quantified using a variety of clinical inventories for depression (45). A larger follow-up study was conducted in 235 patients, however, and results released in 2002 failed to demonstrate a statistically significant difference in outcomes between patients receiving VNS and a control group of patients who had stimulators implanted but not activated, and who received pharmacologic treatment only (46). In light of these negative results, the FDA denied approval of VNS for the treatment of depression in 2004. The following year, however, the agency reversed its decision and granted approval. This unusual reversal was subsequently investigated by the United States Senate Committee on Finance. The findings of the Senate committee are publicly available, and the interested reader is referred directly to the report of the Senate investigation (47).

In spite of the concerns raised during the Senate hearings regarding efficacy and other issues, the FDA approval of VNS for treatment-resistant depression remained in effect, as did the earlier approval for epilepsy. Since FDA approval in 1997, Cyberonics estimates that vagus nerve stimulators have been implanted in more than 72,000 patients with epilepsy (48).

Anatomic and physiologic considerations

Background

Schachter and Saper presented a review of the anatomy and physiology of the vagus nerve in what has since become a highly cited review of VNS, originally published shortly after initial FDA approval (20). The present discussion draws considerably from that review, which, while stating explicitly that 'the mechanism of action of VNS is not known', provides insight into the pathways likely responsible for side-effects, as well as those that might mediate therapeutic effects of VNS.

The possibility of directly modulating cortical activity through stimulation of the vagus nerve arises from the existence of afferent fibres within that nerve. Although the vagus nerve is typically regarded as a parasympathetic efferent nerve, approximately one-fifth of its fibres are visceral sensory afferents. These fibres provide visceral sensation from the heart, lungs, larynx, and gastrointestinal tract from pharynx to transverse colon, as well as some gustatory sensation. The cell bodies of the sensory axons of the vagus nerve lie in the nodose ganglion (the inferior ganglion of the vagus), located just outside and at the outer margin of the jugular foramen. They synapse in the nucleus tractus solitarius (49).

Three main pathways arise from the nucleus tractus solitarius, through which sensory afferent information ascends to the brain: a spinal–medullary pathway, a reticular pathway, and a parabrachial–forebrain pathway.

The solitary nucleus sends feedback signals to preganglionic autonomic and somatic motor neurones in the medulla and spinal cord. These signals contribute to the baroreceptor and Herring–Breuer reflexes. In the former, feedback from carotid sinus afferents in the glossopharyngeal nerve and aortic arch afferents in the vagus nerve causes reflex bradycardia in response to hypertension. In the latter, pulmonary stretch feedback carried by vagal sensory afferents causes inspiration to cease.

The solitary nucleus also projects to the reticular formation of the medulla; Schachter and Saper propose that the medullary projections mediate the respiratory side-effects of VNS (20).

Finally, the solitary nucleus projects to forebrain structures. Most of these projections are relayed through the parabrachial nucleus, located in the dorsal pons, lateral to the locus ceruleus, but some ascend directly into the forebrain. Of these projections, two pathways from parabrachial nucleus to thalamus are of particular relevance. One of these pathways innervates the parvocellular part of the ventroposterior nucleus (VPpc), which conveys visceral sensation to the insular cortex. Insular cortex contains a topographic map of internal organ systems, a visceral analogue of the topographic maps located in somatosensory cortex. Schachter and Saper note that this is likely the pathway that relays sensation from vagal stimulation to conscious perception, and propose that abnormal visceral sensations arising as side-effects of VNS may result from activation of this pathway (20). A second pathway from the parabrachial nucleus projects to the intralaminar nuclei of the thalamus, which in turn have diffuse projections into the cerebral cortex. Schachter and Saper note that these cortical projections may correspond to the pathways through which VNS is believed to control cortical synchronization and desynchronization, exerting a putative effect on epileptiform activity in the cortex (20). In addition, the nucleus tractus solitarius and parabrachial nuclei relay visceral sensory information to the hypothalamus, stria terminalis and amygdala, infralimbic cortex, and basal forebrain; these pathways contribute vagal sensory input to endocrine, emotional, and other processes.

Proposed mechanisms of action

No mechanism for the control of seizures through VNS had been conclusively or convincingly described by 1997 (20), and, no mechanism has been elucidated since that time (50, 51). While the neural circuitry activated during VNS has been mapped in both animal and human studies using a variety of electrophysiologic, biochemical, and functional imaging techniques, the structures activated by VNS correspond to the known anatomic connections of the nerve (52).

Nevertheless, it is interesting to understand the mechanism of action proposed by Zabara and endorsed by Cyberonics at the time VNS was first used therapeutically in patents with epilepsy, and at the time of initial FDA approval. These hypothetical mechanisms are described in the initial patents granted to Zabara in the 1980s (28–30). The following excerpts are taken from his first patent, granted in 1987, 'NeuroCybernetic Prosthesis' (28):

> It is . . . confirmed by experimentation, that the introduction of certain control signals of the proper configuration, intensity and duration can act as a means for discharging or modifying hyperactivity in the brain. The superposition of such corrective measures, whether by the generation of proper interference patterns overriding control pulses or cancelling signals, acts in a way to inhibit the normal progress of the seizure and may prevent it altogether. . . .
>
> The present invention operates utilizing a principle called neurocybernetic spectral discrimination and works in the following way. Since, in general, nerves are of a microscopic diameter and are combined together in a nonhomogeneous mixture of diameters and functional properties, it is not presently possible to adequately control external current to selectively activate a specific group of nerves embedded within a relatively large number of other nerves. Spectral discrimination acts to overcome this fundamental problem by "tuning" the external current (electrical generator) to the electrochemical properties of the selected nerves. . . .
>
> The spectral discriminator acts to selectively activate those inhibitory nerves which can prevent or block the epileptic seizure. . . .
>
> There is a physiological basis for the effectiveness of the selected nerves in blocking or preventing epileptic seizures. The activation of these nerves produces an effect on the reticular system via synaptic transmission. The reticular system has been demonstrated to be important in whatever abnormality leads to epileptic seizures. The reticular system is a relatively large and inhomogeneously constituted structure extending from the hind-brain (medulla) to the mid-brain (thalamus) with neural connections to the cerebral cortex and spinal cord. It is not practical at present to directly electrically activate the reticular system because of its large extent and proximity to vital centers. Thus, it was important to discover what nerves might innervate the reticular system sufficiently to produce a significant effect on the reticular system; the net effect being to produce inhibition of epileptic seizures.
>
> For the purpose of interfacing the prosthesis with the critical processes of the brain, inhibition can also be called by its comparable engineering term of negative feedback. Further, it is possible that the seizure originates due to a temporary lack [or] diminution of negative feedback from the reticular system to seizure sites in the brain. By acting on appropriately selected nerves, the prosthesis results in the replacement of this negative feedback and thus prevents the seizure.
>
> The approach of spectral discrimination is to utilize the basic properties of conduction velocity, diameter, refractory period, threshold, membrane potential, action potential, after potentials, synchronization and synaptic transmission. Based on these properties, the parameters of the pulse generator are chosen in terms of frequency, duration of pulse wave, shape of wave, voltage or current and duration of pulse train. In addition, a time dependent direct current polarization of the membrane can be utilized to produce a "gate" effect.
>
> The "gate" effect is based upon the polarization characteristics of the neural membrane. The membrane potential across the neural membrane can be increased to a point where a block of conduction results. It is a method of separating relatively slower conducting fibers from faster conducting fibers. For example, when the nerve is activated, the action potentials of higher velocity (A) will lead the slower ones (C). A "polarization" block on the nerve membrane will stop A and then the block is removed before C arrives so that the net result is that A, but not C, is prevented from continuing. . . .

Analysis by spectral discrimination has demonstrated that the most desirable extra-cranial sites for all these effects are the cranial nerves. Specific cranial nerves have been determined to be optimum for beneficial effects on neurological problems. In particular, the vagus nerve is the optimum site for control of epileptic seizures.

If the total spectrum of the nerve is not known, it is possible to activate all the nerve fibers by the spectral discriminator and record the response on an oscilloscope. From this total fiber spectrum, it is possible to determine the settings of the spectral discriminator to select the activation of the appropriate subset of nerves. . . .

Choice of left versus right vagus nerve stimulation

The selection of the left as opposed to the right vagus nerve for therapeutic stimulation has some physiologic basis. As noted by Schachter and Saper (20), while the left and right vagi initially develop symmetrically, the right vagus later rotates posteriorly and associates more with the cardiac atria (and with the liver and duodenum in the abdomen), while the left vagus rotates anteriorly and associates more with the cardiac ventricles (and with the fundus of the stomach). It was believed by some that because vagal innervation of the cardiac ventricles is less dense than that of the atria, left vagal stimulation was less likely to have cardiac side effects. In practice, right-sided VNS in humans has received little attention apart from sporadic case reports, and the relative frequencies of cardiac, respiratory, and other side-effects arising from stimulation of one or the other vagus nerve have not been established (53, 54). Some such studies have suggested that right-sided VNS is safe, however, raising the question of whether seizures arising from one hemisphere might respond preferentially to ipsilateral VNS; current practice, in the absence of a mechanism of action, is to stimulate only the left vagus nerve, without regard for the existence or laterality of a seizure focus.

Areas of controversy and uncertainty

In this section we review areas of controversy and uncertainty regarding VNS.

Lack of clear mechanism of action

The scientific literature over the past three decades has seen the publication of thousands of papers dealing with the subject of VNS. In spite of intense interest and focused scientific and clinical attention on the subject, no clear mechanism of action has been elucidated by which peripheral stimulation of the vagus nerve should act to suppress or abort seizures, or reduce the propensity of the brain to seize. In a review published shortly after the initial FDA approval of VNS for intractable epilepsy, Schachter and Saper opened their section on mechanisms of action with the statement: 'The mechanism of action of VNS is unknown, although it is clearly different from that of AEDs [anti-epileptic drugs]' (20). In a review published eight years later, Schachter again wrote: 'The mechanism of action of VNS is unknown' (52). At the time of this writing, the neurosurgical community has had 25 years of experience with VNS in human patients; nevertheless, in a recent review, Fridley and colleagues observed: 'Vagus nerve stimulation has been by far the most prevalent method of stimulation to treat epilepsy, with more than 60,000 patients having received the implant. . . . The mechanism of neuromodulation remains unclear' (50).

In particular, seizures being characterized by synchronous neuronal activity in the cortex, a neural circuit by which stimulation of the vagus nerve exerts a modulatory effect on neuronal activity in the cortex has not been demonstrated, though several hypotheses have been proposed (51, 55), even though the afferent projections of the vagus nerve have been mapped in great detail. Schachter and others have noted that neural pathways activated during VNS have been characterized using a variety of modalities, including electrophysiology, gene expression, and several types of functional imaging, without revealing circuits unknown from neuroanatomic studies of the vagus nerve (52).

Inadequacy of evidence on efficacy of vagus nerve stimulation for treatment of epilepsy

The primary body of evidence used to justify VNS in the management of medically refractory epilepsy was reviewed in an earlier section. Careful reconsideration of the associated clinical trial data, as well as earlier data from animal studies, raises questions as to whether VNS actually does exert clinically meaningful effects in epilepsy.

Animal studies

The most highly cited animal studies concerning the effects of VNS on experimentally induced seizures were conducted in the 1990s, following and concurrently with the human clinical trials discussed earlier (56–59). As such, although some contemporary accounts of the development of VNS suggest that animal studies paved the way for human trials (60), careful review of published findings in the scientific literature brings such histories into doubt. The commonly cited animal studies used a variety of methods to induce seizures in several different species, and differed also in their choices of electrical stimulation parameters. Their findings were in some regards inconsistent, differing as to the effects of VNS on seizure severity, seizure duration, and interictal spikes. Even within individual studies, anti-seizure effects on animal populations were found to be inconsistent, with half to two-thirds of animals exhibiting minimal or no anti-seizure response to VNS in some of the most highly cited studies (56, 59).

It is perhaps worth noting, further, that prior to pilot animal studies by Zabara and colleagues in the 1980s, little in the scientific literature suggested that VNS should directly modulate cortical activity. Two studies are often cited as early evidence in support of VNS for epilepsy, though their implications in this regard have perhaps been overstated by some reviewers. The first, a 1938 report by Bailey and Bremmer, describes a set of experiments using cat 'isolated encephalon' preparations in which the vagus nerves are transected, the spinal cord is transected at the level of the caudal medulla, and eyeball and orbital roof are removed to achieve maximal exposure of cortical surface (25). In this system, the authors observed alteration in the electroencephalogram of the orbital surface of the frontal lobe (increased amplitude and frequency) with stimulation of the vagus nerve: 'Stimulation of the central end of the vagus nerve increases the electrical potentials of the orbital surface of the frontal lobe of the cerebral cortex. No other portion is affected.' However, they conclude:

> Excitation of the central end of the vago-depressor nerve did not diminish cortical activity except when, due to preservation of the cardiomoderator reflex, it lowered blood pressure. Our experiments, therefore, do not support the hypothesis of a direct inhibitory action by depressor nerves on the cortex or diencephalon.

This negative conclusion is typically ignored in reviews of the rational development VNS. The second early study is a 1952 study by Zanchetti (27), which is also one of a small number of references cited in the first patent granted to Zabara, in 1987, for the 'NeuroCybernetic Prosthesis' device used to deliver vagal nerve stimulation in early human trials (28). Also, using a cat isolated encephalon preparation, Zanchetti observed that synchronous cortical activity arose spontaneously in 5 of 15 animals, and could be reduced or eliminated by stimulation of the vagus nerve.

In reconsidering several of the studies most frequently referenced as providing early experimental evidence in support of VNS, one finds that subsequent studies in animals did not uniformly confirm the efficacy of vagal nerve stimulation in treating the various animal models epilepsy. For example, Lockard, Congdon, and DuCharme studied the effects of chronic vagal nerve stimulation in a primate model of epilepsy; their 1990 paper has been referenced more than 70 times by subsequent papers on VNS for epilepsy (56). However, the authors of that study conclude:

> Vagal stimulation had no consistent effects on seizure severity or EEG interictal spikes. . . . Although it appears that chronic vagal stimulation is feasible and that epileptogenic processes are influenced, the safety and efficacy of the procedure are still in question.

Similarly, McLachlan published a study in 1993 entitled 'Suppression of interictal spikes and seizures by stimulation of the vagus nerve' that has since been cited by more than 100 papers (58), yet the manner in which that study qualified its findings is often neglected:

> Interictal spike frequency was reduced by 33% during 20 s of stimulation ($p < 0.001$) and remained low for < or = 3 min. Amplitude of residual spikes was also decreased. Cardiac and respiratory rates were suppressed. . . . *A similar reduction in spike frequency of 39% was obtained by heating the animals' tail ($p < 0.01$).* . . . These findings suggest that vagus nerve stimulation can be a potent *but nonspecific* method to reduce cortical epileptiform activity, probably through an indirect effect mediated by the reticular activating system [emphasis added].

Thus, human trials of VNS for epilepsy moved forward perhaps not in light of evidence from animal studies, but rather in spite of the limited positive evidence from such studies.

Human clinical trials

Several shortcomings of the human clinical trials of VNS for epilepsy will be addressed in subsequent sections. The principal objections associated with these trials are that the magnitude of the treatment effect attributable to VNS was small compared with that of 'placebo' stimulation, and that subjects in both the treatment and control groups had highly variable outcomes. The basis for these objections is clearly illustrated in the original 'Summary of safety and effectiveness data' for the NeuroCybernetic Prosthesis (NCP) Vagus Nerve Stimulation System, one of the principal documents on the basis of which the FDA based its approval of VNS for the treatment of epilepsy. The first data-containing figure from that document is reproduced here (Fig. 19.1), together with a summary table that displays the change in seizure frequency in the 'high-frequency' (treatment) and 'low-frequency' ('placebo') populations enrolled in the early efficacy trials (a total of 196 patients). The figure and accompanying table reveal several weaknesses in the efficacy data submitted to the FDA. The majority of patients in the placebo group improved, and to an extent comparable to the improvements seen in the group that received therapeutic stimulation. Additionally, many of the patients who received therapeutic stimulation experienced increased, rather than decreased, seizure frequency. Indeed, the treatment–response distributions in the figure are very similar, suggesting that VNS modifies the natural history of epilepsy to a small degree relative to placebo stimulation. The absolute difference in median seizures' frequency is small (23% reduction as compared with a 21% reduction in seizure frequency in the placebo group), and that difference is essentially obscured by the wide variance in

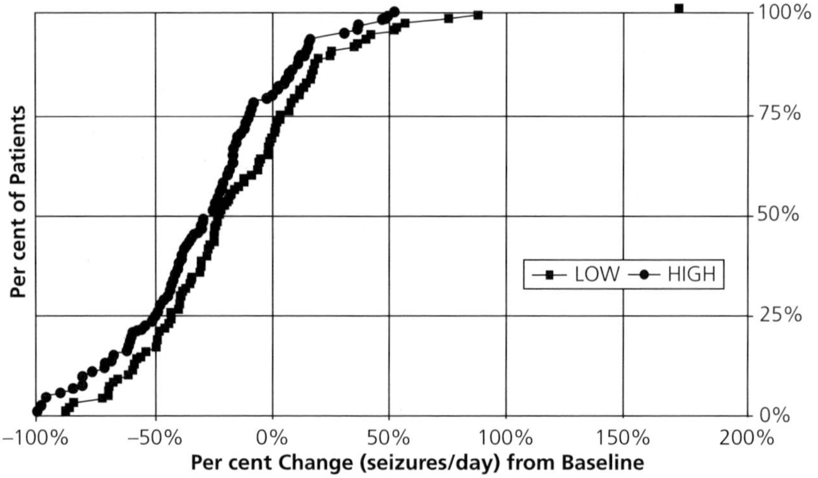

	Per cent Change (seizures/day) from Baseline		
	HIGH	**LOW**	**Difference**
lnl	94	102	196
Median	−23%	−21%	n/a
25%, 75% Quartiles	−8.9%, −49%	4.0%, −43%	n/a
95% confidence intervals	−35%, −21%	−23%, −7.7%	−23%, −2.3%
Range (min,max)	−100%, 52%	−89%, 171%	−23%, −2.3%
Mean ± SD	−28% ± 34%	−15% ± 39%	−13%* ± 37%

*** Difference statistically significant (*p*<0.05) by Analysis of variance (*p* = 0.032) and by Cochran-Mental-Haenszel Aligned Ranks (*p* = 0.040)**

Fig. 19.1 Summary data from the human clinical trial results on the basis of which the FDA approved the use of vagus nerve stimulation in the treatment of epilepsy.

Reproduced from Cyberonics. NeuroCybernetic Prosthesis (NCP) Vagus Nerve Stimulation System Premarket Approval Order and Summary of Safety and Effectiveness Data. Food and Drug Administration Center for Devices and Radiological Health, editor. United States: Department of Health and Human Services; 1997.

outcomes seen in both the treatment and placebo arms (outcomes ranged from a 100% decrease to a 171% increase in seizure frequency).

It may be worth noting that the difference in mean seizure frequency observed in the treatment and placebo arms was clearly influenced by three outliers at the positive tail of the placebo distribution, as the difference in means is much greater than the difference in the medians of the distributions. While the difference in means was found to be statistically significant, the difference in medians was not. Notably, subsequent human clinical trial data were criticized by the Neurological Devices Panel of the FDA in 2004, during its review of VNS for the treatment of depression, and several of these later criticisms were raised on statistical grounds. The objections of the FDA committee are publicly available, and the interested reader is referred directly to its report (61).

Further consideration of the clinical trial results submitted to the FDA for approval of VNS in the treatment of epilepsy reveals a perhaps overly optimistic interpretation of the efficacy data. A subsequent figure from the 'Summary of safety and effectiveness data' reproduced here (Fig. 19.2) is used to support the suggestion that VNS may have increasing efficacy over time, as the median per cent reduction in seizure frequency was observed to increase in those patients who continued therapy beyond the initial phase of the trial, through 3 years of follow-up. Yet even ignoring that patients were permitted to change their anti-epileptic drug regimens during this period, it is impossible also to ignore the high attrition rate of study subjects. The data in the prior figure confirm that many patients were 'non-responders' to VNS, experiencing either increases or small decreases in seizure frequency with therapy. Speculation as to increasing efficacy over time seems disingenuous in that the observed changes could be explained by an expected, disproportionate attrition of non-responders; the report does not comment on this logical possibility, even though the data were clearly available to the investigators.

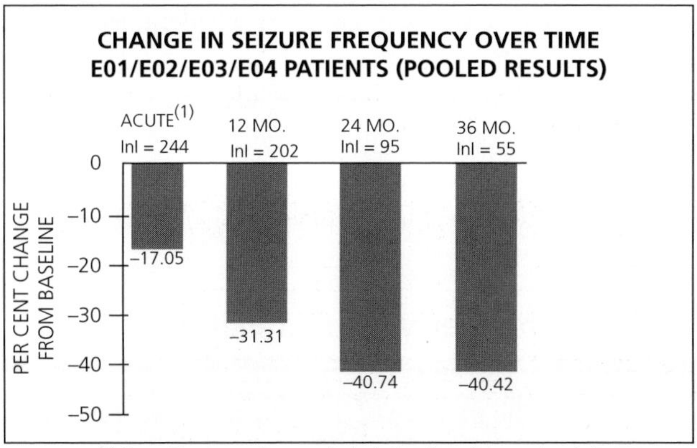

(1) Note: The acute phase results include seizure frequencies of the E03 Study LOW stimulation group, which includes one-half of the E03 patients, N = 57

Patients were permitted to change their AEDs during these studies and these changes may have contributed to the change in seizure frequency.

Fig. 19.2 Data from the human clinical trial results submitted to the FDA by Cyberonics in support of the claim that the efficacy of vagus nerve stimulation might increase over time.

Reproduced from Cyberonics. NeuroCybernetic Prosthesis (NCP) Vagus Nerve Stimulation System Premarket Approval Order and Summary of Safety and Effectiveness Data. Food and Drug Administration Center for Devices and Radiological Health, editor. United States: Department of Health and Human Services; 1997.

Recent reviewers of the efficacy of VNS for epilepsy have differed in their interpretations of these overall results and those of subsequent studies. On one hand, a 2010 Cochrane Collaboration Review on 'Vagus nerve stimulation for partial seizures' (8) concludes that: 'Results of the overall efficacy analysis show that VNS stimulation using the high stimulation paradigm was significantly better than low stimulation ['placebo']. The overall OR (95% confidence interval (CI)) for 50% responders across all studies is 1.93 (95% CI 1.1 to 3.4). . . . VNS for partial seizures appears to be an effective and well tolerated treatment.' On the other hand, a review from the Center for Evidence-Based Policy at Oregon Health and Science University concludes that: 'The true size of the treatment effect of VNS was unknown, as the placebo effect and response to concurrent pharmacologic therapy confounded the interpretation of the study results' (12).

Lack of objective outcome metrics for therapeutic response

It is important to recognize that in all studies of the efficacy of VNS in the treatment of intractable epilepsy, the primary outcome measure has been a subjective one: seizure frequency, as reported by patients and caregivers, and as recorded in seizure diaries periodically reviewed by investigators. Relying on patients and caregivers to record every seizure event exposes seizure frequency data to severe forms of observer bias and recall bias. While the gold-standard method of seizure detection, electroencephalography (EEG), can be applied quite objectively in seizure detection, use of long-term EEG monitoring in many patients over months or years of follow-up would certainly have been challenging, if not entirely impractical. Even so, in no study has there been an attempt to determine the reliability of patients and caregivers in detecting seizures as verified by EEG. Furthermore, caregivers can hardly be expected to observe every seizure for the practical reason that not all patients can be observed at all times. Moreover, partial seizures (the principal seizure type experienced by study subjects) often have only subtle semiologic manifestations and can, therefore, pass unnoticed. On the other hand, twitching, writhing, and other movements not associated with abnormal cortical activity can easily be misidentified as seizures, even by trained observers.

In our experience at a high-volume centre over more than a decade, and as verified recently in a retrospective review of more than 250 consecutive patients receiving VNS for epilepsy at that centre, the quality of patient- and caregiver-reported data on seizure frequency is consistently poor, despite the earnest, well intentioned, best efforts of patients and caregivers (62).

Lack of a dose–response relationship between stimulation parameters and clinical response

Experience in VNS stands in contrast with the practice of other forms of neuromodulation, such as deep-brain stimulation for movement disorders and cochlear implants for deafness and hearing impairment, and in contrast with experience with implantable devices in cardiac electrophysiology, such as pacemakers and implantable defibrillators, in that all of these implantable devices are tuned using rational algorithms for setting device parameters so as to maximize therapeutic effects and minimize side effects (63–69). In VNS, on the other hand, various sets of electrical stimulation parameters have been used in treating epilepsy of various forms and aetiologies, and while human clinical trials have provided strong evidence demonstrating that the side-effects of stimulation increase in frequency and severity with high- (therapeutic) versus low-frequency ('placebo') stimulation (6), no dose–response relationship between stimulation parameters and anti-epileptic efficacy has been demonstrated, and no systematic algorithm for optimizing VNS parameters has been experimentally validated. Indeed, while individual groups have developed heuristic approaches to setting device parameters (70), data from the XE5 study suggested that changing device parameters had little, if any, influence on the efficacy of VNS (18). While Penry and Dean evidently noted that 'a stepwise reduction of seizures was noted with the adjustment of the stimulation parameters' in three of the first four human patients treated in the 1988 pilot trial (9), no data are provided in support of that claim, and that experience has not been replicated in the subsequent quarter-century.

Vagus nerve stimulation is now used to treat epilepsy of various types and diverse aetiologies, and stimulation settings are configured with little, if any, regard for seizure type or anatomic origin. Moreover, even the initial clinical trials, on the basis of which FDA approval was granted, used varying settings of stimulation current, frequency, pulse width, and on- and off-times, as is clear from Fig. 19.3, reproduced from the supporting documents provided to the FDA by Cyberonics in 1997 (6). Studies of the efficacy of VNS have typically not stratified therapeutic efficacy by stimulation settings.

In contrast with the apparent lack of a dose–response relationship between stimulation settings and therapeutic response, dose–response relationships between stimulation settings and side-effects of VNS are well established, and the frequency and intensity of side-effects (including bradyarrhythmias and voice alterations) can, in almost all cases, be eliminated or reduced to tolerable levels by reducing the stimulation current (60, 71).

	STUDY						
Parameter	**E01**	**E02**	**E04**	**E03 HIGH (LOW)**	**E05 HIGH (LOW)**	**XE1–4**	**XE5 3 mo. (Longer)**
CURR (mA)	1–6	0.5 to 5	≤ 1	0.5–3.0	3.5	0–12	0–3.5
FREQ (HZ)	≤ 50	20 to 50	30	20–50 (1 to 2)	30 (1)	1–143	20 (1–30)
PW (μsec)	250	250 to 500	500	500 (130)	500 (130)	130–1000	750 (130–1000)
ON (sec)	60	30 to 60	30	30–90 (30)	30 (30)	7–270	30 (7–60)
OFF (min)	60	5 to 20	10	5 (90)	5 (180)	0.2–180	1.8 (1.1–180)

Fig. 19.3 A variety of different stimulator settings were used in the human clinical trials of vagus nerve stimulation for the treatment of epilepsy.

Reproduced from Cyberonics. NeuroCybernetic Prosthesis (NCP) Vagus Nerve Stimulation System Premarket Approval Order and Summary of Safety and Effectiveness Data. Food and Drug Administration Center for Devices and Radiological Health, editor. United States: Department of Health and Human Services; 1997

Lack of double-blind placebo-controlled trials: ineffective blinding

Vagus nerve stimulation for the treatment of epilepsy has not been studied in well-blinded clinical trials: clinical trials of VNS for the treatment of epilepsy used an 'active control' design in attempt to approach the randomized, double-blinded, placebo-controlled gold standard. In the 'active control' trial design, all patients receive vagus nerve stimulators, and all stimulators provide electrical stimulation to the vagus nerve. However, in the 'therapeutic' or 'high-frequency stimulation' arm, patients received stimulation at 3.5 mA and 20–50 Hz with 500-μs pulse width for 30–90-min intervals separated by 5-min stimulation-free intervals. In the 'active control' or 'low-frequency stimulation' arm, patients received stimulation at 0.5–3 mA and 1–2 Hz with 130-μs pulse width for 30-min intervals separated by 90–180-min stimulation-free intervals (6). The stated goal of this design was to provide vagal stimulation to all patients, as effectively as possible 'blinding' patients with respect to the intended therapeutic or non-therapeutic nature of the stimulation they received. In practice, however, this strategy did not blind patients with respect to the nature of their stimulation, as evidenced by the difference in side-effect profiles experienced by patients in the two arms, shown in the side-effects' table from the 1997 FDA approval documentation reproduced here (Fig. 19.4). Most patients experienced conscious sensations with stimulation of the vagus nerve, rendering the blinding strategy ineffective. Indeed, 72.6% of the 196 patients in the 'HIGH' arm of the E05 trial and 38.6% of the 114 patients in the 'HIGH' arm of the E03 trial experienced voice alterations or hoarseness, as compared to 32.0% and 14.0% of patients in the 'LOW' arms of those trials, respectively (6).

The extent to which clinical trials of VNS for epilepsy have been 'controlled' has been further confounded by concurrent use of anti-epileptic drugs.

Natural history of intractable epilepsy, a relapsing-remitting condition, and implications for assessing efficacy

The efficacy of a therapeutic intervention cannot be established in the absence of an understanding of the natural history of the disease process it is meant to treat. In the case of VNS for 'refractory' epilepsy, establishing efficacy poses a problem that is both practically and statistically difficult, in that doing so requires distinguishing the effects of treatment from the uncertain course of an unpredictable, relapsing-remitting disease.

Epilepsy is characterized by the occurrence of seizures, typically at intervals that appear random. The natural history of epilepsy may vary, depending on the aetiology of the condition, which may remit spontaneously for periods as long as weeks, months, or longer; and may relapse, as well, with an 'unprovoked' and unanticipated seizure. It has been estimated that approximately one-third of epileptic patients remit spontaneously and approximately one-third remit on anti-epileptic drugs, while the remainder of patients, including those considered 'refractory', fail to remit, even with the use of anti-epileptic drugs

Test of Difference between Baseline (12 Weeks) and stimulation (14 Weeks)

Adverse Event	E05					
	HIGH			LOW		
	Baseline	Treatment	*p*-value[C]	Baseline	Treatment	*p*-value[C]
Cough	28.4	52.6	<0.0001	23.3	51.5	<0.0001
Dyspepsia	5.3	21.1	0.0011	13.6	15.5	0.6171
Dyspnea	4.2	27.4	<0.0001	6.8	14.6	0.0114
Infection	4.2	14.7	0.0184	8.7	15.5	.1615
Pain, nonspecific	20.0	33.7	0.0124	19.4	37.9	0.0030
Paresthesia	1.1	24.2	<0.0001	4.9	33.0	<0.000
Throat pain[D]	15.8	42.1	<0.0001	16.5	29.1	0.0236
Voice alteration/hoarseness	6.3	72.6	<0.0001	8.7	32.0	<0.0001
Vomiting	8.4	17.9	0.0389	6.8	14.6	.0325

Adverse Event	E03					
	HIGH			LOW		
	Baseline	Treatment	*p* – value[C]	Baseline	Treatment	*p* – value[C]
Cough	0.0	12.3	0.008	3.5	10.5	.157
Dyspepsia	na	na	na	na	na	na
Dyspnea	1.8	10.5	0.059	0.0	0.0	na
Infection	0.0	3.5	0.157	1.8	3.5	.564
Pain, nonspecific	na	na	na	na	na	na
Paresthesia	0.0	15.8	0.003	0.0	7.0	0.046
Throat pain[D]	0.0	7.0	0.046	0.0	5.3	0.083
Voice alteration/hoarseness	0.0	38.6	<0.0001	0.0	14.0	0.005
Vomiting	1.8	1.8	ns	1.8	1.8	ns

A As reported or observed *Statistically significant* < 0.05

[B] As elicited using Symptoms Checklist, reported or observed Marginally significant 0.05 < *p* < 0.10

[C] Within group analysis

[D] Throat pain is specifically reported as an AE in E03 but not E05. For comparative purposes a separate analysis of E05 data, aggregating neck pain, Pharyngitis and Laryngismus, was done and is presented here

Fig. 19.4 Side-effects experienced by subjects in the large E03 and E05 'active control' trials of vagus nerve stimulation for the treatment of epilepsy. The prevalence of side-effects is consistently higher in the 'HIGH' ('therapeutic,' high-frequency stimulation) group receiving presumed-therapeutic vagus nerve stimulation, than in the 'LOW' ('control,' low-frequency stimulation) group.

Reproduced from Cyberonics. NeuroCybernetic Prosthesis (NCP) Vagus Nerve Stimulation System Premarket Approval Order and Summary of Safety and Effectiveness Data. Food and Drug Administration Center for Devices and Radiological Health, editor. United States: Department of Health and Human Services; 1997

(72). Yet these categorizations are established in hindsight, and although some prognostic factors have been identified (72), there is currently no prospective method for predetermining whether a particular patient will remit, or after what interval, if ever, a patient in apparent remission will ultimately relapse.

In one of the longest studies of the natural history of childhood-onset epilepsy, Sillanpäa and Schmidt (73) prospectively studied a cohort of 144 epileptic patients who experienced first seizures before the age of 16, for a median of 40 years. They concluded that: 'Half the patients with childhood-onset epilepsy will eventually enter terminal remission without relapse [on or off anti-epileptic drugs] and a fifth after relapse. One-third will have a poor long-term outcome in terms of persistent seizures after remission or without any remission ever.' The authors further observe that half of all patients achieved 'late' remission, with a mean delay of 9 years after initiation of treatment; the onset of this 'late' remission, however, was unpredictable. Recently published long-term studies in adults suggest that relapse is common, even after long periods of remission, with a cumulative probability of greater than 80% of relapse 5 years after initial remission (74).

In the clinical trials of VNS, patients in both the 'treatment' and 'control' arms experienced decreasing seizure rates on average. Although the expectation in using VNS to treat epilepsy is not seizure remission, similar considerations apply to establishing responsiveness to VNS in terms of reduction in seizure frequency. Given that in the natural history of epilepsy, the mean delay in time to remission may be as long as 9 years, with episodes of relapse and remission common on shorter timescales, clinical trials several months to one year in duration may not be adequate to distinguish the efficacy of therapy from the natural progression of the disease, when the magnitude of the observed difference between 'therapeutic' and 'control' groups is as small as clinical trials currently suggest.

In the context of disease processes that have become FDA-approved targets for VNS, it may be worth noting that superficial similarities exist between medically refractory epilepsy and medically refractory depression: both are intractable, relapsing-remitting disorders of the central nervous system with diverse aetiologies. Establishing whether vagus nerve therapy alters the natural history of these diseases, and distinguishing small responses to therapy from the naturally relapsing-remitting courses of these diseases, raises similar problems for clinical trials.

Importantly, given the relapsing-remitting natural history of epilepsy, there is reason to believe that standard statistical techniques used to evaluate response to therapy (which may be ideal for chronic or progressive diseases) are not optimal. Berg and colleagues have proposed that the use of a Markovian approach might provide a useful alternative to standard Kaplan–Meier analyses in understanding outcomes in epileptic patients, with the advantage that such techniques permit tracking of individual outcomes over time, even as the underlying condition changes. They further note: 'The technique would also be applicable in virtually any remitting-relapsing disorder' (75).

Summary

While the safety of VNS has been adequately established over the last quarter-century, a careful, comprehensive review of human and animal studies raises questions as to the true efficacy of VNS in the treatment of epilepsy. Nevertheless, as the treatment is safe and may be of some benefit, we describe in Chapter 20 the technical and surgical aspects of VNS that a decade of clinical experience in several hundred patients has suggested reflect optimal clinical practice. We have reviewed some of these aspects of VNS previously (71), and present a similar, updated treatment in Chapter 20.

Appendix

Important studies comprising the evidence base for vagus nerve stimulation in the treatment of intractable epilepsy

E02 study

The first four human patients treated with vagus nerve stimulation for intractable epilepsy:

Penry and Dean, 1990

E01 and E02 studies

Prospective, small, single-blind studies in which patients served as their own controls:

Penry and Dean, 1990

Uthman et al., 1990

Uthman et al., 1993

E03 and E05 studies

Large, randomized, blinded, controlled trials of high-stimulation versus low-stimulation VNS. Conducted by the First International Vagus Nerve Stimulation Study Group in collaboration with Cyberonics Inc., the manufacturer of the NeuroCybernetic Prosthesis device.

Ben-Menachem et al., 1994

George et al., 1994

Handforth et al., 1998

Holder, Wernicke, and Tarver, 1992

Salinsky, Uthman, Ristanovic, Wernicke, and Tarver, 1996

Vagus Nerve Stimulation Study Group, 1995

XE5 study

Open extension of the E05 trial:

Amar, DeGiorgio, Tarver, and Apuzzo, 1999

DeGiorgio et al., 2000

Labar, Murphy, and Tecoma, 1999

E04 study

Uncontrolled, open-label, compassionate use trial:

Labar, D., Murphy, J., and Tecoma, E., 1999 (E04 VNS Study Group)

Retrospective subgroup analyses with registry data from trials E01 through E05

Morris and Mueller, 1999

Murphy, Hornig, and Schallert, 1995

Sirven et al., 2000

Prospective, randomized and non-randomized, controlled or comparative studies

Amar et al., 1998

Ben-Menachem, Hellstrom, Waldton, and Augustinsson, 1999

McGlone et al., 2008

Nei, O'Connor, Liporace, and Sperling, 2006

Scherrmann, Hoppe, Kral, Schramm, and Elger, 2001

Sherman et al., 2008

Prospective uncontrolled studies, case series, and retrospective studies

Amar, Apuzzo, and Liu, 2004

Chavel, Westerveld, and Spencer, 2003

De Herdt et al., 2007

Helmers et al., 2001

Holmes, Silbergeld, Drouhard, Wilensky, and Ojemann, 2004

Hornig, Murphy, Schallert, and Tilton, 1997

Hosain et al., 2000

Huf, Mamelak, and Kneedy-Cayem, 2005

Labar, 2004

Lundgren, Amark, Blennow, Stromblad, and Wallstedt, 1998

Majoie et al., 2001

Mikati et al., 2009

Murphy et al., 1995

Parker et al., 1999

Rossignol et al., 2009

Rychlicki et al., 2006

Vonck et al., 2004

You et al., 2007

References

1 **Baumgartner C, Lurger S, Leutmezer F**. Autonomic symptoms during epileptic seizures. Epileptic disorders: international epilepsy journal with videotape. 2001 Sept;**3**(3):103–16. PubMed PMID: 11679301.

2 **Brodie MJ, Shorvon SD, Canger R et al**. Commission on European Affairs: appropriate standards of epilepsy care across Europe. ILEA. Epilepsia 1997 Nov;**38**(11):1245–50. PubMed PMID: 9579928.

3 **French JA**. Refractory epilepsy: clinical overview. Epilepsia 2007;**48**(Suppl. 1):3–7. PubMed PMID: 17316406.

4 **Madsen JR**. Treatment of intractable epilepsy by electrical stimulation of the vagus nerve. In: Quiñones-Hinojosa A (ed.) Schmidek and Sweet Operative Neurosurgical Techniques: Indications, Methods and Results, 6th edn; Elsevier/Saunders, Philadelphia; 2012;Chapter **113**:1301–1308.

5 **Winn HR**. Section III: Epilepsy. Youmans Neurological Surgery 1. Elsevier/Saunders, Philadelphia; 2011.

6 **Cyberonics**. NeuroCybernetic Prosthesis (NCP) Vagus nerve stimulation system premarket approval order and summary of safety and effectiveness data. Food and Drug Administration Center for Devices and Radiological Health (ed.) United States: Department of Health and Human Services; 1997.

7 **Amar AP, Apuzzo MLJ, Lui CY**. Vagus nerve stimulation therapy after failed cranial surgery for intractable epilepsy: results from the vagus nerve stimulation therapy patient outcome registry. Neurosurgery 2004;**55**:1086–93.

8 **Privitera MD, Welty TTE, Ficker DDM, Welge J**. Vagus nerve stimulation for partial seizures. Cochrane Database of Systematic Reviews 2002, (Issue 1), Art. No.:CD002896. Assessed as up-to-date: 15 June 2010.

9 **Penry JK, Dean JC**. Prevention of intractable partial seizures by intermittent vagal stimulation in humans: preliminary results. Epilepsia 1990;**31**(Suppl. 2):S40–43. PubMed PMID: 2121469.

10 **Uthman BM, Wilder BJ, Penry JK et al**. Treatment of epilepsy by stimulation of the vagus nerve. Neurology 1993 July;**43**(7):1338–45. PubMed PMID: 8327135.

11 **Uthman BM, Wilder BJ, Hammond EJ, Reid SA**. Efficacy and safety of vagus nerve stimulation in patients with complex partial seizures. Epilepsia 1990;**31**(Suppl. 2):S44–50. PubMed PMID: 2226366.

12 **Hayes WS, Inc**. Vagus nerve stimulation for epilepsy (Health Technology Assessment Draft Report). Oregon Health and Science University, Health Technology Assessment Program in Olympia, Washington, USA; 2009.

13 **Ben-Menachem E, Manon-Espaillat R, Ristanovic R et al**. Vagus nerve stimulation for treatment of partial seizures: 1. A controlled study of effect on seizures. First International Vagus Nerve Stimulation Study Group. Epilepsia 1994 May–Jun;**35**(3):616–26. PubMed PMID: 8026408.

14 **George R, Salinsky M, Kuzniecky R et al**. Vagus nerve stimulation for treatment of partial seizures: 3. Long-term follow-up on first 67 patients exiting a controlled study. First International Vagus Nerve Stimulation Study Group. Epilepsia 1994 May–Jun;**35**(3):637–43. PubMed PMID: 8026410.

15 **Labar D, Murphy J, Tecoma E**. Vagus nerve stimulation for medication-resistant generalized epilepsy. E04 VNS Study Group. Neurology 1999 Apr 22;**52**(7):1510–12. PubMed PMID: 10227649.

16 **Handforth A, DeGiorgio CM, Schachter SC et al**. Vagus nerve stimulation therapy for partial-onset seizures: a randomized active-control trial. Neurology 1998 Jul;**51**(1):48–55. PubMed PMID: 9674777.

17 **Amar AP, DeGiorgio CM, Tarver WB, Apuzzo ML**. Long-term multicenter experience with vagus nerve stimulation for intractable partial seizures: results of the XE5 trial. Stereotact Funct Neurosurg 1999;**73**(1–4):104–108. PubMed PMID: 10853111.

18 **DeGiorgio CM, Thompson J, Lewis P et al**. Vagus nerve stimulation: analysis of device parameters in 154 patients during the long-term XE5 study. Epilepsia 2001 Aug;**42**(8):1017–20. PubMed PMID: 11554887.

19 **Lanska DJ. J.L.** Corning and vagal nerve stimulation for seizures in the 1880s. Neurology 2002;**58**(3):452–59.

20 **Schachter SC, Saper CB**. Vagus nerve stimulation. Epilepsia 1998;**39**(7):677–86.

21 **Veach HO**. Studies on the innervation of smooth muscle: I. Vagus effects on the lower end of the esophagus, cardia and stomach of the cat, and the stomach and lung of the turtle in relation to Wedensky inhibition. Am J Physiol 1925;**71**(2):229–64.

22 **Veach HO**. Stimulation of the vagus nerve. Science 1924;**59**(1524):260–61.

23 **Veach HO, Pereira JR**. Effects of variation in frequency of stimulation of skeletal, cardiac and smooth muscle with special reference to inhibition. Am J Physiol 1925;**74**(2):257–84.

24 **Veach HO, Schwartz LL, Weinstein M**. Studies on the innervation of smooth muscle. Am J Physiol 1930;**92**(2):453–56.

25 **Bailey P, Bremer F**. A sensory cortical representation of the vagus nerve: with a note on the effects of low blood pressure on the cortical electrogram. J Neurophysiol 1938;**1**:405–12.

26 **Sachs H, Brendler SJ, Fulton JF**. The orbital gyri. Brain 1949;**72**(2):227–40.

27 **Zanchetti A, Wang SC, Moruzzi G**. The effect of vagal afferent stimulation on the EEG pattern of the cat. EEG Clin Neurophysiol 1952 (4):357–61.

28 **Zabara J, inventor; NeuroCybernetic Prosthesis**. United States of America patent 4,702,254 1987.

29 **Zabara J, inventor; NeuroCybernetic Prosthesis**. United States of America patent 4,867,164 1989.

30 **Zabara J, inventor; NeuroCybernetic Prosthesis**. United States of America patent 5,025,807 1991 June 25, 1991.

31 **Radna RJ, MacLean PD**. Vagal elicitation of respiratory-type and other unit responses in basal limbic structures of squirrel monkeys. Brain Res 1981;**213**:45–61.

32 **Radna RJ, MacLean PD**. Vagal elicitation of respiratory-type and other unit responses in striatopallidum of squirrel monkeys. Brain Res 1981;**213**:29–44.

33 **Zabara J**. Time course of seizure control to brief, repetitive stimuli. Epilepsia 1985;**26**(5):518.

34 **Zabara J**. Peripheral control of hypersynchronous discharge in epilepsy. Electroencephalogr Clin Neurophysiol 1985;**61**(3):S162.

35 **Cyberonics**. VNS Therapy Milestones 2010 Contract No.: EPLPK08–11–7000.

36 **Buras WR, inventor; Cyberonics, Inc.**, assignee. Treatment of reproductive endocrine disorders by vagus nerve stimulation. United States of America patent 7,657,310 2010 February 2, 2010.

37 **Maschino SE, inventor; Cyberonics, Inc.**, assignee. Cranial nerve stimulation to treat eating disorders. United States of America patent 7,620,455 2009 November 17, 2009.

38 **Maschino SE, Buras W, Brannan S, inventors; Cyberonics, Inc.**, assignee. Selective neurostimulation for treating mood disorders. United States of America patent 7,532,935 2009 May 12, 2009.

39 **Maschino SE, Parnis SM, Armstrong SA, inventors; Cyberonics, Inc.**, assignee. Weight loss method and device. United States of America patent 7,835,796 2010 November 16, 2010.

40 **Maschino SE, Parnis SM, Buras WR, Guzman AW, inventors; Cyberonics, Inc.**, assignee. Stimulating cranial nerve to treat disorders associated with the thyroid gland. United States of America patent 7,706,874 2010 April 27, 2010.

41 **Terry RS, Baker RG, Marquette A, inventors; Cyberonics, Inc.**, assignee. Treating refractory hypertension by nerve stimulation. United States of America patent 5,707,400 1998 January 13, 1998.

42 **Wernicke JF, Terry RS, inventors; Cyberonics, Inc.**, assignee. Treatment of dementia by nerve stimulation. United States of America patent 5,269,303 1993 December 14, 1993.

43 **Wernicke JF, Terry RS, Baker RG, inventors; Cyberonics, Inc.**, assignee. Treatment of patients in coma by nerve stimulation. United States of America patent 5,571,150 1996 November 5, 1996.

44 **Zabara J, Barrett BT, Parnis SM, inventors; Nerve stimulation as a treatment for pain**. United States of America patent 6,721,603 2004.

45 **Rush AJ, George MS, Sackeim HA et al**. Vagus nerve stimulation (VNS) for treatment-resistant depressions: a multicenter study. Biol Psychiatr 2000 Feb 15;**47**(4):276–86. PubMed PMID: 10686262.

46 **Rush AJ, Marangell LB, Sackeim HA et al**. Vagus nerve stimulation for treatment-resistant depression: a randomized, controlled acute phase trial. Biol Psychiatr 2005 Sept 1;**58**(5):347–54. PubMed PMID: 16139580.

47 **Grassley CE, Baucus M**. Review of the FDA's approval process for the vagus nerve stimulation therapy system for treatment-resistant depression: Committee Staff Report to the Chairman and Ranking Member. In: US Senators Grassley and Baucus on behalf of the US Senate Committee on Finance, editor. United States: US Government Printing Office; 2006.

48 **Morrison HM, Moore DJ**. Cyberonics 2012 Annual Report. Cyberonics, Inc., 2012.

49 **Kahle W, Frotscher M**. Color Atlas of Human Anatomy: Nervous System and Sensory Organs, 6th edn. Georg Thieme Verlag Stuttgart; 2010.

50 **Fridley J, Thomas JG, Navarro JC, Yoshor D**. Brain stimulation for the treatment of epilepsy. Neurosurg Focus 2012 Mar;**32**(3):E13. PubMed PMID: 22380854.

51 **Beekwilder JP, Beems T**. Overview of the clinical applications of vagus nerve stimulation. J Clin Neurophysiol 2010;**27**(2):130–38.

52 **Schachter SC**. Therapeutic effects of vagus nerve stimulation in epilepsy and implications for sudden unexpected death in epilepsy. Clin Autonom Res 2006 Feb;**16**(1):29–32. PubMed PMID: 16477492.

53 **McGregor A, Wheless J, Baumgartner J, Bettis D**. Right-sided vagus nerve stimulation as a treatment for refractory epilepsy in humans. Epilepsia 2005 Jan;**46**(1):91–96. PubMed PMID: 15660773.

54 **Spuck S, Nowak G, Renneberg A, Tronnier V, Sperner J**. Right-sided vagus nerve stimulation in humans: an effective therapy? Epilepsy Res 2008 Dec;**82**(2–3):232–34. PubMed PMID: 18801642.

55 **Rutecki P**. Anatomical, physiological, and theoretical basis for the antiepileptic effect of vagus nerve stimulation. Epilepsia 1990;**31**(Suppl. 2):S1–6. PubMed PMID: 2226360.

56 **Lockard JS, Congdon WC, DuCharme LL**. Feasibility and safety of vagal stimulation in monkey model. Epilepsia 1990;**31**(Suppl. 2):S20–26. PubMed PMID: 2226362.

57 **Zabara J**. Inhibition of experimental seizures in canines by repetitive vagal stimulation. Epilepsia 1992 Nov–Dec;**33**(6):1005–12. PubMed PMID: 1464256.

58 **McLachlan RS**. Suppression of interictal spikes and seizures by stimulation of the vagus nerve. Epilepsia 1993 Sept–Oct;**34**(5):918–23. PubMed PMID: 8404747.

59 **Takaya M, Terry WJ, Naritoku DK**. Vagus nerve stimulation induces a sustained anticonvulsant effect. Epilepsia 1996 Nov;**37**(11):1111–16. PubMed PMID: 8917063.

60 **Baumgartner JE, Von Allmen GK**. Vagus nerve stimulation for intractable epilepsy. In: Winn HR (ed.) Youmans Neurological Surgery, 6th edn. Saunders; 2011.

61 **Food and Drug Administration Neurological Devices Panel**. Final Statistical Summary Review for PMA P970003/S50 (Original and Various Amendments), Vagus Nerve Stimulator (VNS) Therapy System for Depression, Cyberonics, Inc; 2004.

62 **Yu C, Ramgopal S, Libenson M, Abdelmoumen I et al**. Outcomes of vagal nerve stimulation in a pediatric population: A single center experience. *Seizure: European Journal of Epilepsy*; 2013 Dec; **23**(2):105–111.

63 **Alings M, Vireca E, Bastian D et al**. Clinical use of automatic pacemaker algorithms: results of the AUTOMATICITY registry. Europace 2011 Jul;**13**(7):976–83. PubMed PMID: 21422022.

64 **Wilkoff BL, Auricchio A, Brugada J et al**. HRS/EHRA expert consensus on the monitoring of cardiovascular implantable electronic devices (CIEDs): description of techniques, indications,

personnel, frequency and ethical considerations: developed in partnership with the Heart Rhythm Society (HRS) and the European Heart Rhythm Association (EHRA); and in collaboration with the American College of Cardiology (ACC), the American Heart Association (AHA), the European Society of Cardiology (ESC), the Heart Failure Association of ESC (HFA), and the Heart Failure Society of America (HFSA). Endorsed by the Heart Rhythm Society, the European Heart Rhythm Association (a registered branch of the ESC), the American College of Cardiology, the American Heart Association. Europace 2008 Jun;**10**(6):707–25. PubMed PMID: 18480075.

65 **Trohman RG, Kim MH, Pinski SL**. Cardiac pacing: the state of the art. Lancet 2004 Nov 6–12;**364**(9446):1701–19. PubMed PMID: 15530632.

66 **Volkmann J, Herzog J, Kopper F, Deuschl G**. Introduction to the programming of deep brain stimulators. Mov Disord 2002;**17**(Suppl. 3):S181–87. PubMed PMID: 11948775.

67 **Volkmann J, Moro E, Pahwa R**. Basic algorithms for the programming of deep brain stimulation in Parkinson's disease. Mov Disord 2006 Jun;**21**(Suppl. 14):S284–89. PubMed PMID: 16810675.

68 **Baudhuin J, Cadieux J, Firszt JB, Reeder RM, Maxson JL**. Optimization of programming parameters in children with the advanced bionics cochlear implant. J Am Acad Audiol 2012 May;**23**(5):302–12. PubMed PMID: 22533974. PubMed Central PMCID: 3426836.

69 **Shapiro WH, Bradham TS**. Cochlear implant programming. Otolaryngol Clin North Am 2012 Feb;**45**(1):111–27. PubMed PMID: 22115685.

70 **Heck C, Helmers SL, DeGiorgio CM**. Vagus nerve stimulation therapy, epilepsy, and device parameters: scientific basis and recommendations for use. Neurology 2002 Sep 24;**59**(6)(Suppl. 4):S31–37. PubMed PMID: 12270966.

71 **Madsen JR**. Treatment of intractable epilepsy by electrical stimulation of the vagus nerve. In: Quinones-Hinojosa A (ed.) Schmidek and Sweet: Operative Neurosurgical Techniques: Indications, Methods and Results, 6th edn. Saunders; Elsevier/Saunders, Philadelphia; 2012; Chapter **113**:1301–1308.

72 **Beleza P**. Refractory epilepsy: a clinically oriented review. Eur Neurol 2009;**62**(2):65–71. PubMed PMID: 19521080.

73 **Sillanpäa M, Schmidt D**. Natural history of treated childhood-onset epilepsy: prospective, long-term population-based study. Brain 2006 Mar;**129**(Pt 3):617–24. PubMed PMID: 16401617.

74 **Choi H, Heiman GA, Munger Clary H, Etienne M, Resor SR, Hauser WA**. Seizure remission in adults with long-standing intractable epilepsy: an extended follow-up. Epilepsy Res 2011 Feb;**93**(2–3):115–19. PubMed PMID: 21177075.

75 **Berg AT, Lin J, Ebrahimi N, Testa FM, Levy SR, Shinnar S**. Modeling remission and relapse in pediatric epilepsy: application of a Markov process. Epilepsy Res 2004 Jun;**60**(1):31–40. PubMed PMID: 15279868.

Chapter 20

Vagus nerve stimulation in the treatment of epilepsy II: procedure, evidence, and adverse events

Benjamin I. Rapoport and Joseph R. Madsen

Key points

1 Vagus nerve stimulation is a safe therapeutic alternative for the treatment of patients suffering from medically refractory epilepsy, although its efficacy relative to the natural history of refractory epilepsy remains in question.

2 There are few risks to the procedure, procedure-associated morbidity is low, and known side-effects can usually be tolerated or managed by modifying stimulation parameters.

3 Optimal practices with regard to the technical and surgical aspects of vagus nerve stimulation have been developed by a number of neurosurgeons and neurologists, each with over a decade of clinical experience in several hundred patients, including one of the authors. This chapter describes many of those empirically derived best practices in detail.

4 Understanding the geometry and function of the implanted components, particularly the helical configuration of the electrodes with respect to the vagus nerve, facilitates efficient implantation and effective stimulation.

5 Restrictions on access to MRI scans for patients with implanted vagus nerve stimulators may loom as a significant risk in the future.

Introduction

As we discussed in Chapter 19, while the safety of vagus nerve stimulation has been adequately established over the last quarter-century, a careful, comprehensive review of human and animal studies raises questions as to the true efficacy of vagus nerve stimulation in the treatment of epilepsy. Nevertheless, as the treatment is safe and may be of some benefit, we describe in this companion chapter the technical and surgical aspects of vagus nerve stimulation that a decade of clinical experience in several hundred patients has suggested reflect optimal clinical practice. We have reviewed some of these aspects of vagus nerve stimulation previously (1), and present a similar, updated treatment here.

Patient selection

Vagus nerve stimulation (VNS) is not a first-line treatment for epilepsy, and should be reserved for patients who have failed to achieve adequate seizure control through other treatment modalities. We recommend that all patients considering VNS undergo evaluation by epileptologists and surgeons familiar with all available treatment options. Candidates for vagus nerve stimulation should certainly have epilepsy that is medically refractory, in the sense that their seizures have not been adequately controlled using multiple anti-epileptic drugs, alone or in combination, at maximum tolerable doses. In addition, we consider a potentially curative surgical resection preferable to VNS. Some patients consider trial of VNS preferable to extra-temporal surgery in an eloquent area, corpus callosotomy, or a second craniotomy after failure of a first operation. It is not unreasonable to consider VNS as a low-risk and low-morbidity alternative to a high-risk surgical procedure.

The clinical trials that led to United States Food and Drug Administration (FDA) approval of VNS for intractable epilepsy primarily studied patients with medically refractory partial seizures. Since approval, the efficacy of VNS has been studied in patients with other types of epilepsy. Those studies have found that the efficacy of VNS in treating generalized seizures and Lennox–Gastaut syndrome is comparable to that in partial seizures. VNS may also be used safely in children with intractable epilepsy, though a randomized controlled trial has questioned its efficacy (2). Prognostic factors predicting favourable outcomes in patients receiving VNS have not been identified.

For practical reasons, a candidate for VNS must have a chest wall that is large enough and has enough redundant skin to accommodate the implantable pulse generator. Previous left cervical or bilateral vagotomy is an absolute contraindication for VNS. Upper airway or pharyngeal problems; pulmonary, cardiac, or gastrointestinal problems; dysautonomia; a history of vasovagal syncope; and the presence of a brain stimulator, are all considered relative contraindications for VNS, and stimulator implantation as well as follow-up care in such patients requires particular caution.

Devices used in vagus nerve stimulation

The implantable system used for vagus nerve stimulation is the VNS Therapy System, an updated version of the original NeuroCybernetic Prosthesis, designed and manufactured by Cyberonics Corporation. The two primary implantable components of the system are a stimulating electrode and a pulse generator.

The generator circuitry communicates via radiofrequency telemetry with an external programming device, which can be used to adjust the electrical output of the pulse generator. The stimulation waveform produced by the generator consists of charge-balanced, square-wave pulses, and the full waveform is characterized by five adjustable parameters: current amplitude, stimulation frequency, pulse width, on-time, and off-time. The generator contains a battery, the lifetime of which depends on the power consumption of the stimulator, which in turn depends on the stimulation settings: higher amplitude, higher frequency, and longer on-times consume more power, resulting in shorter battery lifetimes. Software in the external programmer estimates remaining battery life, making it possible to replace a generator before it stops working, and thereby continue stimulation uninterrupted with the same stimulation parameters.

The stimulating electrode is connected to the pulse generator during the implantation procedure via a connector pin that inserts into the generator, is protected by an epoxy resin header, and is secured intra-operatively using a set screw and torque screwdriver. The electrode is insulated by a silicone elastomer coating, and can be used safely in patients allergic to latex. A silicone 'collar' is used to tether the electrode wires to the soft tissue of the neck, and to hold in place a redundant loop of wire (a 'strain relief' loop) that protects the vagus nerve from traction.

The stimulating end of the electrode terminates in three helical coils that are wrapped around the vagus nerve. Distally to proximally, these coils respectively serve as negative electrode, positive electrode, and strain-relieving tether to protect the electrodes themselves from excessive force during stretching of the vagus nerve with positional changes of the head and neck. Each coil makes three loops, and can be manipulated by suture ties extending from its proximal and distal ends. The actual electrode contacts are made from platinum, and are welded to the middle loops of the positive- and negative-electrode coils.

In addition to communicating via radio-frequency telemetry with the external programming device, the implanted generator can also be controlled by a handheld, external magnet. Transiently passing the magnet over the generator produces a signal that the generator interprets as an immediate request for additional stimulation, which is added in real time to the pre-programmed stimulation waveform. Some patients and caregivers have reported that in patients who experience auras or exhibit preictal symptoms or signs, on-demand activation of the vagus nerve stimulator may abort or modify an anticipated seizure. On the other hand, continuously holding the handheld magnet over the surface of the pulse generator turns the generator off; this off-switch mechanism can be useful for patients who wish to stop stimulation for any reason, including a possible stimulator malfunction.

Operative procedure

Peri-operative care

Vagus nerve stimulator implantation is typically performed under general anaesthesia. Prophylactic antibiotics are administered pre- and post-operatively, as they are in other procedures involving device implantation. Post-operatively, patients are observed with particular concern for known side-effects of VNS, including vocal cord dysfunction, dysphagia, bradycardia, and impaired respiration.

Operative technique

The cervical portion of the vagus nerve is located in the carotid sheath, typically between the carotid artery and jugular vein. While it is generally embedded in the connective tissue of the carotid sheath between the carotid artery and jugular vein, the nerve can assume various positions relative to the vascular structures. The cervical portion of the nerve below the carotid bifurcation is generally free of macroscopic branches, so that circumferential dissection of the vagus nerve for placement of the coil electrodes can be performed without damaging or devascularizing branches of the nerve.

As we have described previously (1), the patient should be positioned so as to facilitate exposure of the vagus nerve: supine, with the neck in slight extension and head turned slightly to the right so as to expose a sufficient length of the cervical portion of the vagus nerve. Excessive turning of the head should be avoided, so as to avoid the need for excessive retraction of the sternocleidomastoid muscle.

Two skin incisions will be required: a cervical incision for access to the vagus nerve, and a subpectoral incision for placement of the implantable generator. With contemporary generator models (103 and after, called 'Demipulse') most patients do well with subcutaneous generator placement and no longer require subpectoral generator pockets, as described earlier. The anterior axillary incision requires access to the anterior axillary fold, and will be facilitated by positioning the left arm in slight abduction. The left hand may be taped near the patient's left hip to facilitate ideal arm position ('hand in trousers pocket position'). The surgeon stands on the left side of the patient, and the assistant stands across the table or to the right of the surgeon.

The cervical incision is centred over the anterior border of the sternocleidomastoid, approximately two-thirds of the distance from the angle of the jaw to the clavicle. An incision 2 to 2.5 cm long is adequate in thin patients, but longer incisions may be necessary in muscular or obese patients, or in patients who have had prior surgery. Dissection of the vagus nerve is most straightforward when the exposure remains below the carotid bifurcation. The platysma is divided along the direction of its fibres, at the anterior border of the sternocleidomastoid. That muscular border is then followed in an avascular plane to the carotid sheath, which may be exposed using a Cloward retractor with short, blunt blades. The vagus nerve is identified within the carotid sheath. The carotid sheath fascia must be carefully preserved when it is opened on either side of the vagus nerve, because it must support anchoring sutures that fix the electrodes after they are placed on the nerve. Approximately 3 cm of the vagus nerve must be dissected free of the sheath, and this dissection is facilitated by passing a vessel loop around the nerve to elevate it, while sharply dissecting open the sheath laterally to free the nerve. A further 3 cm within the carotid sheath should be opened inferiorly with blunt dissection, in order to contain the 'strain relief' loop of electrode cable.

The second incision is used for fashioning the sub-cutaneous or subpectoral pocket that will contain the implantable pulse generator. Several techniques have been described for making this incision. An incision about 2.5 cm long in the anterior axillary line, oriented in the direction of the natural skin creases, works well. If a sub-cutaneous pocket is desired, dissection is stopped just above the fascia of the pectoralis; subpectoral placement requires dissecting deep to the pectoralis. The pulse generator is approximately 5 cm in longest dimension, and should be recessed within its pocket by 1 to 2 cm from the skin incision.

Once the pocket has been made, the tunnelling device can be passed in either direction between the pocket and the cervical incision. Tunnelling must be performed with care to avoid injuring deep structures. Ideally, the tunnel should emerge just below the platysma. The electrodes can then be passed through the sub-cutaneous tunnel, with the connectors placed in the plastic sheath of the tunnelling device and then pulled from above to below. The coil electrodes themselves, however, must not be passed through the tunnel, as they may be damaged even by minor trauma.

Next, the coil electrodes must be positioned on the vagus nerve. We recommend pulling the electrode cable inferiorly so as to eliminate redundant cable below the coils. Beginning with the most inferior coil (which serves as an anchor and not as an electrode), the threads at both ends of the coil are grasped and the superior thread is passed below the nerve, in the lateral-to-medial direction, while the assistant retracts the nerve upward using the vessel loop placed earlier. The nerve can then be allowed to lie within the slightly opened coil. Pulling the upper thread laterally and the lower thread medially across the nerve completes a first loop around the nerve, and when the coil is released, it will fall into an appropriate position around the nerve. One to one-and-a-half more revolutions around the nerve are usually required, and they can be accomplished in a similar fashion. The electrode coils are then placed around the nerve using a similar technique.

After the electrodes and anchoring coil are in place around the vagus nerve, their corresponding lead wires must be secured. The two electrode leads are conveniently secured within the carotid sheath using a plastic wing anchor, at the point where they are joined to enter the main cable. The anchor can be secured to the deep neck fascia using a 4–0 braided nylon or silk suture on a fine needle. It is important for these anchors to move as little as possible relative to the vagus, when the patient moves his or her neck. Placement of the anchoring sutures in the deep neck fascia is, therefore, preferable to placement in the muscular fascia. The anchors should also be placed far from large vascular structures, including the carotid artery and jugular vein, to prevent erosion into these structures. One anchoring suture should be placed at the upper limit of the exposure of the deep cervical fascia, and a second should be placed at the lower limit. A third anchoring suture should be placed after passing a length of cable above the exposure and deep to the platysma so as to fasten it onto the sternocleidomastoid fascia, away from the incision. It is important to place all anchoring sutures before manipulating the distal electrode cable, as the anchoring sutures protect the electrodes from tension associated with manipulating the distal cable, which might otherwise displace the electrodes from their positions on the vagus nerve.

After the anchoring sutures are in place, the main electrode cable can be connected to its socket on the implantable pulse generator, where it is secured with set screws placed using a torque screwdriver. Once the electrodes have been connected to the stimulator, the system can run diagnostic testing, ensuring proper connectivity and measuring electrode impedances. The external programmer can be brought onto the field in a sterile plastic drape, and the stimulator can be tested, programmed, and activated intra-operatively.

Finally, the pulse generator is inserted and anchored deeply in the pectoral pocket using a 2–0 suture placed in the pectoralis fascia. The generator should be oriented so as to optimally orient its antenna for communication with the external programmer; in current-generation devices, the manufacturer logo is printed on the side of the device that should be orienting facing outward.

A sterile-draped programming wand is then used to perform diagnostic tests, particularly to verify that the impedance is in normal range, and to have the patient identifiers, including initials and date of implant, entered into the electronics of the device. The manufacturer's recommendation is to then reset the current to zero, though we and others have had the practice of allowing the patient to emerge from anaesthesia with a very low setting: 0.25 mA current amplitude, 250 μs pulse width, 30 s on-time, 5 min off-time. We have not encountered problems with these initial settings, but if a patient were found who did not tolerate them, the device could be set to zero current in the recovery room.

Both incisions can be closed with absorbable sutures in the deep fascia of the pectoral pocket and platysma, sub-cutaneous closure, subcuticular closure, and paper strips or skin adhesive across the skin edges. Dry, sterile dressings are applied, and patients should leave these dressings in place for 7 to 10 days so as to keep the incisions dry.

Generator replacement

Current implantable pulse generators contain batteries that have limited service lifetimes, and a stimulator should be replaced before its battery is exhausted in order to ensure uninterrupted stimulation. The operation to replace the stimulator is similar to the procedure in which it is initially placed. The chest wall incision should be reopened. A Bovie cautery should be used, at low-power coagulation settings, to dissect downward and into the pectoral pocket. It is essential to avoid damaging the electrode cable during this dissection. The generator is then removed from its pocket, the set screws are loosened, the cable is disconnected from the generator, and a replacement generator is connected. Surgical closure is accomplished as in the original procedure.

Lead replacement

Over time, dense fibrous tissue tends to form around the electrodes and exposed portion of the vagus nerve. Nevertheless, the leads can be uncoiled around the nerve, removed, and replaced, if electrical diagnostic testing reveals a lead failure or a high impedance. Surgical replacement of the lead is considerably more difficult than initial placement of the lead, and obviously much more difficult than replacement of the generator unit.

Dissection through the scar tissue to find a clear area of the vagus nerve for placement of the new helices may require a longer incision, and often benefits from use of the operating microscope.

Post-operative follow-up and stimulator programming

Following implantation, the stimulator may be activated at any time. Some groups prefer to leave the stimulator off for several weeks in order to distinguish post-operative symptoms from symptoms related to stimulation. We turn the stimulator on at the time of placement, with initial settings as already mentioned. These initial, minimal settings enable patients to become accustomed to vagus nerve stimulation. Settings can be revised iteratively in an attempt to optimize the therapeutic response, over the weeks and months following implantation. The amplitude of the stimulation current is typically the first parameter adjusted; it can be increased incrementally, with a practical upper limit typically determined by patient tolerance to the emergence of stimulation-related side effects. It is reasonable to begin tapering anti-epileptic medication regimens in patients who exhibit sustained improvements in seizure control in response to vagus nerve stimulation.

Complications and adverse effects of vagus nerve stimulation

Vocal cord and pharyngeal effects

Vocal cord anomalies, which patients often experience as hoarseness or intermittent vibration of the voice during stimulation, are a common side-effect of vagus nerve stimulation. This phenomenon was noted in the initial clinical trials. The effect is a result of the proximity of the recurrent laryngeal nerve to the site of stimulation: the recurrent laryngeal nerve initially travels with the main trunk of the vagus before branching at the aortic arch. The intensity of this adverse effect is, therefore, a function of the stimulation amplitude, and can typically be mitigated or eliminated by reducing the stimulation current.

Less common side-effects, including pharyngeal paresthesias, coughing, increased drooling, and sensation of shortness of breath, may be handled similarly. Other nerves in the region of the vagus, including the phrenic (hemidiaphragm paralysis), have occasionally been affected by vagus nerve stimulation (3).

Cardiac rhythm disturbances

Although rare, ventricular asystole has been observed during intra-operative diagnostic testing of the vagus nerve stimulation electrodes. This incidence of this complication has been estimated at approximately 1 in 800 to 1 in 1000 patients. Treatment consists of administering atropine and immediately switching off the stimulator. With older software versions, the 'lead test' for impedance could only be done at 1 mA, but now testing can be done at any current, and it is possible that the incidence of intra-operative bradycardia, which occurred most frequently during the lead test, has dramatically diminished.

Skin breakdown

Patients with little sub-cutaneous fat in the pectoral region and neck are prone to skin breakdown over implanted components in those regions. Such patients should be considered as having a relative contraindication to implantation.

Sleep-related breathing disorder

Decreased respiratory airflow has been observed in some children after the initiation of vagus nerve stimulation. Patients with obstructive sleep apnoea should be monitored with particular care after implantation. Worsening sleep apnoea may be treated with positive pressure devices and by adjusting the vagus nerve stimulation parameters.

Magnetic resonance imaging of patients with vagus nerve stimulators

Magnetic resonance protocols for patients with vagus nerve stimulators have been developed and used safely in the past. Nevertheless, recent FDA and manufacturer warnings have made many clinicians and institutions reluctant or unwilling to use magnetic resonance imaging in patients with vagus nerve stimulators (3). The current product labelling available on the Cyberonics website suggests that: 'Because heating effects have not been characterized nor safety demonstrated on leads without pulse generators or partial leads, MRI should not be performed on patients who have leads without the pulse generators or partial leads.' Absence of lead interruption should be documented by proof of normal impedance before an MRI is done, according to these guidelines, which could have major implications for the future of all patients treated with VNS (all of whom will presumably eventually have generator failure, and many of whom may have lead issues or partial removal of leads).

Conclusions

Vagus nerve stimulation is a safe therapeutic alternative for the treatment of patients suffering from medically refractory epilepsy. There are few risks to the procedure, procedure-associated morbidity is low, and known side-effects can usually be tolerated or managed by modifying stimulation parameters. Restrictions on access to MRI scans may loom as a significant risk in the future.

Relative to the natural history of refractory epilepsy, however, a clear, unambiguous understanding of the efficacy of vagus nerve stimulation is certainly limited. Moreover, there are neither known predictors of therapeutic efficacy in specific patients, nor validated techniques for tuning stimulation parameters to improve efficacy after implantation. While the afferent autonomic pathways activated by stimulation of the vagus nerve have known targets within the central nervous system, no mechanism of action has been demonstrated by which stimulation of the vagus nerve should act to suppress epileptiform activity in the cerebral cortex, even after a quarter-century of experience with vagus nerve stimulation in human patients.

References

1 **Madsen JR**. Treatment of intractable epilepsy by electrical stimulation of the vagus nerve. In: Quinones-Hinojosa A (ed.) Schmidek and Sweet: Operative Neurosurgical Techniques: Indications, Methods and Results, 6th edn. Saunders; 2012.

2 **Klinkenberg S, Aalbers MW, Vles JS et al**. Vagus nerve stimulation in children with intractable epilepsy: a randomized controlled trial. Develop Med Child Neurol 2012 Sep;**54**(9):855–61. PubMed PMID:22540141.

3 **Baumgartner JE, Von Allmen GK**. Vagus nerve stimulation for intractable epilepsy. In: Winn HR (ed.) Youmans Neurological Surgery, 6th edn. Saunders; 2011.

Index